Case Studies for Contemporary Occupational Therapy Practice

Guiding Critical Thinking for Students

Edited by Donald Auriemma, MS ED, OTR/L; Yves Roseus, OTD, OTR/L;
Clover Hutchinson, OTD, MA, OTR/L; and Vikram Pagpatan, OTR/L, ATP, BCP, CLA

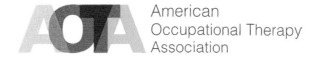

American
Occupational Therapy
Association

AOTA Vision 2025
As an inclusive profession, occupational therapy maximizes health, well-being, and quality of life for all people, populations, and communities through effective solutions that facilitate participation in everyday living.

Mission Statement
The American Occupational Therapy Association advances occupational therapy practice, education, and research through standard-setting and advocacy on behalf of its members, the profession, and the public.

AOTA Staff
Sherry Keramidas, *Executive Director*
Matthew Clark, *Chief Officer, Innovation & Engagement*

Elizabeth Dooley, *Vice President, Strategic Marketing & Communications*
Laura Collins, *Director of Communications and Publications*
Cecelia González, AJOT *Managing Editor*
Ashley Hofmann, *Acquisitions & Development Manager, AOTA Press*
Amy Ricci, *Product Manager & Business Analyst, AOTA Press*

Rebecca Rutberg, *Director, Marketing*
Amanda Goldman, *Marketing Manager*
Jennifer Folden, *Brand Designer*

American Occupational Therapy Association, Inc.
6116 Executive Boulevard, Suite 200
North Bethesda, MD 20852-4929
Phone: 301-652-AOTA (2682)
Fax: 301-652-7711
www.aota.org
To order: 1-877-404-AOTA or store.aota.org

Disclaimers
This publication is designed to provide accurate and authoritative information in regard to the subject matter covered. It is sold or distributed with the understanding that the publisher is not engaged in rendering legal, accounting, or other professional service. If legal advice or other expert assistance is required, the services of a competent professional person should be sought.
—*From the Declaration of Principles jointly adopted by the American Bar Association and a Committee of Publishers and Associations*

It is the objective of the American Occupational Therapy Association to be a forum for free expression and interchange of ideas. The opinions expressed by the contributors to this work are their own and not necessarily those of the American Occupational Therapy Association.

ISBN: 978-1-56900-632-0
eBOOK ISBN: 978-1-56900-633-7
Library of Congress Control Number: 2022948067

Cover art by Darlyn Mora Almonte, Jamaica, NY
Cover design by Steve Parrish, AOTA, North Bethesda, MD
Printed by Automated Graphic Services, Inc., White Plains, MD

Case study photo sources: Chapters 7, 8, and 10 by Unsplash.com. All others by Getty Images. Used under license.

Reference citation: Auriemma, D., Roseus, Y., Hutchinson, C., & Pagpatan, V. (Eds.). (2023). *Case studies for contemporary occupational therapy practice: Guiding critical thinking for students.* AOTA Press.

Dedication

This text is dedicated to Professors Wimberley Edwards, Yvonne Flowers, and Ruth Kriam, the founding faculty of the Occupational Therapy Program at York College of the City University of New York. Their vision, efforts, and foresight have inspired the collaboration of York alumni to create this text.

In Memoriam

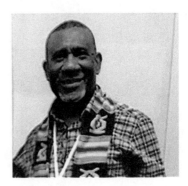

In memory of Dr. Yves Rosesus, co-editor, contributing author, and dear friend. He lost his life in the service of humanity during the COVID-19 pandemic. His memory lives on through his many selfless acts, his contributions, the lives he touched, and this text.

Contents·

Section IV. Subacute Rehabilitation 127

Section V. Skilled Nursing Facility or Long-Term Care 169

Section VI. Home and Community Health...203

Section VII. Inpatient Behavior Health Hospital or Unit 237

Section VIII. Pediatric Services 287

About the Editors

Donald Auriemma, MS ED, OTR/L (he/him), is an Italian American occupational therapist from Southold, New York. He is an associate professor and chair in the Department of Occupational Therapy, at York College of the City University of New York (CUNY). He earned his bachelor of science degree in occupational therapy in 1982 at York College of CUNY and his master of science degree in education from Queens College of CUNY in 1985.

As a clinician, Donald's concentration of practice was adult disabilities. During his career, he earned board certification in both neurorehabilitation and assistive technology. As a scholar, his research has focused on the methods programs have used to admit its students and the impact of the use of those selected tools. As an educator, he has been he has been dedicated to the development of York's students pursuing professional education, and their professional development beyond graduation. The three additional editors and all contributing authors but one are former students.

Yves Roseus, OTD, OTR/L (he/him), was a Haitian American occupational therapist from Queens, New York. He was an adjunct assistant professor at several occupational therapy programs, including York College, CUNY, his alma mater. Yves was a passionate practitioner and delegate at Brookdale Hospital & Medical Center in Brooklyn, New York.

Yves was a board member of and instrumental in the establishment of the only occupational therapy program at Faculté des Sciences de Réhabilitation de Léogâne (FSRL)—Léogâne, Haiti. Yves was an ardent advocate for occupational therapy, a New York State Occupational Therapy Association (NYSOTA) trustee, an Accreditation Council for Occupational Therapy Education evaluator, and a member of the American Occupational Therapy Association (AOTA) and New York State Black Occupational Therapy Caucus (NYSBOTC). He was a recipient of the NYSBOTC Celeste Pasely Merit Award. Yves's service and contribution to the profession has been memorialized by renaming the Dr. Yves Roseus Department of Rehabilitation at Brookdale Hospital & Medical Center and the establishment of the Dr. Yves Roseus Citizen's Award for Service and Advocacy in Occupational Therapy at York College, CUNY, and NYSOTA, and the Dr. Yves Roseus Memorial Lectureship and Practicum that is awarded to an occupational therapy student and practitioner living in Haiti.

Clover Hutchinson, OTD, MA, OTR/L (she/her), is a Jamaican American occupational therapist from Queens, New York. She is an assistant professor at and graduate of York College, CUNY. Formerly, she was the chief of occupational therapy for over 23 years at Brookdale Hospital & Medical Center in Brooklyn, New York, where she established occupational therapy in acute care and expanded its outpatient department. Clover is passionate about the advocacy and mentorship of students, practitioners, and the profession.

Clover's passion is evident in her work as president of NYSBOTC; co-founder of the Coalition of Occupational Therapy Advocates for Diversity, York College Chapter; leadership and committee member of NYSOTA; member of the American Occupational Therapy Association's Accreditation Roster of Evaluators and other local organizations. Clover is a recipient of the NYSOTA distinguished Dr. Jim Hinojosa Memorial Lectureship award, which honors practitioners who exemplify qualities of leadership, mentorship, and contributions to the practice and education in occupational therapy. Additionally, Clover volunteers as an instructor for the Faculté des Sciences de Réhabilitation de Léogâne (FSRL)—Léogâne, Haiti, and facilitates mentorship to occupational therapy practitioners in Kenya.

Vikram Pagpatan, OTR/L, ATP, BCP, CLA (he/him), is an Indian American occupational therapist from Queens, New York. He is an assistant professor and admissions coordinator for the State University of New York (SUNY) Downstate Health Sciences University graduate occupational therapy program and an adjunct assistant professor for the occupational therapy program at York College, CUNY, his distinguished alma mater.

Vikram's clinical specialties are assistive technology, neuromotor pediatric practice, and community reintegration with progressive neurological populations. Vikram's clinical focus is on the integration of assistive technology as an integral and practical part of ADLs and IADLs for individuals throughout the lifespan. Vikram's research interests include investigating concepts of e-professionalism in higher education curriculums, social media integration as a form of professional development for health care professions, exploring holistic higher education admissions best practice to address gender diversity for gender-exclusive professions, and highlighting marginalized populations through reformed admissions procedures.

Vikram's leadership roles includes his service as an AOTA Board Director and AOTA DEI committee member, continued work on statewide policy reform within multiple SUNY-wide University Faculty Senate committees, and his passion for advocacy as the communications chair of the Association of Asian-Americans and Pacific Islanders in Occupational Therapy.

Contributors

Tiffany Almonte, MS, OTR/L
Adjunct Lecturer
York College of the City University of New York
Jamaica, NY
Occupational Therapy Supervisor
Saint Dominic's Family Services/CISS
New York, NY
York College Class of 2016

Donald Auriemma, MS ED, OTR/L
Associate Professor and Chair
Department of Occupational Therapy
York College of the City University of New York
Jamaica, NY
York College Class of 1982

Kerron Blunte, MS, OTR/L, CLT
Adjunct Lecturer
York College of the City University of New York
Jamaica, NY
Northwell Health STARS Rehabilitation
Jamaica, NY
York College Class of 2011

Carol Brown-Wassinger, MS, OTR/L
Senior Occupational Therapist
New York City Department of Education, District 75
New York, NY
York College Class of 2008

Tiffany Cordero-Velez, MS, OTR/L
Adjunct Lecturer
York College of the City University of New York
Jamaica, NY
Senior Occupational Therapist
New York City Department of Education
New York, NY
York College Class of 2016

Mary Devadas, MS, OTR/L, DBA
Adjunct Assistant Professor
York College of the City University of New York
Jamaica, NY
Senior Occupational Therapist
Kingsbrook Jewish Medical Center
Brooklyn, NY
York College Class of 2011

Bebe Haniff, MS, OTR/L
Senior Occupational Therapist
Jamaica Nursing Home
Jamaica, NY
York College Class of 2010

Clover Hutchinson, OTD, MA, OTR/L
Assistant Professor
York College of the City University of New York
Jamaica, NY
York College Class of 1992

Vikram Pagpatan, OTR/L, ATP, BCP, CLA
Adjunct Assistant Professor
York College of the City University of New York
Jamaica, NY
Assistant Professor and Admissions Coordinator
SUNY Downstate Health Sciences University
Brooklyn, NY
York College Class of 2013

Susan Quintin, MS, OTR/L
Senior Occupational Therapist
New York City Department of Education
New York, NY
York College Class of 2001

Ivy Rentz, EdD, MSA, OTR/L
Assistant Professor and Doctoral Capstone Coordinator
Quinnipiac University
Hamden, CT
York College Class of 1998

Eva Rodriguez, PhD, OTR
Associate Professor and Program Director
York College of the City University of New York
Jamaica, NY
York College Class of 1983

Yves Roseus, OTD, OTR/L
Adjunct Assistant Professor
York College of the City University of New York
Jamaica, NY
Senior Occupational Therapist
Brookdale Hospital & Medical Center
Brooklyn, NY
York College Class of 1999

Paula Stewart, MS, OTR/L
Adjunct Lecturer
York College of the City University of New York
Jamaica, NY
Co-Executive Director
Occupational Therapy for Kidz Specializing in Sensory Integration for Kids
Cambria Heights, NY
York College Class of 1997

Frederick Wolodin, MS, OTR/L
Senior Occupational Therapist
Montefiore Medical Center
Bronx, NY
York College Class of 2008

Note From the Artist

For the artwork used on the cover of this text, *Lives and Apples*, the apples represent how diverse yet similar we are as human beings. Just as apples are categorized by color, sweetness, or acidity, human beings are often categorized based on physical appearances, race, ethnicity, culture, sex, gender, physical and mental health, and so forth. Society should approach human beings in a way that promotes and practices social equity. Regardless of individuals' traits, each person deserves to live in an environment that accepts, understands, and respects them and facilitates their participation and engagement in occupations. Occupational therapy is a holistic profession that treats an individual as a whole person—not just the symptoms of their diseases, conditions, or disorders. The occupational therapy profession believes that having a disability does not mean being disabled. Even when participation in an occupation might not be achieved by remediation or restoration approaches, occupational therapy professionals will always work on modifying and adapting the environment to the individual's needs.

In the painting, the book represents education and resources, which give the yellow apple an advantage over the rest. The book gives support and clarity to the individual, who once felt useless and incapable—like a mannequin—to recognize their strengths, find their courage, and chase their dreams. Education, occupational therapy, and many other resources and experiences can affect how one faces and overcomes challenges; the individual is functional in society with or without, in this case, an extremity. The peeled half-apple and the gray apple symbolize role and identity—despite their stage of life or appearance, they remain apples.

No matter the labels, condition, or stage of life, participation in meaningful activities gives people dignity, self-efficacy, and health.

—**Darlyn Mora Almonte, OTS**
York College, City University of New York, Jamaica, NY

Introduction

DONALD AURIEMMA, MS ED, OTR/L; CLOVER HUTCHINSON, OTD, MA, OTR/L; AND VIKRAM PAGPATAN, OTR/L, ATP, BCP, CLA

Case Studies for Contemporary Occupational Therapy Practice: Guiding Critical Thinking for Students was created by the combined efforts of 16 accomplished alumni of the Occupational Therapy Program at York College of the City University of New York. The focus of this group was to create a case-based text that could be used across an occupational therapy curriculum, guide critical thinking, and bridge contemporary practice with the *Occupational Therapy Practice Framework: Domain and Process* (4th ed; American Occupational Therapy Association, 2020) and Accreditation Council on Occupational Therapy Education (2018) standards. It is the desire of the contributors to better prepare students to enter practice in our diverse and rapidly changing world.

This text was envisioned for occupational therapists, occupational therapy assistants, occupational therapy students, and educators through a model of cultural humility, awareness, and competency. It acknowledges the importance of incorporating the various principles and tenets of diversity, equity, justice, inclusion, and belonging through a contemporary and practice based interpretation of occupational therapy.

This text threads various aspects of diversity and cultural humility throughout each case and accompanies the reader through a journey of exploring social determinants of health; problem solving through an array of sociocultural and socioeconomic disparities that exist within communities; and developing analytical, pragmatic, inferential, and clinical reasoning skills through a holistic, case-based lens.

How This Text is Organized

This case text is structured through a discovery and exploration model. Each case begins by presenting the medical and social history of each client, illustrating the individual's past and current occupational identities, and highlighting a potential mechanism of injury or explaining events that brought the individual to occupational therapy.

Readers are guided through a uniformed structure for every case presented in this text, fostering a greater awareness of process throughout a series of practice areas and domains. Readers are presented with a detailed social history that correlates clients' occupational identities to their current need of care while allowing readers to explore other meaningful aspects of clients' identities that can be used to design treatment and services. Additionally, readers are presented with information outlining the occupational therapy initial evaluation findings. This is done through a culturally centered occupational profile and an occupation-centered exploration of the client's cognitive, mental, and physical functions. In the last section of each case study, readers are presented with thought-provoking questions that are designed to address aspects of community reintegration, social determinants of health, and disparities.

Students

Occupational therapy students, occupational therapy assistant students, and postprofessional occupational therapy students can use this text as a resource, tool, and guide to develop clinical reasoning and interpersonal skills through a model of diversity, equity, and justice while fostering a greater awareness of cultural humility and competency building. Students will be confronted with and challenged by ethical dilemmas and disparities within the contexts of culture and community as they develop their professional, interpersonal, and clinical reasoning skills as entry-level practitioners. Students are encouraged to ask questions, challenge notions, discuss their implicit biases, and integrate a holistic perspective throughout each occupational therapy case.

Educators

This text enables students to grow and develop intricate competencies of cultural humility and a greater understanding of diversity, equity, and inclusion at their own pace through guidance and facilitation. Academic and clinical educators can use this comprehensive text as a part of their program curriculums as a pathway text for each major component of the occupational therapy educational process, such as through principles evaluation, treatment planning, and outcome assessment. Each case study also allows educators to select a specific practice population or diagnosis while integrating principles of diversity, equity, inclusion, and cultural humility throughout the entire case—from the occupational profile to the critical guiding questions that directly align with the *OTPF–4*.

REFERENCES

Accreditation Council for Occupational Therapy Education. (2018). 2018 Accreditation Council for Occupational Therapy Education (ACOTE®) standards and interpretive guide (effective July 31, 2020). *American Journal of Occupational Therapy, 72*(Suppl. 2), 7212410005. https://doi.org/10.5014/ajot.2018.72S217

American Occupational Therapy Association. (2020). Occupational therapy practice framework: Domain and process (4th ed.). *American Journal of Occupational Therapy, 74*(2), 7412410010. https://doi.org/10.5014/ajot.2020.74S2001

Acute Care

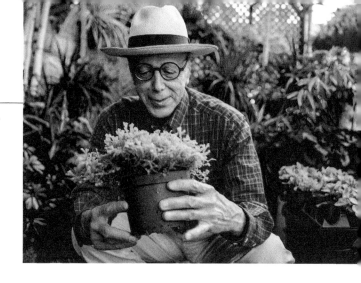

Juan: Myocardial Infarction

DONALD AURIEMMA, MS ED, OTR/L

Juan (he, him, his, himself)

MEDICAL HISTORY

Juan is a 67-year-old Guatemalan American male who is 6' 1" and weighs 190 pounds. He was brought to the emergency department (ED) via emergency medical services after experiencing uncomfortable pressure in his chest, shortness of breath (SOB), and nausea while gardening at home. An electrocardiogram, blood tests, echocardiogram, and chest X-ray were performed, and he received a diagnosis of myocardial infarction (MI) and coronary artery disease. He was then transferred from the ED to the coronary care unit (CCU), where an emergency coronary artery bypass graft ×3 was performed.

His past medical history included treatment for hypertension and high cholesterol. Upon admission, he reported living a sedentary lifestyle, smoking one pack of cigarettes per week, drinking 4 to 5 cups of coffee per day, and consuming 2 to 3 glasses of wine per day. Juan reported no known allergies.

SOCIAL HISTORY

Juan lives with his partner of 25 years, Brian, in a two-story brownstone townhouse that they both own. There are three steps to enter the first floor, which consists of a living room, dining room, and galley kitchen. The second floor has two bedrooms and a full bath. The home is neat and orderly. There is no garage, but there are two dedicated parking spots in front of their home. Their home is just 5 miles from the university where they both work. Juan reported having no blood relatives in the area but having a close group of friends. He and his partner both observe the Catholic religion.

REFERRAL OR PRESCRIPTION

At the CCU, Juan will receive occupational therapy, physical therapy, and registered nursing services for 5 days.

Occupational Therapy Initial Evaluation Findings: Acute Care

OCCUPATIONAL PROFILE

Juan's preadmission occupational history and experiences included being independent in all ADLs and all IADLs. Juan has been employed as a tenured professor of fine arts for the past 27 years and serves as the chair of his department. Juan stated, "Being department chair is extremely stressful," and he felt fortunate that this happened to him during summer break. His patterns of daily living most commonly included having a quick cup of coffee in the morning, arriving on campus by 9:00 a.m., and returning home by 5:00 p.m. He and Brian enjoy dining out for dinner and seldom have dinner at home. After dinner, Juan enjoys reading and sculpting. On the weekends, he loves to work in his garden. When school is out, Juan and Brian love to travel. His interests include art, design, and exploration, and he values how art can affect and shape society. Juan reported that his greatest current need is to understand what happened to him and feel safe enough to return to the life he loves.

ADLs

Regarding self-care, Juan was able to feed himself independently but reported SOB after eating a large meal. While seated, Juan was able to dress both upper extremities independently in a slow spontaneous fashion, but he required minimal assistance to dress his lower extremities. During dressing, his respiration rate elevated to 30 breaths per minute from a baseline of 20; he also complained of SOB. He was able to independently perform the grooming tasks of brushing his hair and teeth. He reported he did not feel he had enough endurance to attempt standing in the tub to shower but was able to sit to manage bowel and bladder care. A score of 4 was achieved on the modified Medical Research Council (mMRC) scale (Mahler & Wells, 1988).

Regarding functional mobility, Juan was able to independently roll and transition between supine and short sit and transferred without a device on and off the bed, chair, and toilet. Tub transfers were not attempted. During the assessment, he required multiple rest periods and verbal cues to maintain a slower pace, because he reported feeling lightheaded.

IADLs

Activities needed that provide day-to-day quality of life and relative independence were explored. Juan can manage his phone and computer communications and handle his finances. Currently, he is not able to maintain his home, prepare meals, or shop.

Regarding rest and sleep, Juan reported having a history of short sleep duration. Currently, he becomes anxious and feels uncomfortable when sleeping in a fully reclined position.

MENTAL FUNCTIONS

Cognitive assessment found Juan to be alert and oriented to person, place, time, and situation, and short- and long-term memory were intact. He is able to follow three-step commands and make his needs known. Affect appeared appropriate, and no gross deficits in perception were observed.

SENSORY FUNCTIONS

No gross deficits were observed with visual, hearing, vestibular, taste, smell, proprioceptive, and cutaneous functions. Juan reported pain and swelling to his right posterior hand at the site of intravenous. Pain was scored as a 4 using a numerical rating scale (0–10) and was described as "throbbing." Edema was assessed using circumferential measurements at the distal palmar crease: 20.3 cm on the right and 17.6 cm on the left.

CARDIOVASCULAR AND RESPIRATORY SYSTEMS FUNCTION

Juan presented with a metabolic equivalent of task (MET) value of 2.5.

MOVEMENT FUNCTIONS

Passive and active range of motion is within functional limits in all extremities. Assessment of muscle strength was contraindicated. Prehension was grossly intact. Juan tolerated standing for 2–3 minutes before reporting fatigue.

NEUROMUSCULAR FUNCTIONS

Static and dynamic sitting balance are both graded as good (G). Static and dynamic standing balance are both graded as fair plus (F+). Muscle tone is normal, and reflex integration is grossly intact.

PLAN FOR DISCHARGE

After 5 days in the CCU, Juan will be discharged home with home health care services, including occupational therapy; physical therapy; and registered nursing, social work, and home health aide services.

Questions and Activities

SAFETY OF CLIENT AND OTHERS: PRECAUTIONS AND CONTRAINDICATIONS

1. While working with Juan, what are the signs and symptoms of cardiac distress you need to be monitoring?
2. Which vital signs should be taken when working with Juan? What are the norms for each? Explain when these vital signs should be taken.
3. The assessment of muscular strength was contraindicated at the time of the initial evaluation. Explain why, and site your source.
4. Create a handout identifying precautions to be taken after a coronary bypass graft.
5. Identify the common psychological reactions associated with an MI that may affect the intervention process.
6. To keep Juan and others safe, what other factors should be considered?

OCCUPATIONS: ADLs, IADLs, EDUCATION, WORK, PLAY, SOCIAL PARTICIPATION, REST AND SLEEP

1. Given the information provided for this case, identify the areas of occupation that will and will not be addressed. Justify your decisions.
2. Identify the MET value for each ADL and IADL that Juan will be engaged in. How could you verify that the values you identified are accurate?
3. Which activities have a value below, at, and above Juan's present MET level? Explain how these values would influence occupational therapy intervention.
4. Identify the areas of education that will be addressed and explain why.

PERFORMANCE SKILLS: MOTOR, PROCESS, AND SOCIAL INTERACTION SKILLS

1. Given the information provided, identify the motor, process, and social interaction skills that affect Juan's occupational performance.
2. Which of these skills would be appropriate to address within this service delivery site? Justify your selection.
3. Which skills would be addressed through remediation, compensation, and education?
4. Which skills would be addressed through the following intervention approaches: create and promote, establish and restore, maintain, modify, and prevent?

PERFORMANCE PATTERNS: HABITS, ROUTINES, ROLES, AND RITUALS

1. Identify Juan's useful habits, routines, roles, and rituals that support his valued occupations. Discuss how you can make use of this information.
2. Identify Juan's impoverished habits, routines, roles, and rituals that do not support his valued occupations. Discuss how can you make use of this information.
3. Identify Juan's dominating habits, routines, roles, and rituals that interfere with his valued occupations. Discuss how can you make use of this information.

CLIENT FACTORS

Values, beliefs, and spirituality
How can the identified values, beliefs, and spirituality be used in this case?

Body structures
Consider the primary and secondary diagnoses and identify the related body structures.

Body functions

1. Identify how the primary and secondary diagnoses have affected the function of the identified body structures.
2. Explain the relationships between the structural and functional factors and Juan's current level of occupational performance.

MENTAL FUNCTIONS: AFFECTIVE, COGNITIVE, AND PERCEPTUAL

1. What common affective issues related to MI may Juan face?
2. How would these issues be addressed in occupational therapy?
3. To address these issues, what other disciplines could you refer Juan to?
4. Identify three tools to assess the level of stress that Juan experienced as department chair. Evaluate them and select one. Justify your selection.
5. How would you assess Juan's ability to cope with the stress of serving as department chair?
6. Identify three stress-reduction techniques that may benefit Juan, evaluate them, select one, and justify your selection.
7. Given the information provided, what additional mental function considerations need to be addressed?

NEUROMUSCULOSKELETAL AND MOVEMENT-RELATED FUNCTIONS

1. Given the information provided, which neuromusculoskeletal or movement-related functions need to be addressed? Justify your selections.
2. If Juan has to perform a sustained activity at 90° shoulder flexion or greater, what would be the effect on myocardial perfusion?
3. If Juan has to perform a sustained activity at 90° shoulder flexion or greater, how could the surgical site be affected?

CARDIOVASCULAR, HEMATOLOGICAL, IMMUNOLOGICAL, AND RESPIRATORY FUNCTIONS

1. Given the information provided, which cardiovascular, hematological, immunological, or respiratory functions need to be addressed?
2. Cardiac rehabilitation has traditionally been divided into three phases; identify and describe each. How can this information serve as a guide to your intervention and discharge plan?
3. Did Juan's MI affect his muscular or cardiovascular endurance? Justify your response.
4. Which type of endurance does MET assess?
5. Compare and contrast MI with chronic heart failure.

SKIN AND RELATED-STRUCTURE FUNCTIONS

1. Create an instruction sheet for Juan to address the edema in his right hand when he is not engaged in his therapy sessions.
2. Given a surgical wound that is not fully healed, when would it be appropriate to initiate shower activity?
3. What other skin and related-structure functions should be considered?

VOICE AND SPEECH FUNCTIONS

Describe how Juan's diagnoses may affect his voice, speech, or occupational performance.

ASSISTIVE TECHNOLOGIES AND DEVICES

1. What assistive technologies or adaptations might be used or made for Juan while he is receiving occupational therapy services on the coronary care floor? Why?
2. What assistive technologies or adaptations might be recommended for when he returns home? Why?

PHARMACOLOGY

Juan is currently taking acebutolol.

1. What is the brand name?
2. Does this drug have a high alert status?
3. What is the classification of this drug?
4. What is the indication for this drug?
5. What is the action of this drug?
6. How may this drug affect client participation during a therapy session?

SOCIOCULTURAL, SOCIOECONOMIC, AND DIVERSITY FACTORS AND LIFESTYLE CHOICES

1. Given Juan's profile, examine how your own culture and beliefs affect your interaction with him.
2. Based on this self-examination, what area of cultural knowledge do you need to pursue?
3. How can this newly acquired cultural knowledge be integrated for effective outcomes?
4. How can you foster cultural interaction and awareness among your coworkers?
5. Discuss how a lack of understanding in the areas of discrimination and stigma, implicit bias, social identity, or racism may contribute to disparities in the delivery of occupational therapy services in this case.

ASSESSMENT TOOLS AND INTERPRETATION OF RESULTS

1. What is the purpose of the mMRC?
2. Which population is this test designed for?
3. How much time is required to administer it?
4. Provide a brief description of this assessment.
5. What is the reliability of the mMRC?
6. What is the validity of the mMRC?
7. What functional inference can be deduced from Juan's score of 4?
8. What additional standardized assessment can be used in this case? Why?

INTERPROFESSIONAL RELATIONSHIPS AND EFFECTIVE INTRAPROFESSIONAL COLLABORATION

1. Identify the other professions that would make up the care team. Explain the focus of each.
2. Identify the roles of the occupational therapy assistant (OTA) that could be used in the occupational therapy process for this case.
3. Identify interventions that can be assigned to the OTA for this case. Justify your selections.

BILLING AND CODING

1. Identify the current *International Classification of Diseases (ICD)* codes for Juan's diagnoses.
2. For this case, identify at least two *Current Procedural Terminology (CPT®)* codes that are most appropriate.

REIMBURSEMENT SYSTEMS AND DOCUMENTATION

1. Who are the authorized individuals you could share the occupational therapy findings with? Explain why.
2. For this case, what forms and frequency of documentation will be required?
3. Which reimbursement system or systems most commonly cover occupational therapy services in this practice setting?

ADVOCACY

1. Which of the following areas of advocacy would be beneficial in this case: patient rights, matters of privacy, confidentiality, informed consent, awareness building, accessing education, and benefits/ resources?
2. Create a plan to advocate for this client based on the selected areas of advocacy.

ETHICAL DECISION MAKING

1. Brian is very concerned about Juan and asks you about the initial evaluation findings. Under what conditions would you be free to share the findings of Juan's evaluation with him?
2. You observe a bruise on Juan's right elbow. He tells you he fell in his room last night but did not report it to any of the staff, and then he asks you not to report it. What should you do?
3. Juan asks you whether he and his partner will be able to resume their sex life when he returns home. Is it the role of occupational therapy to deal with sexual activity? How would you handle this situation?

TELEHEALTH

1. How can telehealth be integrated as a component of the occupational therapy process in this case?
2. Before launching telemedicine services, what questions would be essential to ask Juan to determine whether it is appropriate for him to engage in telemedicine services?
3. What are the challenges you foresee if you attempt to integrate telehealth services with Juan?

Intervention Plan Formulation and Implementation

INTERVENTION PLAN FORMULATION

Create an intervention plan that includes the following:

1. List this individual's **strengths.**
2. List this individual's **barriers** in occupational performance, performance skills, and performance patterns.

3. Based on the individual's goals, health, performance, and service delivery site, **identify the barriers that will be addressed.**
4. From the barriers identified to be addressed, **formulate goals and objectives.**
5. Identify the focus of each goal and objective as either **create, promote, establish, restore, maintain, modify, or prevent.**
6. Identify the **theoretical basis, model(s) of practice, or frame(s) of reference** that will be used to address each goal and objective.
7. For each proposed goal and objective, describe clearly and precisely the **methods** that will be used. This description should include, but not be limited to, safety considerations, environmental considerations, therapeutic use of self, preparatory activities, activity selection, materials, equipment, and flow.
8. Classify the activities selected in the methods description as either **preparatory, enabling, purposeful, or occupation based.**
9. Explain how each activity can be **graded up or down,** creating the just-right challenge.
10. Provide at least two **primary sources of evidence** to support the intervention plan.

INTERVENTION PLAN IMPLEMENTATION

1. Based on your intervention plan, identify which goals and objectives require **more immediate attention.**
2. Describe your proposed **first treatment session.**
3. As the treatment session is progressing, what is **essential to be observed?**

Transition and Discontinuation

Create a plan for discharge from occupational therapy services in collaboration with Juan and members of the interprofessional team. Review the needs of Juan, caregivers, family members, and significant others. The plan must match needs with available resources and the discharge environment.

REFERENCES

American Medical Association. (2019). *CPT® 2020 professional edition.*
World Health Organization. (2019). *International statistical classification of diseases and related health problems* (11th ed.). https://icd.who.int/
Mahler, D. A., & Wells, C. K. (1988). Evaluation of clinical methods for rating dyspnea. *Chest, 93,* 580–586. https://doi.org/10.1378/chest.93.3.580

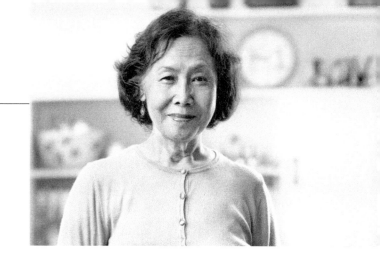

Song: Cerebral Vascular Accident (Right)

DONALD AURIEMMA, MS ED, OTR/L

Song (she, her, hers, herself)

MEDICAL HISTORY

Song is a 69-year-old North Korean refugee female who is 5' 1" and weighs 117 pounds. She was brought to the emergency department by emergency medical services after waking in bed and discovering she was unable to move her left arm and leg. A computed tomography scan of her head, X-rays, magnetic resonance imaging, and blood tests were performed. She received a diagnosis of a right cerebral vascular accident (CVA) of ischemic nature. An emergency endarterectomy was performed. After her surgery, she was transferred to the intensive care unit.

Song reported no previous medical conditions, surgery, or use of medications. She did report the use of a doctor of Chinese medicine for knee and back pain. She reported no substance, nicotine, or caffeine use and an allergic reaction to dairy products.

SOCIAL HISTORY

Song lives with her granddaughter and her granddaughter's family. Six family members share a rented three-bedroom walk-up apartment on the third floor. Song immigrated to the United States just under 2 years ago to assist her granddaughter with child care and care of the home. Her presence allowed her granddaughter to return to work. The children include a 6- and 7-year-old attending school, a 2-year-old, and a newborn at home. The apartment building in which they live is located in a community with many other recent North Korean refugees. Song reports practicing the Taoism religion.

REFERRAL OR PRESCRIPTION

At the acute care hospital, Song will be on the neurological floor, where she will stay for 5 days. She will receive occupational therapy, physical therapy, and social work services.

Occupational Therapy Initial Evaluation Findings: Acute Care

OCCUPATIONAL PROFILE

Song's preadmission occupational history and experiences included being independent in all ADLs and all IADLs. In North Korea, Song and her husband were farmers. After the death of her husband a little more than 2 years ago, she found it impossible to farm on her own. At her daughter's encouragement, she fled North Korea for the United States. Song has the equivalent of primary school education, and her ability to speak English is very limited. Her most common pattern of daily living includes waking up at 5:00 a.m., preparing breakfast for the family, preparing the oldest two children for school, caring for the two younger children at home, shopping, cleaning, preparing dinner, and supervising the two older children after school until their parents return home to assist them with their homework. Her interests include cooking, watching American television, and on occasion socializing with other refugees. She values her family and the opportunity the United States offers her daughter and her daughter's family. Song reported that her greatest current need is not to be a burden to her family.

ADLs

Regarding self-care, while seated, Song was able to don and doff loose-fitting clothing for both upper extremities and both lower extremities. She was unable to effectively manage buttons, zippers, hooks, and laces. Grooming tasks required verbal cues to effectively brush her teeth, comb her hair, and apply makeup on the left side of her body. Regarding functional mobility, Song was able to independently roll and transition between supine and short sitting in bed. She required contact guarding and verbal cuing to transfer with a narrow-base quad cane, on and off the bed, chair, and toilet. Tub transfers were not attempted.

IADLs

Activities that provide day-to-day quality of life and relative independence were explored. Song reported difficulty making voice calls, texting, searching the web, managing money, and caring for her granddaughter's home and her great-grandchildren. Regarding rest and sleep, Song reported difficulty falling asleep and remained asleep for no more than 3–4 hours in the hospital.

MENTAL FUNCTIONS

Cognitive assessment of Song revealed she was alert and oriented to person, place, time, and situation. Short- and long-term memory were intact. She presented with impulsivity and poor insight. She has a tendency to attempt unsupervised transfers, disregarding instructions to use a call bell for assistance. Affect appeared appropriate. A perceptual assessment was performed. The Behavioral Inattention Test (Wilson et al., 1987) indicated mild left visual inattention.

SENSORY FUNCTIONS AND PAIN

No gross deficits were observed with visual, hearing, vestibular, taste, smell, proprioceptive, and cutaneous functions. Use of the Wong-Baker FACES® Pain Rating Scale (Wong-Baker FACES Foundation, 2018) indicated a 2 (*hurts a little bit*) in both knees, with pain described as "achy."

CARDIOVASCULAR AND RESPIRATORY SYSTEMS FUNCTION

No deficits were noted.

MOVEMENT FUNCTIONS

Full passive range of motion and active range of motion were present in all extremities. The manual muscle test indicated scores of 3+ and 5 in left upper extremity (LUE) and left lower extremity (LLE), respectively. Assessment of fine motor (prehension) abilities indicated that Song was able to form gross grasp patterns, lateral pinch, and tripod pinch but was unable to effectively form a palmer and tip-to-tip pinch pattern in the left hand. Additionally, in-hand manipulation skills of tip to palm and palm to tip were slow and awkward. Gross grasp strength was 3 pounds on the left hand and 24 pounds on the right. Standing tolerance was 10–15 minutes.

NEUROMUSCULAR FUNCTIONS

Song was able to sit unsupported without losing her balance and without upper-extremity support. She was able to stand unsupported for 1–2 minutes without losing balance. Any attempt to move either her upper or lower body resulted in her becoming unstable. Muscle tone in the right upper extremity was normal, and coordination was intact. Active isolated movement in the LUE and the LLE was present. Muscle tone appeared normal. Coordination in the LUE and LLE presented with mildly reduced speed and accuracy.

PLAN FOR DISCHARGE

After her 4-day stay on the neurological care floor, Song will be discharged to a subacute rehabilitation facility and will receive occupational therapy, physical therapy, and social worker services.

Questions and Activities

SAFETY OF CLIENT AND OTHERS: PRECAUTIONS OR CONTRAINDICATIONS

1. Identify the components of "standard precautions."
2. Song presents with impulsivity. What safety concerns do you anticipate?
3. Song presents with left-sided visual inattention. What safety concerns do you anticipate?
4. Create a handout identifying precautions to be followed by individuals placed on blood thinners.

5. Identify the common psychological reactions associated with CVA that may affect the treatment process.
6. To keep Song and others safe, what other factors should be considered?

OCCUPATIONS: ADLs, IADLs, EDUCATION, WORK, PLAY, SOCIAL PARTICIPATION, AND REST AND SLEEP

1. Given the information provided for this case, identify the areas of occupation that will and will not be addressed. Justify your decisions.
2. What clothing choices would you recommend to Song to eliminate the need to manage fasteners to dress?
3. What equipment and strategies do you anticipate can be used to increase Song's safety while showering?
4. Which functional mobility skills would be appropriate to address with Song?
5. Identify the areas of education that would be appropriate to engage in with Song, and explain why.

PERFORMANCE SKILLS: MOTOR SKILLS, PROCESS SKILLS, AND SOCIAL INTERACTION SKILLS

1. Given the information provided, identify the motor, process, and social interaction skills that affect Song's occupational performance.
2. Which of these skills would be appropriate to address in this service delivery site? Justify your selection.
3. Which of these skills would be addressed through remediation, compensation, and education?
4. Which of these skills would be addressed through the following intervention approaches: create/promote, establish/restore, maintain, modify, and prevent?

PERFORMANCE PATTERNS: HABITS, ROUTINES, ROLES, AND RITUALS

1. Identify Song's useful habits, routines, roles, and rituals that support valued occupations. How can you make use of this information?
2. Identify Song's impoverished habits, routines, roles, and rituals that do not support valued occupations. How can you make use of this information?
3. Identify Song's dominating habits, routines, roles, and rituals that interfere with valued occupations. How can you make use of this information?

CLIENT FACTORS

Values, beliefs, and spirituality
How can the identified values, beliefs, and spirituality be used in this case?

Body structures
Considering the primary and secondary diagnoses, identify the related body structures.

Body functions
1. Identify how the primary and secondary diagnoses have affected the function of the identified body structures.
2. Explain the relationship between structural and functional factors and Song's current level of occupational performance.

MENTAL FUNCTIONS: AFFECTIVE, COGNITIVE, AND PERCEPTUAL

1. What common affective issues related to CVA may Song face?
2. How would these issues be addressed in occupational therapy?
3. To address these issues, what other disciplines could you refer Song to?
4. What strategies can be used to maximize effective communication with Song?
5. What common strategies are available to assist Song with her impulsiveness?
6. What common strategies are available to assist Song with her left-sided visual inattention?
7. Given the information provided, what additional mental function considerations need to be addressed?

NEUROMUSCULOSKELETAL AND MOVEMENT-RELATED FUNCTIONS

1. Given the information provided, which neuromusculoskeletal and movement-related functions need to be addressed? Justify your selections.
2. Based on the finding that the "patient was able to sit unsupported without losing her balance and without upper-extremity support," should Song's static sitting balance be assigned a grade of fair or fair plus? Justify your selection.
3. Based on the finding that "the patient presented with slightly less than normal speed and skill," should Song's coordination be assigned a grade of 4 or 5? Provide a reference.
4. Compare and contrast neuromusculoskeletal and movement-related functions of CVA and traumatic brain injury.

CARDIOVASCULAR, HEMATOLOGICAL, IMMUNOLOGICAL, AND RESPIRATORY FUNCTIONS

1. Given the information provided, which cardiovascular, hematological, immunological, and respiratory functions need to be addressed? Justify your selection.
2. Which vital signs should be taken when working with Song? What are the norms for each of these vital signs? When should Song's vital signs be taken?

SKIN AND RELATED STRUCTURE FUNCTIONS

1. On arrival at occupational therapy, you noticed an abrasion on Song's lateral aspect of her elbow. Would this abrasion be a concern, and, if so, what possible action would you take?
2. What other skin and related structure functions should be considered?

VOICE AND SPEECH FUNCTIONS

Describe how a CVA may affect the voice and/or speech and their impact on occupational performance.

ASSISTIVE TECHNOLOGIES AND DEVICES

What assistive technologies or adaptations might be used or made for Song while she is receiving occupational therapy services on the neurological care floor? Why?

ETHICAL DECISION MAKING

1. You have only 4 days to provide service to Song before she is transferred to the subacute rehabilitation facility. What factors will you weigh in deciding which of Song's areas of need will and will not be addressed at your service delivery site?
2. It is time for Song's occupational therapy session, but the hospital interpreter has not yet arrived. Identify options to maintain Health Insurance Portability and Accountability Act compliance. Select the most appropriate option and support your decision.
3. You walk past Song's room and observe her walking to the bathroom with her quad cane, but she is unguarded. Identify options of what you should do. Select the most appropriate option and support your decision.
4. Song has exclusively used chopsticks to eat her meals all her life. The hospital supplies only plastic spoons, forks, and knives. Identify options of what you should do. Select the most appropriate option and support your decision.
5. A patient in the occupational therapy gym has made a derogatory statement concerning the Chinese in the presence of Song. Identify options of what you should do. Select the most appropriate option and support your decision.

PHARMACOLOGY

Song is currently taking heparin.

1. What is the brand name?
2. Does this drug have a high alert status?
3. What is the classification of this drug?
4. What is the indication for this drug?
5. What is the action of this drug?
6. How may this drug affect client participation during a therapy session?

SOCIOCULTURAL, SOCIOECONOMIC, AND DIVERSITY FACTORS AND LIFESTYLE CHOICES

1. Given Song's profile, examine how your own culture and beliefs affect your interaction with her.
2. Based on this self-examination, what area of cultural knowledge do you need to pursue?
3. How can this newly acquired cultural knowledge be integrated for effective outcomes?
4. How can you foster cultural interaction and awareness among your coworkers?
5. Discuss how a lack of understanding in the areas of discrimination and stigma, implicit bias, social identity, or racism may contribute to disparities in the delivery of occupational therapy services in this case.

ASSESSMENT TOOLS AND INTERPRETATION OF RESULTS

1. What is the purpose of the Wong-Baker FACES Scale?
2. Which population is this test designed for?
3. How much time is required to administer it?
4. Provide a brief description of this assessment.
5. What is the reliability of this assessment?

6. What is the validity of this assessment?
7. What functional inference can be deduced from a score of 2 on this assessment?

INTERPROFESSIONAL RELATIONSHIP AND EFFECTIVE INTRAPROFESSIONAL COLLABORATION

1. Identify the other professions that would make up the care team. Explain the focus of each.
2. Identify the roles of the occupational therapy assistant (OTA) that could be used in the occupational therapy process for this case.
3. Identify interventions that can be assigned to the OTA for this case. Justify your selections.

BILLING AND CODING

1. Identify the *International Classification of Diseases (ICD)* code for Song's diagnosis.
2. For this case, identify at least two *Current Procedural Terminology (CPT®)* codes that are most appropriate. Justify your selection.

REIMBURSEMENT SYSTEMS AND DOCUMENTATION

1. Who are the authorized individuals you could share the occupational therapy findings with? Explain why.
2. For this case, what forms and frequency of documentation will be required?
3. Which reimbursement system or systems most commonly cover occupational therapy services in this practice setting?

ADVOCACY

1. Which of the following areas of advocacy would be beneficial in this case: patient rights, matters of privacy, confidentiality, informed consent, awareness building, accessing education, and benefits/resources?
2. Create a plan to advocate for this client based on the selected areas of advocacy.

TELEHEALTH

1. How can telehealth be integrated as a component of the occupational therapy process in this case?
2. Before launching telemedicine services, what questions would be essential to ask Song to determine whether it is appropriate for her to engage in telemedicine services?
3. What challenges do you foresee if you attempt to integrate telehealth services with Song?

Intervention Plan Formulation and Implementation

INTERVENTION PLAN FORMULATION

Create an intervention plan that includes the following:

1. List this individual's **strengths.**

2. List this individual's **barriers** in occupational performance, performance skills, and performance patterns.
3. Based on the individual's goals, health, performance, and service delivery site, **identify the barriers that will be addressed.**
4. From the barriers identified to be addressed, **formulate goals and objectives.**
5. Identify the focus of each goal and objective as either **create, promote, establish, restore, maintain, modify, or prevent.**
6. Identify the **theoretical basis, model(s) of practice, or frame(s) of reference** that will be used to address each goal and objective.
7. For each proposed goal and objective, describe clearly and precisely the **methods** that will be used. This description should include, but not be limited to, safety considerations, environmental considerations, therapeutic use of self, preparatory activities, activity selection, materials, equipment, and flow.
8. Classify the activities selected in the methods description as either **preparatory, enabling, purposeful,** or **occupation based.**
9. Explain how each activity can be **graded up or down,** creating the just-right challenge.
10. Provide at least two **primary sources of evidence** to support the intervention plan.

INTERVENTION PLAN IMPLEMENTATION

1. Based on your intervention plan, identify which goals and objectives require **more immediate attention.**
2. Describe your proposed **first treatment session.**
3. As the treatment session is progressing, what is **essential to be observed?**

Transition and Discontinuation

Create a plan for discharge from occupational therapy services in collaboration with Song and members of the interprofessional team. Review the needs of Song, caregivers, family members, and significant others. The plan must match needs with available resources and the discharge environment.

REFERENCES

American Medical Association. (2019). *CPT® 2020 professional edition.*
Wilson, B., Cockburn, J., & Halligan, P. (1987). *Behavioral Inattention Test.* Pearson.
Wong-Baker FACES Foundation. (2018). *Wong-Baker FACES® Pain Rating Scale.* Author.
World Health Organization. (2019). *International statistical classification of diseases and related health problems* (11th ed.). https://icd.who.int/

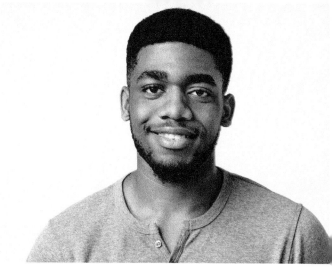

Ethan: Complete C6 Spinal Cord Injury

DONALD AURIEMMA, MS ED, OTR/L

Ethan (he, him, his, himself)

MEDICAL HISTORY

Ethan is a 26-year-old Black male who is 6' 3" and weighs 220 pounds. He was brought to the emergency department by emergency medical services after falling from a roof. Immediately after his fall, Ethan was unable to move and feel both upper extremities and both lower extremities. Medical assessments included testing sensory function and movement, X-rays, computerized tomography scan, and magnetic resonance imaging. Ethan received a diagnosis of a complete C6 spinal cord injury (SCI). In the operating room, he was fitted with a halo brace. After his procedure, he was transferred to the neurological intensive care unit. His past medical history was unremarkable. He reported no drug, alcohol, caffeine, or tobacco use, and a penicillin allergy.

SOCIAL HISTORY

Ethan is an accounting student and part-time roofer. He lives with his wife, Shana, and their 6-month-old daughter, Crystal. Shana is at work and Ethan is at school. They share a one-bedroom basement apartment in Ethan's parents' home. There are 13 steps from the first floor to the basement apartment through a narrow doorway. Ethan has two younger brothers, ages 16 and 19 years, who still live at home. Ethan identifies as a Black Hebrew Israelite.

REFERRAL OR PRESCRIPTION

At the acute care hospital, Ethan will be on the neurological care floor for a 5-day stay. He was referred for occupational therapy, physical therapy, registered nursing, and social work services.

Occupational Therapy Initial Evaluation Findings: Acute Care

OCCUPATIONAL PROFILE

Ethan's preadmission occupational history and experiences included being independent in all ADLs and all IADLs. Ethan had been employed as a roofer for the past 6 months and viewed roofing as a temporary career until he could complete his accounting degree. His patterns of daily living most commonly included having a quick breakfast in the morning, arriving on a job site by 7:00 a.m., and returning home by 8:00 p.m. He frequently worked weekends when overtime was available. During his limited free time, he liked to be home with Shana and his daughter and, when a babysitter was available, to go to the gym or dinner with Shana. His interests include exercise, camping, and finance. He values his family, education, and ability to support his family. Ethan reported that his greatest current need is to do everything possible—not to be a burden on his family.

ADLs

Regarding self-care, Ethan was dependent in his ability to feed, dress, groom, bathe, and toilet himself. Regarding functional mobility, Ethan was dependent on his ability to roll, sit up, scoot, and transfer. When placed in a short sitting position, he immediately complained of being lightheaded, dizzy, and feeling as if he was going to pass out. The Canadian Occupational Performance Measure (COPM; Law et al., 2019) was administered and a score of 73 was obtained.

IADLs

Activities needed that provide day-to-day quality of life and relative independence were explored. Ethan is dependent for using electronic communications, handling his finances, maintaining his home, preparing meals, performing cleanup tasks, and the ability to shop.

Regarding rest and sleep, Ethan reported poor sleep quality and not being able to sleep more than 1–2 hours before waking up. Before his SCI, he primarily slept in prone and had no problem sleeping through the night.

MENTAL FUNCTIONS

Cognitive assessment found Ethan to be alert and oriented to person, place, time, and situation. Short- and long-term memory were intact. Affect assessment revealed mixed emotions. At times, he was soft-spoken and tearful as he verbalized optimism about his recovery, and other times he expressed anger toward his employer for not providing safe working conditions. No gross deficits in perception were observed.

SENSORY FUNCTIONS AND PAIN

No gross deficits were observed with visual, hearing, vestibular, taste, and olfactory functions. There was an absence of cutaneous sensation below dermatome C6; vision, hearing, olfactory, and vestibular senses were intact. He reported no pain.

CARDIOVASCULAR AND RESPIRATORY SYSTEMS FUNCTIONS

Ethan was able to breathe without a ventilator but exhibited low stamina. He presented with a weak cough. Assessment of cardiovascular and respiratory systems function indicated a decrease in blood pressure from 132/75 to 82/47 when transitioned from supine to short sitting.

MOVEMENT FUNCTIONS

Ethan was within normal limits for passive range of motion in both upper and both lower extremities. Active range of motion was within normal limits for all shoulder movements, elbow flexion, forearm supination, and radial wrist extension. Elbow extension, wrist flexion, and hand movements were absent. Total paralysis of the trunk and lower extremities was present. Assessment of muscle strength and endurance was contraindicated at the time of evaluation.

NEUROMUSCULAR FUNCTIONS

Ethan was intact for involuntary and voluntary reactions and movements at the level of C6 and above and absent below. The assessment of sitting and standing balance was contraindicated at the time of evaluation. Muscle tone in innervated musculature was intact, and below the level of injury, flaccid. Deep tendon reflexes in both lower extremities were absent.

PLAN FOR DISCHARGE

After his stay on the neurological care floor, Ethan will be transferred to a rehabilitation center that specializes in SCIs. He will receive occupational therapy, physical therapy, and social work and registered nursing services.

Questions and Activities

SAFETY OF CLIENT AND OTHERS: PRECAUTIONS AND CONTRAINDICATIONS

1. What are the signs and symptoms of orthostatic hypotension and postural hypotension?
2. If Ethan experiences an episode of orthostatic hypotension or postural hypotension, identify the actions that need to be taken.
3. What are the signs and symptoms of autonomic dysreflexia to be aware of while working with Ethan?
4. If Ethan experiences an episode of autonomic dysreflexia, what immediate actions need to be taken?
5. Create a handout identifying the signs and symptoms of deep vein thrombosis (DVT).
6. If Ethan develops a DVT, what immediate actions need to be taken?
7. Ethan is at risk to acquire a pressure ulcer. Explain why.
8. What are the most common sites in which pressure ulcers form? How can occupational therapy play a role in the prevention of pressure ulcers?
9. Which vital signs should be taken when working with Ethan? What are their norms? When should they be taken?

10. Performing the manual muscle test was contraindicated at the time of the initial evaluation. Why?
11. After his SCI, Ethan presents with a weak cough. What risks does this symptom pose?
12. Identify the common psychological reactions associated with a SCI that may affect the treatment process.
13. To keep Ethan and others safe, what other factors should be considered?

OCCUPATIONS: ADLs, IADLs, EDUCATION, WORK, PLAY, SOCIAL PARTICIPATION, AND REST AND SLEEP

1. Given the information provided for this case, identify the areas of occupation that will and will not be addressed. Justify your decisions.
2. What activities can be introduced to Ethan for him to begin feeding himself? Which assistive devices would be needed? Explain why.
3. Ethan wishes to be able to use a phone so he can communicate with his family while he is hospitalized. How can his phone use be facilitated?
4. You receive orders that Ethan is cleared to begin out-of-bed-to-wheelchair activities. Which wheelchair choice and features would be best suited for him? Explain why.
5. What would be a reasonable schedule to increase Ethan's sitting tolerance in a wheelchair? Provide support for your choice of schedule.
6. Ethan wishes to have the ability to contact the floor nurse from his hospital bed; currently, he is unable to use the call bell. What options are available?
7. Which areas of patient education should be given priority? Why?
8. Briefly describe what Ethan's first occupational therapy treatment session would look like.

PERFORMANCE SKILLS: MOTOR SKILLS, PROCESS SKILLS, AND SOCIAL INTERACTION SKILLS

1. Given the information provided, identify the motor, process, and social interaction skills that affect Ethan's occupational performance.
2. Which of these skills would be appropriate to address within this service delivery site? Justify your selection.
3. Which of these skills would be addressed through remediation, compensation, and education?
4. Which of these skills would be addressed through the following intervention approaches: create/promote, establish/restore, maintain, modify, and prevent?

PERFORMANCE PATTERNS: HABITS, ROUTINES, ROLES, AND RITUALS

1. Identify Ethan's useful habits, routines, roles, and rituals that support valued occupations. How can you make use of this information?
2. Identify Ethan's impoverished habits, routines, roles, and rituals that do not support valued occupations. How can you make use of this information?
3. Identify Ethan's dominating habits, routines, roles, and rituals that interfere with valued occupations. How can you make use of this information?

CLIENT FACTORS

Values, beliefs, and spirituality
How can the identified values, beliefs, and spirituality be used in this case?

Body structures
Considering the primary diagnosis, identify the related body structures.

Body functions
1. How has the primary diagnosis affected the function of the identified body structures?
2. Explain the relationships between the structural and functional factors and Ethan's current level of occupational performance.

MENTAL FUNCTIONS: AFFECTIVE, COGNITIVE, AND PERCEPTUAL

1. What common affective issues related to SCI may Ethan face?
2. How would these issues be addressed in occupational therapy?
3. To address these issues, what other disciplines could you refer Ethan to?
4. What common affective issues related to SCI may Ethan's family experience?
5. What support would be available to recommend to Ethan's family to address these issues?
6. Given the information provided, what additional mental function considerations need to be addressed?

NEUROMUSCULOSKELETAL AND MOVEMENT-RELATED FUNCTIONS

1. Given the information provided, which neuromusculoskeletal or movement-related functions need to be addressed? Justify your selections.
2. What early steps should be taken to prevent atrophy from disuse in Ethan's innervated muscle groups?
3. What early steps should be taken to prevent the shortening of soft tissues and the development of contracture?
4. Create an exercise program for Ethan based on occupational performance.
5. Compare and contrast paraplegia with quadriplegia.

CARDIOVASCULAR, HEMATOLOGICAL, IMMUNOLOGICAL, AND RESPIRATORY FUNCTIONS

1. Given the information provided, which cardiovascular, hematological, immunological, and respiratory functions need to be addressed? Justify your selections.
2. Would it be expected that the energy costs of performing a given ADL be the same for Ethan before his injury? Explain why.
3. Identify the metabolic equivalent of task value for upper-body dressing in a person without dysfunction. How would Ethan's value differ?

SKIN AND RELATED STRUCTURE FUNCTIONS

1. Which pressure relief strategies would be the best match for Ethan? Explain why.
2. What other skin and related structure functions should be considered?

VOICE AND SPEECH FUNCTIONS

Describe how Ethan's diagnosis may affect his voice, speech, and occupational performance.

ASSISTIVE TECHNOLOGIES AND DEVICES

What assistive technologies or adaptations might be used or made for Ethan while he is receiving occupational therapy services on the neurological care unit? Why?

ETHICAL DECISION MAKING

1. During your first session with Ethan, he asked you how long it usually takes for patients like him to regain their ability to walk. How can his question be best addressed?
2. You arrive at Ethan's room for his scheduled treatment session, and it becomes apparent to you that he has had a bowel movement that has not yet been attended to. How can this situation be best addressed?
3. During a treatment session, you observe that Ethan presents with an abrasion over his left lateral malleolus that was not previously observed or documented. How should this observation be addressed?

PHARMACOLOGY

Ethan is currently taking codeine.

1. What is the brand name?
2. Does this drug have a high alert status?
3. What is the classification of this drug?
4. What is the indication for this drug?
5. What is the action of this drug?
6. How may this drug affect client participation during a therapy session?

SOCIOCULTURAL, SOCIOECONOMIC, DIVERSITY FACTORS, AND LIFESTYLE CHOICES

1. Given Ethan's profile, examine how your own culture and beliefs affect your interaction with him.
2. Based on this self-examination, what area of cultural knowledge do you need to pursue?
3. How can this newly acquired cultural knowledge be integrated for effective outcomes?
4. How can you foster cultural interaction and awareness among your coworkers?
5. Discuss how a lack of understanding in the areas of discrimination and stigma, implicit bias, social identity, or racism may contribute to disparities in the delivery of occupational therapy services in this case.

ASSESSMENT TOOLS AND INTERPRETATION OF RESULTS

1. What is the purpose of the COPM?
2. Which population is this test designed for?
3. How much time is required to administer it?
4. Provide a brief description of this assessment.
5. What is the reliability of the COPM?
6. What is the validity of the COPM?
7. What functional inference can be deduced from Ethan's score of 73?
8. What additional standardized assessment can be used in this case? Why?

INTERPROFESSIONAL RELATIONSHIP AND EFFECTIVE INTRAPROFESSIONAL COLLABORATION

1. Identify the other professions that would make up the care team. Explain the focus of each.
2. Identify the roles of the occupational therapy assistant (OTA) that could be used in the occupational therapy process for this case.
3. Identify interventions that can be assigned to the OTA for this case. Justify your selections.

BILLING AND CODING

1. Identify the *International Classification of Diseases (ICD)* codes for Ethan's diagnosis.
2. For this case, identify at least two *Current Procedural Terminology (CPT®)* codes that are most appropriate. Justify your selection.

REIMBURSEMENT SYSTEMS AND DOCUMENTATION

1. Who would be the authorized individuals you could share the occupational therapy findings with? Explain why.
2. For this case, what forms and frequency of documentation will be required?
3. Which reimbursement system or systems most commonly cover occupational therapy services in this practice setting?

ADVOCACY

1. Which of the following areas of advocacy would be beneficial in this case: patient rights, matters of privacy, confidentiality, informed consent, awareness building, accessing education, and benefits/resources?
2. Create a plan to advocate for this client based on the selected areas of advocacy.

TELEHEALTH

1. How can telehealth be integrated as a component of the occupational therapy process in this case?
2. Before launching telemedicine services, what questions would be essential to ask Ethan to determine whether it is appropriate for him to engage in telemedicine services?
3. What are the barriers, obstacles, or challenges you foresee if attempting to integrate telehealth services with Ethan?

Intervention Plan Formulation and Implementation

INTERVENTION PLAN FORMULATION

Create an intervention plan that includes the following:

1. List this individual's **strengths.**
2. List this individual's **barriers** in occupational performance, performance skills, and performance patterns.

3. Based on the individual's goals, health, performance, and service delivery site, **identify the barriers that will be addressed.**
4. From the barriers identified to be addressed, **formulate goals and objectives.**
5. Identify the focus of each goal and objective as either **create, promote, establish, restore, maintain, modify, or prevent.**
6. Identify the **theoretical basis, model(s) of practice, or frame(s) of reference** that will be used to address each goal and objective.
7. For each proposed goal and objective, describe clearly and precisely the **methods** that will be used. This description should include, but not be limited to, safety considerations, environmental considerations, therapeutic use of self, preparatory activities, activity selection, materials, equipment, and flow.
8. Classify the activities selected in the methods description as either **preparatory, enabling, purposeful, or occupation based.**
9. Explain how each activity can be **graded up or down,** creating the just-right challenge.
10. Provide at least two **primary sources of evidence** to support the intervention plan.

INTERVENTION PLAN IMPLEMENTATION

11. Based on your intervention plan, identify which goals and objectives require **more immediate attention.**
12. Describe your proposed **first treatment session.**
13. As the treatment session is progressing, what is **essential to be observed?**

Transition and Discontinuation

Create a plan for discharge from occupational therapy services in collaboration with Ethan and members of the interprofessional team. Review the needs of Ethan, caregivers, family members, and significant others. The plan must match needs with available resources and the discharge environment.

REFERENCES

American Medical Association. (2019). *CPT® 2020 professional edition.*
Law, M., Baptiste, S., Carswell, A., McColl, M., Polatajko, H., & Pollock, N. (2019). *Canadian Occupational Performance Measure* (5th ed., rev.). COPM Inc.
World Health Organization. (2019). *International statistical classification of diseases and related health problems* (11th ed.). https://icd.who.int/

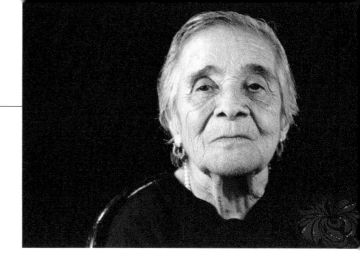

Hannah: Congestive Heart Failure

DONALD AURIEMMA, MS ED, OTR/L

Hannah (she, her, hers, herself)

MEDICAL HISTORY

Hannah is an 81-year-old Chippewa Native American who is 5' 2" and weighs 90 pounds. She was brought to the emergency department (ED) by emergency medical services after reporting shortness of breath and presenting with bilateral rales, jugular venous distension, bilateral lower-extremity edema, and the following vital signs: heart rate 103 beats/minute, respiratory rate 32 breaths per minute, blood pressure 154/92 mm hg, and oxygen saturation 88%. Blood tests, urinalysis, echocardiogram, and chest radiography were performed, and she received a diagnosis of congestive heart failure (CHF). From the ED she was transferred to the coronary care unit (CCU) where she received nitrates to decrease preload, myocardial oxygen consumption, systemic vascular resistance, and supplementary oxygen.

Her medical history included hypertension, myocardial infarct atrial arrhythmia, and two previous admissions for CHF episodes. Upon admission, she reported living a sedentary lifestyle, drinking 3 to 4 cups of coffee per day, and no alcohol, drug, or nicotine use. Hannah reported no known allergies.

SOCIAL HISTORY

Hannah lives alone in a one-bedroom garden apartment on the ground floor. At home, she uses a straight cane only for outside ambulation. Her daughter, Eva, lives in the apartment above her with two adult grandchildren. All three are dedicated to Hannah and are employed full time, working weekdays. There are three steps to enter Hannah's apartment, which consists of a living room, bathroom, bedroom, dinette, and small kitchen. Hannah follows the Ojibwa religion.

REFERRAL OR PRESCRIPTION

At the acute care hospital, Hannah will be in the CCU for a 5-day stay. She has been referred for occupational therapy, physical therapy, social work, and registered nursing services.

Occupational Therapy Initial Evaluation Findings: Acute Care

OCCUPATIONAL PROFILE

Hannah's preadmission occupational history and experiences included being independent in all ADLs, although performing them in a slow and effortful manner. Regarding IADLs, her daughter prepared meals that Hannah reheated. Additionally, she shopped and cleaned Hannah's apartment on weekends. Hannah has been retired for 6 years. Her patterns of daily living most commonly included spending the day at home watching television and being taken to church on Sundays by her granddaughter. At least three evenings per week, one of her grandchildren eats dinner with her in her apartment. Her interests include following the local baseball team and reading her bible. She values her family, church, and Native American heritage. Hannah reported that her current goal is to return home and be able to attend church on Sundays.

ADLs

Regarding self-care, Hannah was able to feed herself independently, but consumption of a large meal left her feeling short of breath. While seated, Hannah was able to dress both her upper extremities independently in a slow spontaneous fashion but required moderate assistance to dress both lower extremities secondary to becoming noticeably short of breath. Her respiration rate elevated to 29 breaths per minute from a baseline of 20 breaths per minute during lower-extremity dressing. Hannah was able to independently perform the grooming tasks of brushing her hair and teeth while seated but reported that she did not feel she had enough endurance to attempt standing in the tub to shower. Regarding functional mobility, Hannah was able to independently roll and move between supine and short sit with contact guarding. She required minimal assistance to transfer with her adult rolling walker on and off the bed, chair, hospital wheelchair, and toilet in a very slow and mindful manner. Tub transfers were not attempted.

IADLs

Activities needed that provide day-to-day quality of life and relative independence were explored. Hannah can manage her communications and her checkbook but is dependent on others to prepare meals using the stove, clean up, and shop. Regarding rest and sleep, Hannah reported that she is unable to sleep unless she is propped up by three or four pillows. She has been diagnosed with central sleep apnea with Cheyne-Stokes breathing. The Satisfaction, Alertness, Timing, Efficiency and Duration (SATED) questionnaire (Buysse, 2014) was administered, and a score of 5 was obtained.

MENTAL FUNCTIONS

Cognitive assessment found Hannah to be alert and oriented to person, place, time, and situation, and short- and long-term memory were intact. She was able to follow three-step commands and make her needs known. Affect appeared appropriate, and no gross deficits in perception were observed.

SENSORY FUNCTIONS AND PAIN

No gross deficits were observed with visual, hearing, vestibular, taste, smell, proprioceptive, and cutaneous functions. Hannah did report using reading glasses. No pain was reported.

CARDIOVASCULAR AND RESPIRATORY SYSTEM FUNCTIONS

Edema in both ankles was 2+ using a pitting edema scale. Assessment of cardiovascular and respiratory systems function indicated a metabolic equivalent of task (MET) value of 2.0. At the time of evaluation, Hannah was receiving 2 liters of supplemental oxygen through a nasal cannula.

MOVEMENT FUNCTIONS

Passive range of motion and active range of motion in all four extremities were within normal limits. Manual muscle testing was performed and revealed a gross muscle strength of 3+/5 in both upper and both lower extremities. Gross grasp strength in both right and left hands was 17 pounds. No gross deficits in prehension and coordination were observed. Standing tolerance was 3–5 minutes.

NEUROMUSCULAR FUNCTIONS

Static and dynamic sitting balance were both 5/5, static standing balance was 3+/5, and dynamic standing balance was 3/5. Muscle tone was normal, and no gross deficits in reflex integration were observed.

PLAN FOR DISCHARGE

After her stay on the medical floor, Hannah will be discharged home with home health care services. She will be receiving occupational therapy; physical therapy; and social work, registered nursing, and home health aide services.

Questions and Activities

SAFETY OF CLIENT AND OTHERS: PRECAUTIONS AND CONTRAINDICATIONS

1. What are the signs and symptoms of respiratory distress to be aware of while working with Hannah?
2. If Hannah experiences respiratory distress, what immediate actions must be taken?
3. Which vital signs should be taken when working with Hannah? What are the norms for each? When should they be taken?
4. Create a handout identifying precautions that need to be followed when using supplemental oxygen.
5. Describe the correct guarding method to be used during transfer-training sessions.
6. Identify the common psychological reactions associated with CHF that may affect the treatment process.
7. To keep Hannah and others safe, what other factors should be considered?

OCCUPATIONS: ADLs, IADLs, EDUCATION, WORK, PLAY, SOCIAL PARTICIPATION, AND REST AND SLEEP

1. Given the information provided for this case, identify the areas of occupation that will and will not be addressed. Justify your decisions.
2. Identify the MET value for each ADL and IADL that Hannah will be engaged in during her intervention sessions.
3. Which activities have a value below, at, and above Hannah's present MET level? Explain how these values would influence occupational therapy intervention.
4. Identify the areas of education that would be appropriate to engage in with Hannah and explain why.
5. Briefly describe what Hannah's first occupational therapy treatment session would look like.

PERFORMANCE SKILLS: MOTOR SKILLS, PROCESS SKILLS, AND SOCIAL INTERACTION SKILLS

1. Given the information provided, identify the motor, process, and social interaction skills that affect Hannah's occupational performance.
2. Which of these skills would be appropriate to address within this service delivery site? Justify your selection.
3. Which of these skills would be addressed through remediation, compensation, and education?
4. Which of these skills would be addressed through the following intervention approaches: create/promote, establish/restore, maintain, modify, and prevent?

PERFORMANCE PATTERNS: HABITS, ROUTINES, ROLES, AND RITUALS

1. Identify Hannah's useful habits, routines, roles and rituals that support valued occupations. How can you make use of this information?
2. Identify Hannah's impoverished habits, routines, roles, and rituals that do not support valued occupations. How can you make use of this information?
3. Identify Hannah's dominating habits, routines, roles, and rituals that interfere with valued occupations. How can you make use of this information?

CLIENT FACTORS

Values, beliefs, and spirituality
How can the identified values, beliefs, and spirituality be used in this case?

Body structures
Considering Hannah's primary and secondary diagnoses, identify the related body structures.

Body functions
1. How have the primary and secondary diagnoses affected the function of the identified body structures?
2. Explain the relationships between the structural and functional factors and Hannah's current level of occupational performance.

MENTAL FUNCTIONS: AFFECTIVE, COGNITIVE, AND PERCEPTUAL

1. What common affective issues related to CHF may Hannah face?

2. How would these issues be addressed in occupational therapy?
3. To address these issues, what other disciplines could you refer Hannah to?
4. How might the social worker address these issues with Hannah?
5. Given the information provided, what additional mental function considerations need to be addressed?

NEUROMUSCULOSKELETAL AND MOVEMENT-RELATED FUNCTIONS

1. Given the information provided, which neuromusculoskeletal or movement-related functions need to be addressed? Justify your selections.
2. What is disuse atrophy? Explain how it relates to Hannah's current condition.
3. How can 3+/5 muscle strength in Hannah's four extremities be best addressed?
4. Create an exercise program for Hannah based on occupational performance.

CARDIOVASCULAR, HEMATOLOGICAL, IMMUNOLOGICAL, AND RESPIRATORY FUNCTIONS

1. Given the information provided, which cardiovascular, hematological, immunological, and respiratory functions need to be addressed? Justify your selections.
2. Identify energy conservation principles and describe how Hannah could apply these concepts while performing her ADLs.
3. Compare and contrast central sleep apnea with Cheyne-Stokes breathing and obstructive sleep apnea.

SKIN AND RELATED STRUCTURE FUNCTIONS

1. How can Hannah address the edema in her right hand when she is not actively engaged in therapy sessions?
2. What other skin and related structure functions should be considered?

VOICE AND SPEECH FUNCTIONS

Describe how Hannah's diagnoses may affect her voice, speech, and occupational performance.

ASSISTIVE TECHNOLOGIES AND DEVICES

1. What assistive technologies or adaptations might be used or made for Hannah while she is receiving occupational therapy services on the coronary care floor? Why?
2. What assistive technologies or adaptations might be recommended for when she returns home? Why?

ETHICAL DECISION MAKING

1. Hannah informs you that her dentures were accidentally thrown out by the morning hospital staff. What should you do?
2. You observe Hannah walking to use the bathroom without the use of oxygen or a walker. What do you do?
3. Hannah informs you she is behind in paying her utility bills and does not wish her family to know. What should you do? Explain your decision.

PHARMACOLOGY

Hannah is currently taking acebutolol.

1. What is the brand name?
2. Does this drug have a high alert status?
3. What is the classification of this drug?
4. What is the indication for this drug?
5. What is the action of this drug?
6. How may this drug affect client participation during a therapy session?

SOCIOCULTURAL, SOCIOECONOMIC, AND DIVERSITY FACTORS AND LIFESTYLE CHOICES

1. Given Hannah's profile, examine how your own culture and beliefs affect your interaction with her.
2. Based on this self-examination, what area of cultural knowledge do you need to pursue?
3. How can this newly acquired cultural knowledge be integrated for effective outcomes?
4. How can you foster cultural interaction and awareness among your coworkers?
5. Discuss how a lack of understanding in the areas of discrimination and stigma, implicit bias, social identity, or racism may contribute to disparities in the delivery of occupational therapy services in this case.

ASSESSMENT TOOLS AND INTERPRETATION OF RESULTS

1. What is the purpose of the SATED?
2. Which population is this test designed for?
3. How much time is required to administer it?
4. Provide a brief description of this assessment.
5. What is the reliability of the SATED?
6. What is the validity of the SATED?
7. What functional inference can be deduced from Hannah's score of 5?
8. What additional standardized assessment can be used in this case? Why?

INTERPROFESSIONAL RELATIONSHIP AND EFFECTIVE INTRAPROFESSIONAL COLLABORATION

1. Identify the other professions that would make up the care team. Explain the focus of each.
2. Identify the roles of the occupational therapy assistant (OTA) that could be used in the occupational therapy process for this case.
3. Identify interventions that can be assigned to the OTA for this case. Justify your selections.
4. What other professionals would be part of this patient's care and what would be their primary focus?

BILLING AND CODING

1. Identify the *International Classification of Diseases (ICD)* codes for Hannah's diagnoses.
2. For this case, identify at least two *Current Procedural Terminology (CPT®)* codes that are most appropriate. Justify your selection.

REIMBURSEMENT SYSTEMS AND DOCUMENTATION

1. Who would be the authorized individuals you could share the occupational therapy findings with? Explain why.
2. For this case, what forms and frequency of documentation will be required?
3. Which reimbursement system or systems most commonly cover occupational therapy services in this practice setting?

ADVOCACY

1. Which of the following areas of advocacy would be beneficial in this case: patient rights, matters of privacy, confidentiality, informed consent, awareness building, accessing education, and/or benefits/resources?
2. Create a plan to advocate for this client based on the selected areas of advocacy.

TELEHEALTH

1. How can telehealth be integrated as a component of the occupational therapy process in this case?
2. Before launching telemedicine services, what questions would be essential to ask Hannah to determine whether it is appropriate for her to engage in telemedicine services?
3. What are the barriers, obstacles, or challenges you foresee if attempting to integrate telehealth services with Hannah?

Intervention Plan Formulation and Implementation

INTERVENTION PLAN FORMULATION

Create an intervention plan that includes the following:

1. List this individual's **strengths.**
2. List this individual's **barriers** in occupational performance, performance skills, and performance patterns.
3. Based on the individual's goals, health, performance, and service delivery site, **identify the barriers that will be addressed.**
4. From the barriers identified to be addressed, **formulate goals and objectives.**
5. Identify the focus of each goal and objective as either **create, promote, establish, restore, maintain, modify, or prevent.**
6. Identify the **theoretical basis, model(s) of practice, or frame(s) of reference** that will be used to address each goal and objective.
7. For each proposed goal and objective, describe clearly and precisely the **methods** that will be used. This description should include, but not be limited to, safety considerations, environmental considerations, therapeutic use of self, preparatory activities, activity selection, materials, equipment, and flow.
8. Classify the activities selected in the methods description as either **preparatory, enabling, purposeful, or occupation based.**
9. Explain how each activity can be **graded up or down,** creating the just-right challenge.
10. Provide at least two **primary sources of evidence** to support the intervention plan.

INTERVENTION PLAN IMPLEMENTATION

1. Based on your intervention plan, identify which goals and objectives require **more immediate attention.**
2. Describe your proposed **first treatment session.**
3. As the treatment session is progressing, what is **essential to be observed?**

Transition and Discontinuation

Create a plan for discharge from occupational therapy services in collaboration with Hannah and members of the interprofessional team. Review the needs of Hannah, caregivers, family members, and significant others. The plan must match needs with available resources and the discharge environment.

REFERENCES

American Medical Association. (2019). *CPT® 2020 professional edition.*

Buysse, D. J. (2014). Sleep health: Can we define it? Does it matter? *Sleep, 37*(1), 9–17. https://doi.org/10.5665/sleep.3298

World Health Organization. (2019). *International statistical classification of diseases and related health problems* (11th ed.). https://icd.who.int/

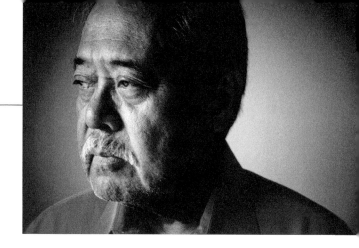

Howie: Right Distal Radius and Ulna Fracture

YVES ROSEUS, OTD, OTR/L

Howie (he, him, his, himself)

MEDICAL HISTORY

Howie is an 84-year-old Filipino male, living in the United States, who is 5′10″ and weighs 185 pounds. He was brought to the emergency department (ED) by emergency medical services after slipping in his bathtub, which resulted in pain, swelling, and deformity of his distal right forearm. After X-rays were taken, he received a diagnosis of comminuted fractures of his right distal radius and ulna bones. From the ED, he was taken to the operating room, where an open reduction and internal fixation (ORIF) was performed to stabilize the fracture sites. A postsurgical volar fiberglass splint was applied to protect the surgical site. Howie was transferred to the orthopedic care unit after his surgery.

Howie's medical history includes hypertension, high cholesterol, and insulin-dependent diabetes mellitus. He reported living an active lifestyle and no nicotine, drug, or caffeine use, but he consumes between three and six cans of beer per day. He reported being allergic to shellfish.

SOCIAL HISTORY

Howie has recently been widowed after 52 years of marriage. He lives alone in a three-bedroom ranch-style home. His suburban home is located just 15 miles from the city. There is a ramp to enter the first floor, which consists of a living room, dining room, den, eat-in kitchen, and one-and-a-half baths. There is a detached garage. Howie reported having one daughter who lives out of state with her husband and two children. He reports following the Catholic religion.

REFERRAL OR PRESCRIPTION

At the acute care hospital, Howie is currently in the orthopedic care unit for a 3-day stay. He has been referred for occupational therapy, registered nursing services, and social work services.

Occupational Therapy Initial Evaluation Findings: Acute Care

OCCUPATIONAL PROFILE

Howie's preadmission occupational history and experiences included being independent in all ADLs and all IADLs. Howie is a retired baggage handler from a major international airline. His former career had allowed him and his wife to travel to every continent. His patterns of daily living most commonly included attending his local senior citizen center Monday through Friday. He usually drove himself to the center and stayed for both breakfast and lunch and participated in its variety of groups. He typically returned home between 3:30 and 4:00 p.m. and prepared and ate dinner alone. After dinner, he enjoyed watching the evening news and would be in bed by 9:00 p.m. Weekends were usually filled with grocery shopping and working around his home. Each Christmas, he travels and stays with his daughter and her family and returns home after New Year's Day; in turn, they spend 1 week each summer with him. His interests include spending time with his many friends at the senior citizen center and traveling. He values independence, community, and his family. Howie reported his greatest current need is to return home and be able to care for himself.

ADLs

Howie was evaluated in the occupational therapy gym. Regarding self-care, he was able to feed himself using his left hand when food was presented precut. While seated, Howie was able to don and doff all his clothing for his upper and lower body but required assistance managing fasteners (buttons, zippers, and laces). Howie was able to wash at the sink but required assistance to wash and dry his left upper extremity. He was able to independently perform the grooming tasks of brushing his hair and teeth. Regarding functional mobility, Howie is able to independently roll and move between supine and short sit in bed. He transfers and ambulates without a device.

IADLs

Activities needed that provide day-to-day quality of life and relative independence were explored. Howie can manage his communications, handle his finances, and perform simple cleanup tasks. He is aware that he currently is not able to maintain his home, prepare meals, and shop without assistance. Regarding rest and sleep, Howie reports waking up every 1 to 2 hours because of pain at the fracture site.

MENTAL FUNCTIONS

Cognitive assessment found Howie to be alert and oriented to person, place, time, and situation, and short- and long-term memory were intact. He is able to follow three-step commands and make his needs known. Affect appeared appropriate, and no gross deficits in perception were observed.

SENSORY FUNCTIONS AND PAIN

No gross deficits were observed with visual, hearing, vestibular, taste, smell, proprioceptive, and cutaneous functions. Pain in the right distal forearm and hand was scored as a 7 on the numerical rating scale (0–10). The pain was described as "continuous." Circumferential measurements were taken at the distal palmar crease: 21.3 cm on the right and 17.6 cm on the left.

CARDIOVASCULAR AND RESPIRATORY SYSTEMS FUNCTIONS

Howie is able to perform all self-care and functional ambulation without report of or noticeable signs of fatigue.

MOVEMENT FUNCTIONS

Passive range of motion and active range of motion are intact in all four extremities except the right forearm, wrist, and digits (Table 5.1). Active range of motion for right forearm supination is 0–15° and for forearm pronation is 0–65°. Wrist flexion and extension were not assessed secondary to immobilization with a splint.

TABLE 5.1. Active Range of Motion (Degrees) of Right Digits

Joint	Digit 1	Digit 2	Digit 3	Digit 4	Digit 5
Metacarpophalangeal joint	0–50	5–52	0–55	0–55	10–70
Interphalangeal joint	0–15				
Proximal interphalangeal joint		5–43	0–46	0–46	0–55
Distal interphalangeal joint		0–10	0–14	0–15	0–20
Total active motion	**65**	**95**	**115**	**116**	**135**

Assessment of muscle strength in the left upper extremity and right shoulder groups through a functional muscle test (FMT) indicated all tested groups to be 5/5. Muscle strength testing of the right forearm, wrist, and digits were contraindicated. Gross grasp strength in the left hand is 37 pounds, and the right hand was not evaluated. Prehension in the left hand is grossly intact, and the right hand was not evaluated.

NEUROMUSCULAR FUNCTIONS

Static and dynamic sitting balance are 5/5, and static and dynamic standing balance are 4/5. Muscle tone is normal, and reflex integration is grossly intact.

PLAN FOR DISCHARGE

After his stay on the orthopedic care floor, Howie will be discharged home and receive outpatient occupational therapy services.

Questions and Activities

SAFETY OF CLIENT AND OTHERS: PRECAUTIONS AND CONTRAINDICATIONS

1. Create a precaution sheet identifying the risks of a poorly fitted hand splint.
2. Which vital signs should be taken when working with Howie? What are the norms for each? When should they be taken?
3. Using the FMT to assess his right forearm, wrist, and digits was contraindicated at the time of the initial evaluation. Why?
4. What are the precautions to be followed for an ORIF?
5. Would it be contraindicated for Howie to remove his splint to bathe? Support your decision.
6. To keep Howie and others safe, what other factors should be considered?

OCCUPATIONS: ADLs, IADLs, EDUCATION, WORK, PLAY, SOCIAL PARTICIPATION, AND REST AND SLEEP

1. Given the information provided for this case, identify the areas of occupation that will and will not be addressed. Justify your decisions.
2. Identify the areas of education that would be appropriate to engage in with Howie and explain why.
3. Briefly describe what the first treatment session with Howie would be like.

PERFORMANCE SKILLS: MOTOR SKILLS, PROCESS SKILLS, AND SOCIAL INTERACTION

1. Given the information provided, identify the motor, process, and social interaction skills that affect Howie's occupational performance.
2. Which of these skills would be appropriate to address in this service delivery site? Justify your selection.
3. Which of these skills would be addressed through remediation, compensation, and education?
4. Which of these skills would be addressed through the following intervention approaches: create/promote, establish/restore, maintain, modify, and prevent?

PERFORMANCE PATTERNS: HABITS, ROUTINES, ROLES, AND RITUALS

1. Identify Howie's useful habits, routines, roles, and rituals that support valued occupations. How can you make use of this information?
2. Identify Howie's impoverished habits, routines, roles, and rituals that do not support valued occupations. How can you make use of this information?
3. Identify Howie's dominating habits, routines, roles, and rituals that interfere with valued occupations. How can you make use of this information?

CLIENT FACTORS

Values, beliefs, and spirituality
How can the identified values, beliefs, and spirituality be used in this case?

Body structures
Considering the primary and secondary diagnoses, identify the related body structures.

Body Functions

1. Identify how the primary and secondary diagnoses have affected the function of the identified body structures.
2. Explain the relationships between the structural and functional factors and Howie's current level of occupational performance.

MENTAL FUNCTIONS: AFFECTIVE, COGNITIVE, AND PERCEPTUAL

1. What common affective issues related to fracture and surgical treatment may Howie face?
2. How would these issues be addressed in occupational therapy?
3. To address these issues, what other disciplines could you refer Howie to?
4. Given the information provided, what additional mental function considerations need to be addressed?

NEUROMUSCULOSKELETAL AND MOVEMENT-RELATED FUNCTIONS

1. Given the information provided, which neuromusculoskeletal or movement-related functions need to be addressed? Justify your selections.
2. Identify the theory for reducing edema.
3. According to the evidence, which is the best edema reduction technique or techniques that should be implemented to address the edema in Howie's right hand? Justify your selection.
4. Identify the theory for remediation of shortened soft tissue.
5. According to the evidence, which intervention selection would be the best choice? Explain why.
6. Compare and contrast ORIF with closed reduction and external fixation.
7. Create an exercise program for Howie based on occupational performance.

CARDIOVASCULAR, HEMATOLOGICAL, IMMUNOLOGICAL, AND RESPIRATORY FUNCTIONS

1. Given the information provided, identify cardiovascular, hematological, immunological, or respiratory functions that need to be addressed. Justify your selections.
2. As an 84-year-old patient, Howie is susceptible to cardiorespiratory risks associated with being in bed for 3 days. What are these risks? What preventive measures should be considered?
3. As you evaluate Howie in his bed, you notice he is wearing a cuff around each of his lower legs attached to a pneumatic device. What is the name and purpose of this medical device?

SKIN AND RELATED STRUCTURE FUNCTIONS

1. As a result of the trauma that Howie experienced, an inflammatory response was triggered resulting in the accumulation of fluids to his right upper extremity. Explain the physiological process of an inflammatory response.
2. List the most common types of edema.
3. Which type of edema is Howie most likely experiencing? Support your selection.
4. What are the signs and symptoms of an infected surgical wound?
5. What precautions must be followed during the treatment session to prevent an infection?
6. What other skin and related structure functions should be considered?

VOICE AND SPEECH FUNCTIONS

Describe how Howie's diagnoses may affect his voice, speech, and occupational performance.

ASSISTIVE TECHNOLOGIES AND DEVICES

1. Which assistive technologies or adaptations can be implemented to allow Howie to manage fasteners (buttons, zippers, and laces) independently?
2. Which assistive technologies or adaptations can be implemented to allow Howie to cut his food independently?
3. Which assistive technologies or adaptations can be implemented to allow Howie to prepare a simple meal independently?
4. What assistive technologies or adaptations might be recommended for use at home?

ETHICAL DECISION MAKING

Howie revealed that he typically drinks three to six cans of beer per day. Should this habit be addressed? Why or why not?

PHARMACOLOGY

Howie is currently taking Motrin®.

1. What is the generic name?
2. Does this drug have a high alert status?
3. What is the classification of this drug?
4. What is the indication for this drug?
5. What is the action of this drug?
6. How may this drug affect client participation during a therapy session?

SOCIOCULTURAL, SOCIOECONOMIC, AND DIVERSITY FACTORS AND LIFESTYLE CHOICES

1. Given Howie's profile, examine how your own culture and beliefs affect your interaction with him.
2. Based on this self-examination, what area of cultural knowledge do you need to pursue?
3. How can this newly acquired cultural knowledge be integrated for effective outcomes?
4. How can you foster cultural interaction and awareness among your coworkers?
5. Discuss how a lack of understanding in the areas of discrimination and stigma, implicit bias, social identity, or racism may contribute to disparities in the delivery of occupational therapy services in this case.

ASSESSMENT TOOLS AND INTERPRETATION OF RESULTS

1. What is the purpose of goniometric measurement?
2. Which population is this test designed for?
3. How much time is required to administer it?

4. Provide a brief description of this assessment.
5. What is the reliability of goniometric measurement?
6. What is the validity of goniometric measurement?
7. What functional inference can be deduced from the active range of motion in Howie's right hand?
8. What additional standardized assessment can be used in this case? Why?

INTERPROFESSIONAL RELATIONSHIP AND EFFECTIVE INTRAPROFESSIONAL COLLABORATION

1. Identify the other professions that would make up the care team. Explain the focus of each.
2. Identify the roles of the occupational therapy assistant (OTA) that could be used in the occupational therapy process for this case.
3. Identify interventions that can be assigned to the OTA for this case. Justify your selections.

BILLING AND CODING

1. Identify the *International Classification of Diseases (ICD)* codes for Howie's diagnoses.
2. For this case, identify at least two *Current Procedural Terminology (CPT)* codes that are most appropriate. Justify your selection.

REIMBURSEMENT SYSTEMS AND DOCUMENTATION

1. Who would be the authorized individuals you could share the occupational therapy findings with? Explain why.
2. For this case, what forms and frequency of documentation will be required?
3. Which reimbursement system or systems most commonly cover occupational therapy services in this practice setting?

ADVOCACY

1. Which of the following areas of advocacy would be beneficial in this case: patient rights, matters of privacy, confidentiality, informed consent, awareness building, accessing education, and benefits/resources?
2. Create a plan to advocate for this client based on the selected areas of advocacy.

TELEHEALTH

1. How can telehealth be integrated as a component of the occupational therapy process in this case?
2. Before launching telemedicine services, what questions would be essential to ask Howie to determine whether it is appropriate for him to engage in telemedicine services?
3. What are the barriers, obstacles, or challenges you foresee if attempting to integrate telehealth services with Howie?

Intervention Plan Formulation and Implementation

INTERVENTION PLAN FORMULATION

Create an intervention plan that includes the following:

1. List this individual's **strengths.**
2. List this individual's **barriers** in occupational performance, performance skills, and performance patterns.
3. Based on the individual's goals, health, performance, and service delivery site, **identify the barriers that will be addressed.**
4. From the barriers identified to be addressed, **formulate goals and objectives.**
5. Identify the focus of each goal and objective identify as either **create, promote, establish, restore, maintain, modify, or prevent.**
6. Identify the **theoretical basis, model(s) of practice, or frame(s) of reference** that will be used to address each goal and objective.
7. For each proposed goal and objective, describe clearly and precisely the **methods** that will be used. This description should include, but not be limited to, safety considerations, environmental considerations, therapeutic use of self, preparatory activities, activity selection, materials, equipment, and flow.
8. Classify the activities selected in the methods description as either **preparatory, enabling, purposeful,** or **occupation based.**
9. Explain how each activity can be **graded up or down,** creating the just-right challenge.
10. Provide at least two **primary sources of evidence** to support the intervention plan.

INTERVENTION PLAN IMPLEMENTATION

1. Based on your intervention plan, identify which goals and objectives require **more immediate attention.**
2. Describe your proposed **first treatment session.**
3. As the treatment session is progressing, what is **essential to be observed**?

Transition and Discontinuation

Create a plan for discharge from occupational therapy services in collaboration with Howie and members of the interprofessional team. Review the needs of Howie, caregivers, family members, and significant others. The plan must match needs with available resources and the discharge environment.

REFERENCES

American Medical Association. (2019). *CPT® 2020 professional edition.*
World Health Organization. (2019). *International statistical classification of diseases and related health problems* (11th ed.). https://icd.who.int/

Outpatient Rehabilitation

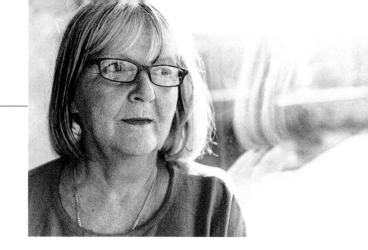

Florence: Rheumatoid Arthritis

YVES ROSEUS, OTD, OTR/L

Florence (she, her, hers, herself)

MEDICAL HISTORY

Florence is a 69-year-old Irish-American female who is 5' 0" and weighs 127 pounds. She was electively admitted to the orthopedic service with a diagnosis of rheumatoid arthritis (RA). She underwent a left total shoulder arthroplasty (TSA). Her medical history included RA for 35 years, pleurisy, osteoporosis, hypertension, Sjogren's syndrome, and gastrointestinal bleeding. Surgical history included bilateral (B/L) total knee replacements, B/L wrist synovectomy, and B/L metacarpal phalangeal arthroplasty of Digits 2–5. She reported living a sedentary lifestyle and no alcohol, drug, or tobacco use. Florence reported drinking 4 to 5 cups of tea per day. She has no known allergies.

SOCIAL HISTORY

Florence worked as a high school food service worker until age 52, when her condition did not allow her to work any longer. She qualified and received Social Security disability. Florence lives alone in a city-subsidized one-bedroom accessible apartment located just 2 miles from the hospital. Her building is elevator equipped and is compliant with the Americans with Disabilities Act (P. L. 101-336). Her apartment has an open floor plan for its living room, dining room, and kitchen. Florence reported never being married and having only one close friend, Mary, who also has a disability. Florence identifies as a follower of the Anglican Church. She identifies as asexual.

REFERRAL OR PRESCRIPTION

Florence was referred for outpatient services. She is to receive occupational therapy services 2 times per week for 10 weeks. Occupational therapy services are to progress the patient to Phase 2 of the TSA protocol.

Occupational Therapy Initial Evaluation Findings: Outpatient Rehabilitation

OCCUPATIONAL PROFILE

Florence's preadmission occupational history and experiences included requiring the assistance of a home health aide (HHA) for the past 5 years to bathe and perform her hair care. She reported being independent with modifications in dressing, toileting, and feeding. Shopping, care of the home, and meal preparation were completed by her HHA. Her patterns of daily living most commonly included being washed by her HHA by 9:30 a.m. and eating her prepared breakfast by 10:30 a.m. Her days are usually filled with escorted trips to local stores, medical appointments, and the senior citizens club. The club is located in the building where she resides, and it is where she commonly eats lunch with her friend Mary; dinner is eaten at home. Her interests include reading romance novels, collecting figurines, and spending time with her cat. She values honesty and cleanliness. Florence reported her greatest current need is to be able to stay in her own home and receive needed outpatient services. She reported being very afraid of placement in a nursing home.

ADLs

Regarding self-care, Florence was able to feed herself using her right upper extremity when foods were cut first and presented to her. Florence required maximal assistance to dress both upper extremities and both lower extremities and to don and doff her left shoulder immobilizer support brace. She was able to independently perform the grooming tasks of brushing her hair and teeth. The Quick Disability Arm Shoulder Hand (DASH) Questionnaire (Hudak et al., 1996) was administered, and she obtained a score of 63.7%.

Regarding functional mobility, Florence was able to independently roll, bridge, and move between supine and short sit in bed. Florence transferred on and off the bed, chair, and raised toilet using a wide-base quad cane. She required moderate assistance to transfer in and out of the tub using a transfer tub bench similar to the one in her home.

IADLs

Activities needed that provide day-to-day quality of life and relative independence were explored. Florence can manage her communications and handle her finances, but she is dependent in maintaining her home, preparing meals, cleaning up, and shopping.

In regard to rest and sleep, Florence reports not being able to find a comfortable position to sleep.

MENTAL FUNCTIONS

Cognitive assessment found Florence to be alert and oriented to person, place, time, and situation, and short- and long-term memory were intact. She was able to follow three-step commands and make her needs known. Affect appeared appropriate, and no gross deficits in perception were observed.

SENSORY FUNCTIONS AND PAIN

No gross deficits were observed with hearing, vestibular, taste, smell, proprioceptive, and cutaneous functions. Florence reported being nearsighted and required eyeglasses. Use of the numerical rating scale (0–10) indicated 7/10 pain in her left shoulder. The pain was described as "miserable." No edema was noted.

CARDIOVASCULAR AND RESPIRATORY SYSTEMS FUNCTION

Florence presented with a metabolic equivalent of task value of 2.5–3.0.

MOVEMENT FUNCTIONS

Passive range of motion, active range of motion, and muscle strength in both upper extremities were within functional limits, except for the left shoulder. The left shoulder was positioned in a soft immobilizing shoulder adduction sling that was not removed. Flexible, swan neck deformities in Digits 2–5 and Boutonniere deformities of Digit 1 in both hands were observed. Gross grasp strength was not assessed.

NEUROMUSCULAR FUNCTIONS

Static and dynamic sitting balance were 5/5, and static and dynamic standing balance were 4/5. Muscle tone was normal, and reflex integration was grossly intact.

PLAN FOR DISCHARGE

At the conclusion of her 10 weeks of outpatient occupational therapy services, Florence will be discharged with a home exercise program.

Questions and Activities

SAFETY OF CLIENT AND OTHERS: PRECAUTIONS AND CONTRAINDICATIONS

1. Provide a summary of the Phase 2 TSA postsurgical protocol.
2. At the time of the evaluation, what precautions must be observed after her TSA?
3. Create a handout identifying precautions needed to be followed by patients with an unhealed surgical wound.
4. It is initially contraindicated for Florence to shower. Why?
5. To maintain safety, what other factors should be considered?

OCCUPATIONS: ADLs, IADLs, EDUCATION, WORK, PLAY, SOCIAL PARTICIPATION, AND REST AND SLEEP

1. Given the information provided for this case, identify the areas of occupation that will and will not be addressed. Justify your decisions.

2. What strategies can be used to improve Florence's ability to dress?
3. What strategies can be used to improve Florence's ability to cut her own food?
4. When would it be appropriate for Florence to once again shower in her bathroom?
5. What strategies can be used to improve Florence's ability to have a more continuous and restful sleep?
6. What strategies can be used to improve Florence's ability to prepare a simple light meal when the HHA is absent?
7. Briefly describe what the first treatment session with Florence would be like.

PERFORMANCE SKILLS: MOTOR SKILLS, PROCESS SKILLS, AND SOCIAL INTERACTION SKILLS

1. Given the information provided, identify the motor, process, and social interaction skills that affect Florence's occupational performance.
2. Which of these skills would be appropriate to address within this service delivery site? Justify your selection.
3. Which of these skills would be addressed through remediation, compensation, and education?
4. Which of these skills would be addressed through the following intervention approaches: create/promote, establish/restore, maintain, modify and/or prevent?

PERFORMANCE PATTERNS: HABITS, ROUTINES, ROLES, AND RITUALS

1. Identify Florence's useful habits, routines, roles, and rituals that support valued occupations. How can you make use of this information?
2. Identify Florence's impoverished habits, routines, roles, and rituals that do not support valued occupations. How can you make use of this information?
3. Identify Florence's dominating habits, routines, roles, and rituals that interfere with valued occupations. How can you make use of this information?

CLIENT FACTORS

Values, beliefs, and spirituality
How can the identified values, beliefs, and spirituality be used in this case?

Body structures
Considering the primary and secondary diagnoses, identify the related body structures.

Body functions
1. Identify how the primary and secondary diagnoses have affected the function of the identified body structures.
2. Explain the relationships between the structural and functional factors and Florence's current level of occupational performance.

MENTAL FUNCTIONS: AFFECTIVE, COGNITIVE, AND PERCEPTUAL

1. What common affective issues related to TSA may Florence face?
2. How would these issues be addressed in occupational therapy?

3. To address these issues, what other disciplines could you refer Florence to?
4. What strategies or techniques would be available to help minimize the postsurgical pain Florence is experiencing?
5. Given the information provided, which additional mental function considerations need to be addressed?

NEUROMUSCULOSKELETAL AND MOVEMENT-RELATED FUNCTIONS

1. Given the information provided, identify neuromusculoskeletal and movement-related functions that need to be addressed. Justify your selections.
2. What are the exercises identified to be performed with the left upper extremity during Phase 2 of the TSA?
3. Explain how these exercises match Florence's current level of postsurgical healing.
4. Identify and summarize all previous and subsequent phases of the TSA protocol.
5. Compare and contrast total shoulder replacement with a reverse shoulder replacement.
6. Create an exercise program for Florence based on occupational performance.

CARDIOVASCULAR, HEMATOLOGICAL, IMMUNOLOGICAL, AND RESPIRATORY FUNCTIONS

1. Given the information provided, identify cardiovascular, hematological, immunological, and respiratory functions that need to be addressed. Justify your selections.
2. What are common cardiovascular and respiratory conditions that have been associated with the later stages of RA?

SKIN AND RELATED STRUCTURE FUNCTIONS

1. What are common trophic changes that have been associated with the later stages of RA?
2. What other skin and related structure functions should be considered?

VOICE AND SPEECH FUNCTIONS

Describe how Florence's diagnoses may affect her voice, speech, and occupational performance.

ASSISTIVE TECHNOLOGIES AND DEVICES

1. What assistive technologies and adaptations might be used or made for Florence while she is receiving outpatient occupational therapy services? Why?
2. Florence has Medicaid and Medicare; which one would serve as the primary payer for her outpatient occupational therapy services?

ETHICAL DECISION MAKING

1. Florence confides in you that her HHA leaves 1 hour early every day, during her assigned time, to pick up her son. How should this situation be addressed?
2. Florence confides in you that she was so desperate for a good night's sleep that she slept two evenings not wearing her left shoulder immobilizer support brace. How should this situation be addressed?

PHARMACOLOGY

Florence is currently taking Celebrex.

1. What is the generic name?
2. Does this drug have a high alert status?
3. What is the classification of this drug?
4. What is the indication for this drug?
5. What is the action of this drug?
6. How may this drug affect client participation during a therapy session?

SOCIOCULTURAL, SOCIOECONOMIC, AND DIVERSITY FACTORS AND LIFESTYLE CHOICES

1. Given Florence's profile, examine how your own culture and beliefs affect your interaction with her.
2. Based on this self-examination, what area of cultural knowledge do you need to pursue?
3. How can this newly acquired cultural knowledge be integrated for effective outcomes?
4. How can you foster cultural interaction and awareness among your coworkers?
5. Discuss how a lack of understanding in the areas of discrimination and stigma, implicit bias, social identity, or racism may contribute to disparities in the delivery of occupational therapy services in this case.

ASSESSMENT TOOLS AND INTERPRETATION OF RESULTS

1. What is the purpose of the Quick DASH?
2. Which population is this test designed for?
3. How much time is required to administer it?
4. Provide a brief description of this assessment.
5. What is the reliability of the Quick DASH?
6. What is the validity of the Quick DASH?
7. What functional inference can be deduced from Florence's score of 63.7%?
8. What additional standardized assessment can be used in this case? Why?

INTERPROFESSIONAL RELATIONSHIP AND EFFECTIVE INTRAPROFESSIONAL COLLABORATION

1. Identify the other professions that would make up the care team. Explain the focus of each.
2. Identify roles of the occupational therapy assistant (OTA) that could be used in the occupational therapy process for this case.
3. Identify interventions that can be assigned to the OTA for this case. Justify your selections.

BILLING AND CODING

1. Identify the *International Classification of Diseases (ICD)* codes for Florence's diagnoses.
2. For this case, identify at least two *Current Procedural Terminology (CPT®)* codes that are most appropriate. Justify your selection.

REIMBURSEMENT SYSTEMS AND DOCUMENTATION

1. Who would be the authorized individuals you could share the occupational therapy findings with? Explain why.
2. For this case, what forms and frequency of documentation will be required?
3. Which reimbursement system or systems most commonly cover occupational therapy services in this practice setting?

ADVOCACY

1. Which of the following areas of advocacy would be beneficial in this case: patient rights, matters of privacy, confidentiality, informed consent, awareness building, accessing education, and benefits/ resources?
2. Create a plan to advocate for this client based on the selected areas of advocacy.

TELEHEALTH

1. How can telehealth be integrated as a component of the occupational therapy process in this case?
2. Before launching telemedicine services, what questions would be essential to ask Florence to determine whether it is appropriate for her to engage in telemedicine services?
3. What are the challenges you foresee if attempting to integrate telehealth services with this client?

Intervention Plan Formulation and Implementation

INTERVENTION PLAN FORMULATION

Create an intervention plan that includes the following:

1. List this individual's **strengths.**
2. List this individual's **barriers** in occupational performance, performance skills, and performance patterns.
3. Based on the individual's goals, health, performance, and service delivery site, **identify the barriers that will be addressed.**
4. From the barriers identified to be addressed, **formulate goals and objectives.**
5. Identify the focus of each goal and objective as either **create, promote, establish, restore, maintain, modify, or prevent.**
6. Identify the **theoretical basis, model(s) of practice, or frame(s) of reference** that will be used to address each goal and objective.
7. For each proposed goal and objective, describe clearly and precisely the **methods** that will be used. This description should include, but not be limited to, safety considerations, environmental considerations, therapeutic use of self, preparatory activities, activity selection, materials, equipment, and flow.
8. Classify the activities selected in the methods description as either **preparatory, enabling, purposeful, or occupation based.**
9. Explain how each activity can be **graded up or down,** creating the just-right challenge.
10. Provide at least two **primary sources of evidence** to support the intervention plan.

INTERVENTION PLAN IMPLEMENTATION

1. Based on your intervention plan, identify which goals and objectives require **more immediate attention.**
2. Describe your proposed **first treatment session.**
3. As the treatment session is progressing, what is **essential to be observed**?

Transition and Discontinuation

Create a plan for discharge from occupational therapy services in collaboration with Florence and members of the interprofessional team. Review the needs of Florence, her caregiver, family members, and significant others. The plan must match needs with available resources and the discharge environment.

REFERENCES

American Medical Association. (2019). *CPT® 2020 professional edition.*

Americans with Disabilities Act of 1990, Pub. L. 101-336, 42 U.S.C. §§ 12101–12213 (2000).

Hudak, P. L., Amadio, P. C., Bombardier, C., Beaton, D., Cole, D., Davis, A., . . . Wright, J. (1996). Development of an upper extremity outcome measure: The DASH (Disabilities of the Arm, Shoulder, and Head). *American Journal of Industrial Medicine, 29,* 602–608. https://doi.org/10.1002/(SICI)1097-0274(199606)29:6<602::AID-AJIM4>3.0.CO;2-L

World Health Organization. (2019). *International statistical classification of diseases and related health problems* (11th ed.). https://icd.who.int/

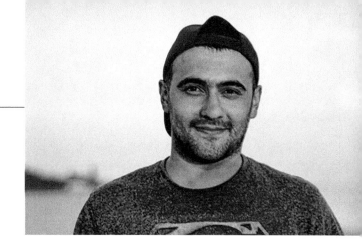

Brian: Traumatic Above-Elbow Amputation

YVES ROSEUS, OTD, OTR/L

Brian (he, him, his, himself)

MEDICAL HISTORY

Brian is a 31-year-old native Hawaiian male who is 6' 2" and weighs 180 pounds. He was brought to the emergency department by emergency medical services after being attacked by a great white shark while recreational surfing. He presented with a severed right upper limb, multiple lacerations, and severe blood loss. He was stabilized by the administration of isotonic fluids and 4 units of blood. Once stabilized, he was sent to the operating room, where vascular and plastic surgeons addressed his lacerations and performed an emergency closed above-elbow amputation (AEA). Brian's medical history was unremarkable. He reported no tobacco, caffeine, or drug use. He reported commonly having three to four alcoholic drinks over the course of a weekend. Brian has no known allergies. After his surgery, Brian spent 1 week on the medical-surgical floor. From there, he completed 2 weeks in in-patient rehabilitation, where he received wound care, self-care retaining, preprosthetic training, and assessment by a prosthetist.

SOCIAL HISTORY

Brian lives with his girlfriend Asia in their beachfront apartment. Brain and Asia met while both worked as accountants at the same firm. Their apartment is located on the seventh floor of an elevator-equipped building. It has a living room, dinette, kitchen, bathroom, and small balcony with ocean views. Currently, Brian's family lives in California, and he has no close relatives on the island. Brian and Asia both have a large network of friends. Asia has two brothers and parents who live within an hour's drive. Brian's goal is to get back home to Asia and return to his career and the lifestyle that he loves. He wishes to be able to use his myoelectric arm with enough skill to be able to perform his ADLs, prepare a meal, and use his computer. He is scheduled to return to work after his 6 weeks of outpatient occupational therapy services. Brian reports that his parents are devout Buddhists; however, he does not identify with any religion.

REFERRAL OR PRESCRIPTION

Brian was referred for outpatient services. He is to receive occupational therapy services 2 times per week for 10 weeks.

Occupational Therapy Initial Evaluation Findings: Outpatient Rehabilitation

OCCUPATIONAL PROFILE

Brian's preadmission occupational history and experiences included being independent in all ADLs and all IADLs. Brian has been employed as a tax accountant for the past 6 years and was recently promoted to manager of the tax department. He holds a bachelor's degree in accounting and a master's in business administration. During the tax season, he typically worked 60–70 hours per week. His most common patterns of daily living include being up and out of his home by 6:00 a.m. and returning home by 8:00 p.m. His interests include mountain biking, surf sailing, hiking, climbing, and rappelling. Brian values his relationship with Asia, an active and healthy lifestyle, and professional and financial success. He reported his greatest current need is to return to his job as an accountant and be able to support himself and Asia.

ADLs

Regarding self-care, Brian was able to feed, dress, groom, and toilet independently using one-hand techniques. Brian required moderate assistance to wash his right upper extremity. Regarding functional mobility, Brian was able to independently roll, bridge, scoot, and transition between supine and sitting. Brian transferred independently from all surfaces without using a device.

IADLs

Activities needed that provide day-to-day quality of life and relative independence were explored. Brian can manage his communications, handle his finances, perform simple household chores, and shop using his left upper extremity. He reports being hesitant to cook because of concern that he will burn his uninjured arm. Regarding rest and sleep, Brian reported frequently waking up in the middle of the night reliving the horrors of the shark attack.

MENTAL FUNCTIONS

Cognitive assessment found Brian to be alert and oriented to person, place, time, and situation, and short- and long-term memory were intact. He is able to follow three-step commands and make his needs known. Affect appeared appropriate, and no gross deficits in perception were observed.

SENSORY FUNCTIONS AND PAIN

No gross deficits were observed with visual, hearing, vestibular, taste, smell, and proprioceptive functions. Using the Numeric Rating Scale (0–10), Brian reported pain at a 4. Cutaneous sensation assessment using a calibrated paper clip indicated that two-point discrimination was 10 mm at the distal end of the residual limb. Brian reported experiencing phantom limb sensation in his right residual limb. He stated, "It feels like my arm is still there."

CARDIOVASCULAR AND RESPIRATORY SYSTEMS FUNCTION

There were no deficits with cardiovascular and respiratory systems function.

MOVEMENT FUNCTIONS

Passive range of motion (PROM) and active range of motion (AROM) in all joints of Brian's left upper extremity and both lower extremities are within normal limits (WNL). At his right shoulder, PROM and AROM are WNL. Muscle strength of all groups of both lower extremities and the left upper extremity were 5/5. Muscle strength to the right shoulder was 4/5. His residual limb is well shaped and adequately healed to accommodate the prosthetic socket. Gross grasp strength in Brian's left hand was 88 pounds, and left gross grasp, pinch, and in-hand manipulation abilities were within defined limits.

NEUROMUSCULAR FUNCTIONS

Static and dynamic sitting and standing balance were 5/5. Muscle tone was normal, and reflex integration was intact.

PLAN FOR DISCHARGE

After the completion of 10 weeks of outpatient rehabilitation, Brian will be discharged and return to work.

Questions and Activities

SAFETY OF CLIENT AND OTHERS: PRECAUTIONS AND CONTRAINDICATIONS

1. During the first session, it is customary to check out and evaluate the prosthesis before initiating training. What should be evaluated? Explain why.
2. Create a handout indicating the signs of a poorly fitted prosthesis and actions that need to be taken if one is identified.
3. What has Brian reported that could an indication he may be experiencing posttraumatic stress disorder (PTSD)?
4. If you have a concern that Brian may be experiencing PTSD, what should you do?
5. To maintain safety, what other factors should be considered?

OCCUPATIONS: ADLs, IADLs, EDUCATION, WORK, PLAY, SOCIAL PARTICIPATION, AND REST AND SLEEP

1. Given the information provided for this case, identify the areas of occupation that will and will not be addressed. Justify your decisions.
2. Identify goals that would reflect Brian's ability to care for his prosthesis.
3. Identify goals that would reflect Brian's ability to manage the controls of the prosthesis.

4. Brian wishes to perform his ADLs in a bilateral manner. Identify a progression of dressing tasks he can perform, from simple to complex, while integrating the use of his prosthesis. Provide an explanation for your choices.
5. Brian wishes to be able to prepare a meal. Describe a treatment session that takes into consideration the basic use of his prosthesis and his concern about burning his left upper extremity.

PERFORMANCE SKILLS: MOTOR SKILLS, PROCESS SKILLS, AND SOCIAL INTERACTION SKILLS

1. Given the information provided, identify the motor, process, and social interaction skills that affect Brian's occupational performance.
2. Which of these skills would be appropriate to address in this service delivery site? Justify your selection.
3. Which of these skills would be addressed through remediation, compensation, and education?
4. Which of these skills would be addressed through the following intervention approaches: create/promote, establish/restore, maintain, modify, and prevent?

PERFORMANCE PATTERNS: HABITS, ROUTINES, ROLES, AND RITUALS

1. Identify Brian's useful habits, routines, roles, and rituals that support valued occupations. How can you make use of this information?
2. Identify Brian's impoverished habits, routines, roles, and rituals that do not support valued occupations. How can you make use of this information?
3. Identify Brian's dominating habits, routines, roles, and rituals that interfere with valued occupations. How can you make use of this information?

CLIENT FACTORS

Values, beliefs, and spirituality
How can the identified values, beliefs, and spirituality be used within this case?

Body structures
Considering the primary and secondary diagnoses, identify the related body structures.

Body functions
1. Identify how the primary and secondary diagnoses have affected the function of the identified body structures.
2. Explain the relationships between the structural and functional factors and current level of occupational performance.

MENTAL FUNCTIONS: AFFECTIVE, COGNITIVE, AND PERCEPTUAL

1. What common affective issues related to Brian's amputation may he have to face?
2. How would these issues be addressed in occupational therapy?
3. To address these issues, what other disciplines could you refer Brian to?
4. Given the information provided, which additional mental function considerations need to be addressed?

NEUROMUSCULOSKELETAL AND MOVEMENT-RELATED FUNCTIONS

1. Given the information provided, identify neuromusculoskeletal and movement-related functions that need to be addressed. Justify your selections.
2. Given that Brian has undergone a right AEA, which muscle groups were likely lost, and which were retained?
3. How can the retained muscle groups be strengthened?
4. A myoelectric prosthesis was selected over a body-powered prosthesis. Identify the pros and cons of this selection.
5. Given Brian's lifestyle, what would be the best choice for a terminal device?
6. Compare and contrast open amputation with closed amputation.
7. Create an exercise program for Brian based on occupational performance.

CARDIOVASCULAR, HEMATOLOGICAL, IMMUNOLOGICAL, AND RESPIRATORY FUNCTIONS

1. Given the information provided, identify cardiovascular, hematological, immunological, and respiratory functions that need to be addressed. Justify your selections.
2. How can the use of a myoelectric prosthesis influence the energy cost of an activity?

VOICE AND SPEECH FUNCTIONS

Describe how Brian's diagnosis may affect his voice, speech, and occupational performance.

SKIN AND RELATED STRUCTURE FUNCTIONS

1. Identify two adjunctive modalities that can be used to reduce the hypersensitivity to light touch in the distal portion of Brian's residual limb. Describe both the precautions and recommended application for each.
2. Create a handout identifying the wearing schedule for Brain to build up his tolerance of his upper-extremity prosthesis.
3. What are the components of a myoelectric prosthesis?
4. How often should Brian's prosthesis be cleaned? How should it be cleaned?
5. What other skin and related structure functions should be considered?

ASSISTIVE TECHNOLOGIES AND DEVICES

What assistive technologies or adaptations might be used or made for Brian while he is receiving occupational therapy services as an outpatient?

ETHICAL DECISION MAKING

1. Asia informs you that immediately after his discharge from the rehabilitation center Brian has returned to driving his car. Based on your state's Department of Motor Vehicle laws, how should this information be addressed?
2. Asia informs you that the previous night Brian screamed for more than 10 minutes because he believed the shark was attacking him. How should this situation be addressed?

3. Brian privately informs you that he has not been intimate with Asia since he has returned home. He is concerned that she may no longer find him attractive. How should his concerns be addressed?

PHARMACOLOGY

Brian is currently taking amoxicillin.

1. What is the brand name?
2. Does this drug have a high alert status?
3. What is the classification of this drug?
4. What is the indication for this drug?
5. What is the action of this drug?
6. How may this drug affect client participation during a therapy session?

SOCIOCULTURAL, SOCIOECONOMIC, AND DIVERSITY FACTORS AND LIFESTYLE CHOICES

1. Given Brian's profile, examine how your own culture and beliefs affect your interaction with him.
2. Based on this self-examination, what area of cultural knowledge do you need to pursue?
3. How can this newly acquired cultural knowledge be integrated for effective outcomes?
4. How can you foster cultural interaction and awareness among your coworkers?
5. Discuss how a lack of understanding in the areas of discrimination and stigma, implicit bias, social identity, or racism may contribute to disparities in the delivery of occupational therapy services in this case.

ASSESSMENT TOOLS AND INTERPRETATION OF RESULTS

1. What is the purpose of the two-point discrimination test?
2. Which population is this test designed for?
3. How much time is required to administer it?
4. Provide a brief description of this assessment.
5. What is the reliability of the two-point discrimination test?
6. What is the validity of the two-point discrimination test?
7. What functional inference can be deduced from Brian's score of 10 mm?
8. What additional standardized cutaneous assessments could have been used in this case? Why?

INTERPROFESSIONAL RELATIONSHIP AND EFFECTIVE INTRAPROFESSIONAL COLLABORATION

1. Identify the other professions that would make up the care team. Explain the focus of each.
2. Identify the roles of the occupational therapy assistant (OTA) that could be used in the occupational therapy process for this case.
3. Identify interventions that can be assigned to the OTA for this case. Justify your selections.

BILLING AND CODING

1. Identify the *International Classification of Diseases (ICD)* code for Brian's diagnosis.

2. For this case, identify at least two *Current Procedural Terminology (CPT®)* codes that are most appropriate. Justify your selection.

REIMBURSEMENT SYSTEMS AND DOCUMENTATION

1. Who would be the authorized individuals you could share the occupational therapy findings with? Explain why.
2. For this case, what forms and frequency of documentation will be required?
3. Which reimbursement system or systems most commonly cover occupational therapy services in this practice setting?

ADVOCACY

1. Which of the following areas of advocacy would be beneficial in this case: patient rights, matters of privacy, confidentiality, informed consent, awareness building, accessing education, and/or benefits/ resources?
2. Create a plan to advocate for this client based on the selected areas of advocacy.

TELEHEALTH

1. How can telehealth be integrated as a component of the occupational therapy process in this case?
2. Before launching telemedicine services, what questions would be essential to ask Brian to determine whether it is appropriate for him to engage in telemedicine services?
3. What challenges do you foresee if attempting to integrate telehealth services with this client?

Intervention Plan Formulation and Implementation

INTERVENTION PLAN FORMULATION

Create an intervention plan that includes the following:

1. List this individual's **strengths.**
2. List this individual's **barriers** in occupational performance, performance skills, and performance patterns.
3. Based on the individual's goals, health, performance, and service delivery site, **identify the barriers that will be addressed.**
4. From the barriers identified to be addressed, **formulate goals and objectives.**
5. Identify the focus of each goal and objective as either **create, promote, establish, restore, maintain, modify, or prevent.**
6. Identify the **theoretical basis, model(s) of practice, or frame(s) of reference** that will be used to address each goal and objective.
7. For each proposed goal and objective, describe clearly and precisely the **methods** that will be used. This description should include, but not be limited to, safety considerations, environmental considerations, therapeutic use of self, preparatory activities, activity selection, materials, equipment, and flow.

8. Classify the activities selected in the methods description as either **preparatory, enabling, purposeful, or occupation based.**
9. Explain how each activity can be **graded up or down,** creating the just-right challenge.
10. Provide at least two **primary sources of evidence** to support the intervention plan.

INTERVENTION PLAN IMPLEMENTATION

1. Based on your intervention plan, identify which goals and objectives require **more immediate attention.**
2. Describe your proposed **first treatment session.**
3. As the treatment session is progressing, what is **essential to be observed?**

Transition and Discontinuation

Create a plan for discharge from occupational therapy services in collaboration with Brian and members of the interprofessional team. Review the needs of Brian, caregivers, family members, and significant others. The plan must match needs with available resources and the discharge environment.

REFERENCES

American Medical Association. (2019). *CPT® 2020 professional edition.*
World Health Organization. (2019). *International statistical classification of diseases and related health problems* (11th ed.). https://icd.who.int/

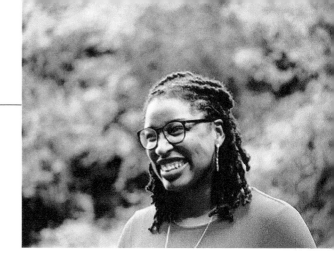

Yvonne: Breast Cancer

YVES ROSEUS, OTD, OTR/L

Yvonne (she, her, hers, herself)

MEDICAL HISTORY

Yvonne is a 44-year-old Black female who is 5' 11" and weighs 209 pounds. She was electively admitted to the surgical service with a diagnosis of Stage 2 breast cancer. She underwent a left radical mastectomy. Her medical history included being diagnosed with lupus 24 years ago and having a herniated disc between the second and third lumbar vertebrae. Past medical procedures included decompression and fusion of the second and third lumbar vertebra 10 years ago. She reported living an active lifestyle, with occasional use of alcohol and tobacco and no drug use. Yvonne reported drinking 2 to 3 large cups of coffee per day. She reported being allergic to pollen.

SOCIAL HISTORY

Yvonne lives with her spouse Tiffany in a one-bedroom apartment in a full-service high-rise building in the city center. Her apartment has an open floor plan for its living room, dining room, and kitchen. Yvonne and her spouse have been together for 15 years and married for 2 years. She reports being a member of the African Methodist Episcopal Church.

REFERRAL OR PRESCRIPTION

Yvonne was referred for outpatient services. She is to receive occupational therapy services 2 times per week for 8 weeks.

Occupational Therapy Initial Evaluation Findings: Outpatient Rehabilitation

OCCUPATIONAL PROFILE

Yvonne's occupational history and experiences included being a police officer for the past 21 years. She reported being independent in all ADLs and IADLs before surgery. Her patterns of daily living most commonly included picking up breakfast on the way to work, working the day shift from 9:00 a.m. to 5:00 p.m., and picking up dinner for herself and her spouse on the way home. During the week, they go to the gym or pool in their building. Weekends are dedicated to friends, day trips, and a busy schedule of social events. Yvonne's interests include Tae Kwon Do, microbrewing, and motorcycle riding. She values love, honesty, and acceptance. Yvonne reported that her greatest current need is to get her arm moving well and to prepare for retirement from her job.

ADLs

Regarding self-care, Yvonne was independent in feeding, grooming, toileting, and bathing. She was able to dress but required assistance to don and doff her bra. Regarding functional mobility, Yvonne was able to independently roll, bridge, and transition between supine and short sit in bed. Yvonne transferred to and from all surfaces independently. Yvonne was able to ambulate independently but was observed with postural guarding of her left upper extremity.

IADLs

Activities needed that provide day-to-day quality of life and relative independence were explored. Yvonne's spouse has taken over full responsibility of cooking, shopping, and care of the home while Yvonne recovers. Regarding rest and sleep, Yvonne reported waking up each night, going to the bathroom, and looking at the surgical site.

MENTAL FUNCTIONS

Cognitive assessment found Yvonne to be alert and oriented to person, place, time, and situation, and her short- and long-term memory were intact. She is able to follow three-step commands and make her needs known. Regarding affect, Yvonne reported frequently crying when she looked at the surgical site. No gross deficits in perception were observed.

SENSORY FUNCTION AND PAINS

No gross deficits were observed with visual, hearing, vestibular, taste, smell, and proprioceptive functions. Use of the numerical rating scale (NRS; 0–10) for pain indicated a score of 7 for Yvonne's left shoulder before taking pain medication and a 4 after taking pain medication. She also reports having a sensation of her left breast still being present. Her surgical incision was fully closed, staples were removed, and the scar was flat. Light touch and localization were impaired; edema was unremarkable.

CARDIOVASCULAR AND RESPIRATORY SYSTEMS FUNCTION

Assessment of cardiovascular and respiratory systems function indicated no deficits.

MOVEMENT FUNCTIONS

Passive range of motion (PROM), active range of motion (AROM), and muscle strength in Yvonne's right upper extremity and both lower extremities were within normal limits. Her AROM was within normal limits throughout the left upper extremity (LUE) except to the shoulder. PROM at the left shoulder was as follows: shoulder flexion, 0–102°; abduction, 0–88°; external rotation, 0–60°; and internal rotation, 0–80°. AROM at the left shoulder was as follows: shoulder flexion, 0–102°; abduction, 0–88°; external rotation, 0–60°; and internal rotation, 0–80°. Muscle strength in the LUE was not evaluated. Yvonne held her LUE in a guarded position. No gross defects were found in prehension.

NEUROMUSCULAR FUNCTIONS

Static and dynamic sitting and standing balance were 5/5. Muscle tone was normal, and reflex integration was intact.

PLAN FOR DISCHARGE

After completion of outpatient occupational therapy services, Yvonne will be discharged to a home program.

Questions and Activities

SAFETY OF CLIENT AND OTHERS: PRECAUTIONS AND CONTRAINDICATIONS

1. Create a precaution handout identifying the precautions and contraindications after a radical mastectomy.
2. Compare and contrast radical mastectomy with general postsurgical precautions.
3. Identify the common emotional reactions associated with mastectomy that may affect the treatment process.

OCCUPATIONS: ADLs, IADLs, EDUCATION, WORK, PLAY, SOCIAL PARTICIPATION, AND REST AND SLEEP

1. Given the information provided for this case, identify the areas of occupation that will and will not be addressed. Justify your decisions.
2. What strategies or assistive devices can be used to improve Yvonne's ability to dress?
3. What strategies or assistive devices can be used to improve Yvonne's ability to have a more restful sleep?

4. What strategies or assistive devices can be used to improve Yvonne's ability to prepare a simple meal?
5. Briefly describe what the first treatment session with Yvonne would be like.

PERFORMANCE SKILLS: MOTOR SKILLS, PROCESS SKILLS, AND SOCIAL INTERACTION SKILLS

1. Given the information provided, identify the motor, process, and social interaction skills that affect Yvonne's occupational performance.
2. Which of these skills would be appropriate to address within this service delivery site? Justify your selection.
3. Which of these skills would be addressed through remediation, compensation, and education?
4. Which of these skills would be addressed through the following intervention approaches: create/promote, establish/restore, maintain, modify, and prevent?

PERFORMANCE PATTERNS: HABITS, ROUTINES, ROLES, AND RITUALS

1. Identify Yvonne's useful habits, routines, roles, and rituals that support valued occupations. How can you make use of this information?
2. Identify Yvonne's impoverished habits, routines, roles, and rituals that do not support valued occupations. How can you make use of this information?
3. Identify Yvonne's dominating habits, routines, roles, and rituals that interfere with valued occupations. How can you make use of this information?

CLIENT FACTORS

Values, beliefs, and spirituality
How can the identified values, beliefs, and spirituality be used in this case?

Body structures
Considering the primary and secondary diagnoses, identify the related body structures.

Body functions
1. Identify how the primary and secondary diagnoses have affected the function of the identified body structures.
2. Explain the relationships between the structural and functional factors and Yvonne's current level of occupational performance.

MENTAL FUNCTIONS: AFFECTIVE, COGNITIVE, AND PERCEPTUAL

1. What common affective issues related to her radical mastectomy may Yvonne have to face?
2. How would these issues be addressed in occupational therapy?
3. To address these issues, what other disciplines could you refer Yvonne to?
4. Given the information provided, which additional mental function considerations need to be addressed?

NEUROMUSCULOSKELETAL AND MOVEMENT-RELATED FUNCTIONS

1. Given the information provided, identify neuromusculoskeletal and movement-related functions that need to be addressed. Justify your selections.
2. Identify the structural changes that have led to the limited range of motion (ROM) in Yvonne's left shoulder girdle.
3. Which model or frame of reference would be the best choice to address Yvonne's limitation of ROM?
4. Which type of exercise would be the best choice to address Yvonne's limitation in ROM? Justify your selection?
5. During a subsequent visit, you noticed that Yvonne's right hand had become swollen. What would be your concern? How should her hand be assessed?
6. Create an exercise program for Yvonne based on occupational performance.

CARDIOVASCULAR, HEMATOLOGICAL, IMMUNOLOGICAL, AND RESPIRATORY FUNCTIONS

1. Given the information provided, identify cardiovascular, hematological, immunological, and respiratory functions that need to be addressed. Justify your selections.
2. How may the radical mastectomy affect Yvonne's respiratory function?

SKIN AND RELATED STRUCTURE FUNCTIONS

1. Compare and contrast a simple mastectomy with a radical mastectomy.
2. What phenomena would explain Yvonne's continued sensation of her left breast being present? How may this situation be addressed?
3. What are common trophic changes to be expected along and around her surgical site?
4. Does Yvonne's ethnicity pose an increased risk for these changes?
5. What intervention would you select to minimize or prevent these changes?
6. What other skin and related structure functions should be considered?

VOICE AND SPEECH FUNCTIONS

Describe how the diagnosis may affect Yvonne's voice, speech, and occupational performance.

ASSISTIVE TECHNOLOGIES AND DEVICES

1. Yvonne chose to have a prosthesis versus reconstructive surgery. What are the advantages and disadvantages of each?
2. Identify and discuss the various breast forms or prosthesis that may be available to Yvonne.
3. Yvonne's insurance is a health maintenance organization. Would it cover the cost of her prosthesis?

ETHICAL DECISION MAKING

1. Yvonne has arrived for her occupational therapy session, and you observe the occupational therapy assistant (OTA) taking Yvonne's blood pressure in her LUE. Identify what is wrong and the best manner to address the situation.

2. During a treatment session, you observed that Yvonne's surgical site is red and warm to the touch. Identify what your concern would be and the best manner to address this situation.
3. Yvonne informs you that she has become aware of a mass in her right breast but pleads with you not to tell anyone. What are your ethical and legal responsibilities in this situation?
4. During a treatment session, an associate from housekeeping looks at Yvonne and makes a disparaging remark concerning her sexual orientation. How would you address this behavior?
5. Yvonne has confided in you that her spouse is reluctant to resume sexual intimacy with her. How can you best address this situation?

PHARMACOLOGY

Yvonne is currently using Voltaren.

1. What is the generic name?
2. Does this drug have a high alert status?
3. What is the classification of this drug?
4. What is the indication for this drug?
5. What is the action of this drug?
6. How may this drug affect client participation during a therapy session?

SOCIOCULTURAL, SOCIOECONOMIC, AND DIVERSITY FACTORS AND LIFESTYLE CHOICES

1. Given Yvonne's profile, examine how your own culture and beliefs affect your interaction with her.
2. Based on this self-examination, what area of cultural knowledge do you need to pursue?
3. How can this newly acquired cultural knowledge be integrated for effective outcomes?
4. How can you foster cultural interaction and awareness among your coworkers?
5. Discuss how a lack of understanding in the areas of discrimination and stigma, implicit bias, social identity, or racism may contribute to disparities in the delivery of occupational therapy services in this case.

ASSESSMENT TOOLS AND INTERPRETATION OF RESULTS

1. What is the purpose of NRS?
2. What are the psychometric properties of this instrument?
3. For which population were the norms developed?
4. Provide a brief description of this assessment.
5. What is the reliability of the NRS?
6. What is the validity of the NRS?
7. What functional inference can be deduced from Yvonne's score of 7/10?
8. What additional standardized assessment can be used in this case? Why?

INTERPROFESSIONAL RELATIONSHIP AND EFFECTIVE INTRAPROFESSIONAL COLLABORATION

1. Identify the other professions that would make up the care team. Explain the focus of each.
2. Identify the roles of the occupational therapy assistant (OTA) that could be used in the occupational therapy process for this case.

3. Identify interventions that can be assigned to the OTA for this case. Justify your selections.

BILLING AND CODING

1. Identify the *International Classification of Diseases (ICD)* codes for Yvonne's diagnoses.
2. For this case, identify at least two *Current Procedural Terminology (CPT®)* codes that are most appropriate. Justify your selection.

REIMBURSEMENT SYSTEMS AND DOCUMENTATION

1. Who would be the authorized individuals you could share the occupational therapy findings with? Explain why.
2. For this case, what forms and frequency of documentation will be required?
3. Which reimbursement system or systems most commonly cover occupational therapy services in this practice setting?

ADVOCACY

1. Which of the following areas of advocacy would be beneficial in this case: patient rights, matters of privacy, confidentiality, informed consent, awareness building, accessing education and/or benefits/resources?
2. Create a plan to advocate for this client based on the selected areas of advocacy.

TELEHEALTH

1. How can telehealth be integrated as a component of the occupational therapy process in this case?
2. Before launching telemedicine services, what questions would be essential to ask Yvonne to determine whether it is appropriate for her to engage in telemedicine services?
3. What challenges do you foresee if attempting to integrate telehealth services with this client?

Intervention Plan Formulation and Implementation

INTERVENTION PLAN FORMULATION

Create an intervention plan that includes the following:

1. List this individual's **strengths.**
2. List this individual's **barriers** in occupational performance, performance skills, and performance patterns.
3. Based on the individual's goals, health, performance, and service delivery site, **identify the barriers that will be addressed.**
4. From the barriers identified to be addressed, **formulate goals and objectives.**
5. Identify the focus of each goal and objective as either **create, promote, establish, restore, maintain, modify, or prevent.**

6. Identify the **theoretical basis, model(s) of practice, or frame(s) of reference** that will be used to address each goal and objective.
7. For each proposed goal and objective, describe clearly and precisely the **methods** that will be used. This description should include, but not be limited to, safety considerations, environmental considerations, therapeutic use of self, preparatory activities, activity selection, materials, equipment, and flow.
8. Classify the activities selected in the methods description as either **preparatory, enabling, purposeful, or occupation based.**
9. Explain how each activity can be **graded up or down,** creating the just-right challenge.
10. Provide at least two **primary sources of evidence** to support the intervention plan.

INTERVENTION PLAN IMPLEMENTATION

1. Based on your intervention plan, identify which goals and objectives require **more immediate attention.**
2. Describe your proposed **first treatment session.**
3. As the treatment session is progressing, what is **essential to be observed?**

Transition and Discontinuation

Create a plan for discharge from occupational therapy services in collaboration with Yvonne and members of the interprofessional team. Review the needs of Yvonne, caregivers, family members, and significant others. The plan must match needs with available resources and the discharge environment.

REFERENCES

American Medical Association. (2019). *CPT® 2020 professional edition.*
World Health Organization. (2019). *International statistical classification of diseases and related health problems* (11th ed.). https://icd.who.int/

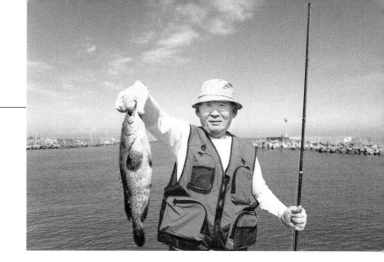

Chin: Carpal Tunnel Syndrome

CLOVER HUTCHINSON, OTD, MA, OTR/L

Chin (he, him, his, himself)

MEDICAL HISTORY

Chin is a 62-year-old Chinese American male who is 5' 4" and weighs 140 pounds. Recently, he received a diagnosis of carpal tunnel syndrome (CTS). He was seen by the orthopedic service for an ambulatory right endoscopic carpal tunnel release. After surgery, he was fitted with an anterior wrist splint. He was scheduled to begin occupational therapy at the outpatient department 10 days postsurgery. He reported no alcohol, tobacco, caffeine, or drug use and being allergic to sulfa-based medications.

SOCIAL HISTORY

Chin lives with his wife, son, daughter-in-law, and three grandchildren. His apartment is located on the fourth floor of a walk-up building. The apartment consists of a living room, kitchen, bathroom, three bedrooms, and a dining room that has been converted into two additional bedrooms. His building is in a part of a town in which many recent Chinese immigrants reside. Chin identifies as a Confucianist.

REFERRAL OR PRESCRIPTION

Chin was referred for outpatient services. He is to receive occupational therapy services 2 times per week for 6 weeks.

Occupational Therapy Initial Evaluation Findings: Outpatient Rehabilitation

OCCUPATIONAL PROFILE

Chin's preadmission occupational history and experiences included being independent in all ADLs and all IADLs. He has been employed as a waiter in a well-known Chinese restaurant for the past 18 years. His patterns of daily living most commonly included arriving to work at 11:00 a.m. and returning home by 12:00 a.m. Chin works 6 days per week to support his family and was traditionally off only on Mondays. He is deeply concerned that if he does not return to work in 6 weeks he will lose his job. His interests include fishing and walking about his community. He values providing his children and grandchildren with the opportunity to pursue college-level education and allow them to achieve the American dream. Chin reported his greatest current need is to return to work in no later than 6 weeks.

ADLs

Regarding self-care, Chin reported no difficulties except for opening a variety of containers. Regarding functional mobility, Chin reported no difficulties with bed mobility and transfers.

IADLs

Activities needed that provide day-to-day quality of life and relative independence were explored. Chin's wife has taken on the responsibility to maintain the home, prepare meals, clean up, and shop while her husband is recovering. Regarding rest and sleep, Chin reported sleeping comfortably and uninterrupted.

MENTAL FUNCTIONS

Cognitive assessment found Chin to be alert and oriented to person, place, time, and situation, and his short- and long-term memory were intact. He is able to follow three-step commands and make his needs known. Chin has a fair command of the English language but reported difficulty understanding technical medical terms. Affect appeared appropriate, and no gross deficits in perception were observed.

SENSORY FUNCTIONS AND PAIN

No gross deficits were observed with visual, hearing, vestibular, taste, smell, and proprioceptive functions. Impaired light touch, deep pressure, and thermal senses were identified in distal volar portions of the thumb, dorsal portions of the index and middle fingers, and a radial portion of the ring finger. Edema was observed in his right hand. Circumferential measurements taken at the distal palmar crease indicated 19.5 cm for the right hand and 17.8 cm for the left. Use of the numerical rating scale (0–10) for pain indicated a score of 2 for Chin's right anterior wrist. The pain was described as "tolerable."

CARDIOVASCULAR AND RESPIRATORY SYSTEMS FUNCTION

No deficits were noted in cardiovascular and respiratory systems function.

MOVEMENT FUNCTIONS

Passive range of motion (PROM) and active range of motion (AROM) in all four extremities except right wrist and digits were within normal limits. The PROM of the digits of the right hand was within normal limits. Goniometric measurements of the AROM of the digits of the right hand are shown in Table 9.1. In addition, strength was measured in both hands (Table 9.2). Chin scored a 73 on the Jebsen–Taylor Hand Function Test (Jebsen et al., 1969). Observation of the surgical site revealed the presence of two closed flat and dry incision sites, covered in scabs. Sutures were still present.

TABLE 9.1. Active Range of Motion (Degrees) of Right-Hand Digits

Joint	Digit 1	Digit 2	Digit 3	Digit 4	Digit 5
Metacarpophalangeal joint	0–46	0–70	0–76	0–76	0–90
Interphalangeal joint	0–68				
Proximal interphalangeal joint		0–83	0–85	0–85	0–100
Distal interphalangeal joint		0–40	0–40	0–52	0–60
Total active motion	**114**	**193**	**201**	**213**	**250**

TABLE 9.2. Hand Strength Measurements (lb)

Test	Right Hand	Left Hand
Gross grasp	46	70
Tripod pinch	12	17
Lateral pinch	15	20
Tip pinch	10	15

NEUROMUSCULAR FUNCTIONS

Static and dynamic sitting and standing balance were 5/5. Muscle tone was normal, and reflex integration was intact.

PLAN FOR DISCHARGE

Chin will be discharged from outpatient occupational therapy services with a home exercise program and plans to return to work.

Questions and Activities Guiding Critical Thinking

SAFETY OF CLIENT AND OTHERS: PRECAUTIONS AND CONTRAINDICATIONS

1. Create a handout identifying the postsurgical precautions after a carpal tunnel procedure.
2. Identify and explain the splint-wearing schedule and precautions that Chin must follow.
3. What are the common signs and symptoms of an infected wound?
4. If you have a concern that Chin's wound is infected, what actions must be taken?
5. Identify the common emotional reactions associated with not being able to work that may affect the treatment process.
6. To maintain safety, what other factors should be considered?

OCCUPATIONS: ADLs, IADLs, EDUCATION, WORK, PLAY, SOCIAL PARTICIPATION, AND REST AND SLEEP

1. Given the information provided for this case, identify the areas of occupation that will and will not be addressed. Justify your decisions.
2. Identify assistive devices or strategies that will allow Chin to open containers.
3. Identify the areas of education that would be appropriate to engage in with Chin and explain why.
4. Briefly describe what the first treatment session with Chin would be like.

PERFORMANCE SKILLS: MOTOR SKILLS, PROCESS SKILLS, AND SOCIAL INTERACTION SKILLS

1. Given the information provided, identify the motor, process, and social interaction skills that affect Chin's occupational performance.
2. Which of these skills would be appropriate to address in this service delivery site? Justify your selection.
3. Which of these skills would be addressed through remediation, compensation, and education?
4. Which of these skills would be addressed through the following intervention approaches: create/promote, establish/restore, maintain, modify, and prevent?

PERFORMANCE PATTERNS: HABITS, ROUTINES, ROLES, AND RITUALS

1. Identify Chin's useful habits, routines, roles, and rituals that support valued occupations. How can you make use of this information?
2. Identify Chin's impoverished habits, routines, roles, and rituals that do not support valued occupations. How can you make use of this information?
3. Identify Chin's dominating habits, routines, roles, and rituals that interfere with valued occupations. How can you make use of this information?

CLIENT FACTORS

Values, beliefs, spirituality
How can the identified values, beliefs, and spirituality be used in this case?

Body structures
Considering the primary and secondary diagnoses, identify the related body structures.

Body functions

1. Identify how the primary and secondary diagnoses have affected the function of the identified body structures.
2. Explain the relationships between the structural and functional factors and Chin's current level of occupational performance.

MENTAL FUNCTIONS: AFFECTIVE, COGNITIVE, AND PERCEPTUAL

1. What common affective issues related to his surgery may Chin have to face?
2. What does the literature identify as common concerns of people who must miss work for an extended period of time?
3. How would these issues be addressed in occupational therapy?
4. To address these issues, what other disciplines could you refer Chin to?
5. Given the information provided, which additional mental function considerations need to be addressed?

NEUROMUSCULOSKELETAL AND MOVEMENT-RELATED FUNCTIONS

1. Given the information provided, identify neuromusculoskeletal and movement-related functions that need to be addressed. Justify your selections.
2. Locate an occupational therapy protocol for clients who have undergone an endoscopic carpal tunnel release procedure. Identify and explain each phase of intervention.
3. What are the expected norms for AROM at the wrist and digits?
4. Which assessment tools should be used to assess gross grasp and pinch strength?
5. When should tools to assess gross grasp and pinch strength be used?
6. Are the gross grasp and pinch strength for Chin's right and left hands within the normative range for his age and gender?
7. Compare and contrast CTS with cervical radiculopathy.
8. Create an exercise program for Chin based on occupational performance.

CARDIOVASCULAR, HEMATOLOGICAL, IMMUNOLOGICAL, AND RESPIRATORY FUNCTIONS

1. Given the information provided, identify cardiovascular, hematological, immunological, and respiratory functions that need to be addressed. Justify your selections.
2. How can pain affect an individual's vital signs?

SKIN AND RELATED STRUCTURE FUNCTIONS

1. How can the edema in Chin's right hand be best addressed during his therapy sessions?
2. How can Chin address the edema in his right hand when he is not actively engaged in his therapy sessions?
3. Identify an alternative edema assessment tool or method other than circumferential measurements.
4. What are the risks and benefits of an endoscopic release versus an open surgical release?
5. What other skin and related structure functions should be considered?

VOICE AND SPEECH FUNCTIONS

Describe how Chin's diagnosis may affect his voice, speech, and occupational performance.

ASSISTIVE TECHNOLOGIES AND DEVICES

What assistive technologies or adaptations might be used or made for Chin while he is receiving occupational therapy services? Why?

ETHICAL DECISION MAKING

1. Chin frequently asks to take a break during the therapy session to smoke a cigarette. How would you address smoking and its effect on wound healing?
2. Chin informs you that he missed his follow-up appointment with the surgeon because he did not have the copayment. How can you best address this situation?
3. Chin shows you a recent photograph of him lifting his 4-year-old grandson with both hands. How can you best address this situation?

PHARMACOLOGY

Chin is currently taking Naprosyn.

1. What is the generic name?
2. Does this drug have a high alert status?
3. What is the classification of this drug?
4. What is the indication for this drug?
5. What is the action of this drug?
6. How may this drug affect client participation during a therapy session?

SOCIOCULTURAL, SOCIOECONOMIC, AND DIVERSITY FACTORS AND LIFESTYLE CHOICES

1. Given Chin's profile, examine how your own culture and beliefs affect your interaction with him.
2. Based on this self-examination, what area of cultural knowledge do you need to pursue?
3. How can this newly acquired cultural knowledge be integrated for effective outcomes?
4. How can you foster cultural interaction and awareness among your coworkers?
5. Discuss how a lack of understanding in the areas of discrimination and stigma, implicit bias, social identity, or racism may contribute to disparities in the delivery of occupational therapy services in this case.

ASSESSMENT TOOLS AND INTERPRETATION OF RESULTS

1. What is the purpose of the Jebsen–Taylor Hand Function Test?
2. Which population is this test designed for?
3. How much time is required to administer it?
4. Provide a brief description of this assessment.
5. What is the reliability of the Jebsen–Taylor Hand Function Test?
6. What is the validity of the Jebsen–Taylor Hand Function Test?

7. What functional inference can be deduced from Chin's score of 73?
8. What additional standardized assessment can be used in this case? Why?

INTERPROFESSIONAL RELATIONSHIP AND EFFECTIVE INTRAPROFESSIONAL COLLABORATION

1. Identify the other professions that would make up the care team. Explain the focus of each.
2. Identify the roles of the occupational therapy assistant (OTA) that could be used in the occupational therapy process for this case.
3. Identify interventions that can be assigned to the OTA for this case. Justify your selections.

BILLING AND CODING

1. Identify the *International Classification of Diseases (ICD)* code for Chin's diagnosis.
2. For this case, identify at least two *Current Procedural Terminology (CPT®)* codes that are most appropriate. Justify your selection.

REIMBURSEMENT SYSTEMS AND DOCUMENTATION

1. Who would be the authorized individuals that you could share the occupational therapy findings with? Explain why.
2. For this case, what forms and frequency of documentation will be required?
3. Which reimbursement system or systems most commonly cover occupational therapy services in this practice setting?

ADVOCACY

1. Which of the following areas of advocacy would be beneficial in this case: patient rights, matters of privacy, confidentiality, informed consent, awareness building, accessing education, and benefits/resources?
2. Create a plan to advocate for this client based on the selected areas of advocacy.

TELEHEALTH

1. How can telehealth be integrated as a component of the occupational therapy process in this case?
2. Before launching telemedicine services, what questions would be essential to ask Chin to determine whether it is appropriate for him to engage in telemedicine services?
3. What challenges do you foresee if attempting to integrate telehealth services with this client?

Intervention Plan Formulation and Implementation

INTERVENTION PLAN FORMULATION

Create an intervention plan that includes the following:

1. List this individual's **strengths.**

2. List this individual's **barriers** in occupational performance, performance skills, and performance patterns.
3. Based on the individual's goals, health, performance, and service delivery site, **identify the barriers that will be addressed.**
4. From the barriers identified to be addressed, **formulate goals and objectives.**
5. Identify the focus of each goal and objective as either **create, promote, establish, restore, maintain, modify, or prevent.**
6. Identify the **theoretical basis, model(s) of practice, or frame(s) of reference** that will be used to address each goal and objective.
7. For each proposed goal and objective, describe clearly and precisely the **methods** that will be used. This description should include, but not be limited to, safety considerations, environmental considerations, therapeutic use of self, preparatory activities, activity selection, materials, equipment, and flow.
8. Classify the activities selected in the methods description as either **preparatory, enabling, purposeful, or occupation based.**
9. Explain how each activity can be **graded up or down,** creating the just-right challenge.
10. Provide at least two **primary sources of evidence** to support the intervention plan.

INTERVENTION PLAN IMPLEMENTATION

1. Based on your intervention plan, identify which goals and objectives require **more immediate attention.**
2. Describe your proposed **first treatment session.**
3. As the treatment session is progressing, what is **essential to be observed?**

Transition and Discontinuation

Create a plan for discharge from occupational therapy services in collaboration with Chin and members of the interprofessional team. Review the needs of Chin, caregivers, family members, and significant others. The plan must match needs with available resources and the discharge environment.

REFERENCES

American Medical Association. (2019). *CPT® 2020 professional edition.*
Jebsen, R. H., Taylor, N., Trieschmann, R. B., Trotter, M. J., & Howard, L. A. (1969). An objective and standardized test of hand function. *Archives of Physical Medicine and Rehabilitation, 50,* 311–319.
World Health Organization. (2019). *International statistical classification of diseases and related health problems* (11th ed.). https://icd.who.int/

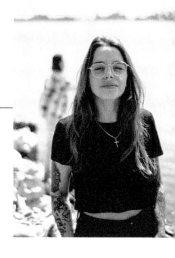

Patricia: Laceration of Flexor Digitorum Profundus and Superficialis Tendons

CLOVER HUTCHINSON, OTD, MA, OTR/L

Patricia (she, her, hers, herself)

MEDICAL HISTORY

Patricia is a 36-year-old Danish American female who is 5' 11" and weighs 140 pounds. She was brought in by emergency medical services to the emergency department after lacerating her left index finger with a box cutter while working as a sales associate. Physical examination and X-rays were performed, and Patricia received a diagnosis of complete tendon laceration to her left second flexor digitorum profundus and flexor digitorum superficialis. She was taken to the operating room, where the tendons were surgically repaired. She was placed in a protective posterior fiberglass splint and discharged from the hospital the same day. Her medical history was unremarkable. She reported no alcohol, drug, tobacco, or coffee use and has no known allergies.

SOCIAL HISTORY

Patricia lives as a single mother with her 8-year-old son in the basement apartment of her parents' home. There are 12 steps to descend to enter her apartment from the hallway. Her apartment includes a kitchenette, a combined living room and dinette space, two small bedrooms, and a bathroom. Patricia does not own a car. Her home is a 15-minute bus ride to work and is 20 minutes from the medical center. Patricia reported just ending a 6-month relationship with her last boyfriend, and her parents have been active in watching her son while she is at work. Patricia identifies as an Evangelical Lutheran.

REFERRAL OR PRESCRIPTION

Patricia was referred for outpatient services. She is to receive occupational therapy services 2 times per week for 10 weeks.

Occupational Therapy Initial Evaluation Findings: Outpatient Rehabilitation

OCCUPATIONAL PROFILE

Patricia's preadmission occupational history and experiences included being independent in all ADLs and all IADLs. Patricia has been employed full time for the past 8 months as a sales associate for a national chain store. She reported that this job has been her first with a comprehensive benefits package. Her patterns of daily living most commonly included having breakfast with her son, putting him on the school bus, and then going to work. Her mother usually picked up her son from the bus and assisted him with his homework. Once Patricia arrived home, she usually cooked dinner, helped her son complete his homework, and then chatted to friends on social media. Weekends usually included playdates for her son on Saturdays and church on Sundays. Her interests include spending time on social media and going out with friends on occasion. She values the love of her parents and the gift of her son. Patricia reported her greatest current need is to get her hand better and get back to work.

ADLs

Regarding self-care, Patricia is able to feed herself but requires assistance to cut her food. She is able to don and doff all garments but requires assistance with fasteners. She is not able to blow dry her hair without assistance. Regarding functional mobility, Patricia is able to be independent in all bed mobility, transfer, and ambulation.

IADLs

Activities needed that provide day-to-day quality of life and relative independence were explored. Patricia can manage her communications, handle her finances, prepare simple meals, and perform light cleanup tasks and light shopping. Regarding rest and sleep, Patricia reported that she frequently awakes at night secondary to the presence of "throbbing pain" in her surgically repaired finger.

MENTAL FUNCTIONS

Cognitive assessment found Patricia to be alert and oriented to person, place, time, and situation, and her short- and long-term memory were intact. She is able to follow three-step commands and make her needs known. Regarding affect, she reported feeling anxious because of not having money coming in to pay her bills. She scored 58 out of 100 on the Zung Self-Rating Anxiety Scale (Zung, 1971). No gross deficits in perception were observed.

SENSORY FUNCTIONS AND PAIN

No gross deficits were observed with visual, hearing, vestibular, taste, smell, proprioceptive, and cutaneous functions. A 2.5-cm scabbed incision with six external stitches was observed over the anterior base of Patricia's left index finger. Circumferential measurements were taken over the proximal phalanx; the left was 8.0 cm, and the right was 7.2 cm. Use of the numerical rating scale (0–10) for pain indicated a score of 3 for Patricia's left index finger, and she described the surgical area as "sensitive to touch."

CARDIOVASCULAR AND RESPIRATORY SYSTEMS FUNCTION

No deficits were noted in cardiovascular and respiratory systems function. Patricia reported that she performs all ADLs and IADLs without experiencing fatigue.

MOVEMENT FUNCTIONS

All four extremities are intact for passive range of motion, active range of motion, and muscular strength. Movement of the left wrist and digits was contraindicated and not assessed at the time of evaluation. Patricia has a left dorsal protective fiberglass splint with a bulky dressing and ace bandage wrap.

NEUROMUSCULAR FUNCTIONS

Static and dynamic sitting and standing balance were both 5/5. Muscle tone was normal, and reflex integration was intact.

PLAN FOR DISCHARGE

Following completion of outpatient occupational therapy services, Patricia will be discharged to a home program.

Questions and Activities

SAFETY OF CLIENT AND OTHERS: PRECAUTIONS AND CONTRAINDICATIONS

1. Create a handout that identifies and explains precautions and contraindications to be followed after tendon repair.
2. Patricia has an unhealed wound. Identify and explain the precautions to be followed.
3. Identify and explain the splint-wearing schedule and the precautions that Patricia must follow.
4. Identify the common emotional reactions associated with hand injuries that may affect the treatment process.
5. To maintain safety, what other factors should be considered?

OCCUPATIONS: ADLs, IADLs, EDUCATION, WORK, PLAY, SOCIAL PARTICIPATION, AND REST AND SLEEP

1. Given the information provided for this case, identify the areas of occupation that will and will not be addressed. Justify your decisions.

2. What strategies or assistive devices can Patricia use that can lead her to independent dressing?
3. What strategies or assistive devices can Patricia use that can lead her to independently blow dry her hair?

PERFORMANCE SKILLS: MOTOR SKILLS, PROCESS SKILLS, AND SOCIAL INTERACTION

1. Given the information provided, identify the motor, process, and social interaction skills that affect Patricia's occupational performance.
2. Which of these skills would be appropriate to address in this service delivery site? Justify your selection.
3. Which of these skills would be addressed through remediation, compensation, and education?
4. Which of these skills would be addressed through the following intervention approaches: create/promote, establish/restore, maintain, modify, and prevent?

PERFORMANCE PATTERNS: HABITS, ROUTINES, ROLES, AND RITUALS

1. Identify Patricia's useful habits, routines, roles, and rituals that support valued occupations. How can you make use of this information?
2. Identify Patricia's impoverished habits, routines, roles, and rituals that do not support valued occupations. How can you make use of this information?
3. Identify Patricia's dominating habits, routines, roles, and rituals that interfere with valued occupations. How can you make use of this information?

CLIENT FACTORS

Values, beliefs, and spirituality
How can the identified values, beliefs, and spirituality be used in this case?

Body structures
Considering the primary and secondary diagnoses, identify the related body structures.

Body functions
1. Identify how the primary and secondary diagnoses have affected the function of the identified body structures.
2. Explain the relationships between the structural and functional factors and Patricia's current level of occupational performance.

MENTAL FUNCTIONS: AFFECTIVE, COGNITIVE, AND PERCEPTUAL

1. What common affective issues related to her laceration and repair may Patricia have to face?
2. How would these issues be addressed in occupational therapy?
3. To address these issues, what other disciplines could you refer Patricia to?
4. To address Patricia's anxiety, what other disciplines could you refer Patricia to?
5. Which stress reduction techniques may benefit Patricia? Why?
6. Patricia is concerned about the cost of all her medical services. What service may assist her with this concern?
7. Given the information provided, which additional mental function considerations need to be addressed?

NEUROMUSCULOSKELETAL AND MOVEMENT-RELATED FUNCTIONS

1. Given the information provided, identify neuromusculoskeletal and movement-related functions that need to be addressed. Justify your selections.
2. Identify two sources to obtain a protocol for a flexor tendon repair. Select one and apply it to Patricia's zone of injury.
3. Identify biweekly time frames for the following: required splint wearing, exercises, and allowed activities. Explain why.
4. Create an exercise program for Patricia based on occupational performance.

CARDIOVASCULAR, HEMATOLOGICAL, IMMUNOLOGICAL, AND RESPIRATORY FUNCTIONS

1. Given the information provided, identify cardiovascular, hematological, immunological, and respiratory functions that need to be addressed. Justify your selections.
2. Identify the physical manifestation of anxiety on cardiovascular and respiratory functions. Explain the physiological mechanisms.

SKIN AND RELATED STRUCTURE FUNCTIONS

1. Compare and contrast laceration and abrasion.
2. What is the expected time frame for the sutures to be removed?
3. How long does it take for a tendon to heal after surgery?
4. What other skin and related structure functions should be considered?

VOICE AND SPEECH FUNCTIONS

Describe how Patricia's diagnosis may affect her voice, speech, and occupational performance.

ASSISTIVE TECHNOLOGIES AND DEVICES

Explain the function of the protective splint that the surgeon placed on Patricia after her surgery.

ETHICAL DECISION MAKING

1. You observed a male aide ask Patricia out on a date. Identify what would be your concern, and explain the best manner to address this situation.
2. During the session, you became aware that Patricia smelled of marijuana. Identify what would be your concern, and explain the best manner to address this situation.
3. At the end of the session, Patricia asked to borrow bus fare to return home. Identify what would be your concern, and explain the best manner to address this situation.
4. During Week 2, Patricia confides to you that she removes her protective splint for hours at a time. Identify what would be your concern, and explain the best manner to address this situation.

PHARMACOLOGY

Patricia is currently taking Amcill.

1. What is the generic name?
2. Does this drug have a high alert status?
3. What is the classification of this drug?
4. What is the indication for this drug?
5. What is the action of this drug?
6. How may this drug affect client participation during a therapy session?
7. To maintain safety, what other factors should be considered?

SOCIOCULTURAL, SOCIOECONOMIC, AND DIVERSITY FACTORS AND LIFESTYLE CHOICES

1. Given Patricia's profile, examine how your own culture and beliefs affect your interaction with her.
2. Based on this self-examination, what area of cultural knowledge do you need to pursue?
3. How can this newly acquired cultural knowledge be integrated for effective outcomes?
4. How can you foster cultural interaction and awareness among your coworkers?

ASSESSMENT TOOLS AND INTERPRETATION OF RESULTS

1. What is the purpose of the Zung Self-Rating Anxiety Scale?
2. Which population is this test designed for?
3. How much time is required to administer it?
4. Provide a brief description of this assessment.
5. What is the reliability of the Zung Self-Rating Anxiety Scale?
6. What is the validity of the Zung Self-Rating Anxiety Scale?
7. What functional inference can be deduced from Patricia's score of 58?
8. What additional standardized assessment can be used in this case? Why?

INTERPROFESSIONAL RELATIONSHIP AND EFFECTIVE INTRAPROFESSIONAL COLLABORATION

1. Identify the other professions that would make up the care team. Explain the focus of each.
2. Identify the roles of the occupational therapy assistant (OTA) that could be used in the occupational therapy process for this case.
3. Identify interventions that can be assigned to the OTA for this case. Justify your selections.

BILLING AND CODING

1. Identify the *International Classification of Diseases (ICD)* codes for Patricia's diagnosis.
2. For this case, identify at least two *Current Procedural Terminology (CPT®)* codes that are most appropriate. Justify your selection.

REIMBURSEMENT SYSTEMS AND DOCUMENTATION

1. Who would be the authorized individuals you could share the occupational therapy findings with? Explain why.

2. For this case, what forms and frequency of documentation will be required?
3. Which reimbursement system or systems most commonly cover occupational therapy services in this practice setting?
4. Which insurance covers individuals injured during the performance of their duties at work?

ADVOCACY

1. Which of the following areas of advocacy would be beneficial in this case: patient rights, matters of privacy, confidentiality, informed consent, awareness building, accessing education and/or benefits/resources?
2. Create a plan to advocate for this client based on the selected areas of advocacy.

TELEHEALTH

1. How can telehealth be integrated as a component of the occupational therapy process into this case?
2. Before launching telemedicine services, what questions would be essential to ask Patricia to determine whether it is appropriate for her to engage in telemedicine services?
3. What are the challenges you foresee if attempting to integrate telehealth services with this client?

Intervention Plan Formulation and Implementation

INTERVENTION PLAN FORMULATION

Create an intervention plan that includes the following:

1. List this individual's **strengths.**
2. List this individual's **barriers** in occupational performance, performance skills, and performance patterns.
3. Based on the individual's goals, health, performance, and service delivery site, **identify the barriers that will be addressed.**
4. From the barriers identified to be addressed, **formulate goals and objectives.**
5. Identify the focus of each goal and objective as either **create, promote, establish, restore, maintain, modify, or prevent.**
6. Identify the **theoretical basis, model(s) of practice, or frame(s) of reference** that will be used to address each goal and objective.
7. For each proposed goal and objective, describe clearly and precisely the **methods** that will be used. This description should include, but not be limited to, safety considerations, environmental considerations, therapeutic use of self, preparatory activities, activity selection, materials, equipment, and flow.
8. Classify the activities selected in the methods description as either **preparatory, enabling, purposeful, or occupation based.**
9. Explain how each activity can be **graded up or down,** creating the just-right challenge.
10. Provide at least two **primary sources of evidence** to support the intervention plan.

INTERVENTION PLAN IMPLEMENTATION

1. Based on your intervention plan, identify which goals and objectives require **more immediate attention.**
2. Describe your proposed **first treatment session**.
3. As the treatment session is progressing, what is **essential to be observed?**

Transition and Discontinuation

Create a plan for discharge from occupational therapy services in collaboration with Patricia and members of the interprofessional team. Review the needs of Patricia, caregivers, family members, and significant others. The plan must match needs with available resources and the discharge environment.

REFERENCES

American Medical Association. (2019). *CPT® 2020 professional edition.*

World Health Organization. (2019). *International statistical classification of diseases and related health problems* (11th ed.). https://icd.who.int/

Zung, W. W. (1971). A rating instrument for anxiety disorders. *Psychosomatics, 12,* 371–379. https://doi.org/10.1016/S0033-3182(71)71479-0

Rehabilitation Unit or Rehabilitation Hospital

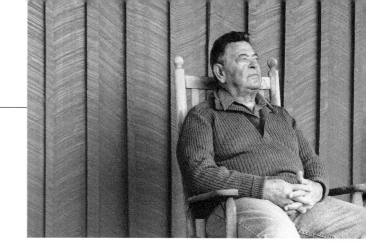

Fetu: Cerebral Vascular Accident

CLOVER HUTCHINSON, OTD, MA, OTR/L

Fetu (he, him, his, himself)

MEDICAL HISTORY

Fetu is a 71-year-old New Zealander male living in the United States who is 5' 11" and weighs 235 pounds. He was brought by emergency medical services to the emergency department (ED) after being found by his wife on the bathroom floor. He was unable to move his right side and had difficulty speaking. A computed axial tomography scan, magnetic resonance imaging, and electrocardiogram were performed. He was diagnosed with a left ischemic cerebral vascular accident (CVA) of the middle cerebral artery. Fetu received acute treatment with thrombolytic agents and was stabilized. From the ED, he was transferred to the stroke unit. His medical history included treatment for hypertension, diabetes mellitus, and high cholesterol. Upon admission, he reported living a sedentary lifestyle and drinking 4–5 cups of coffee per day. He reported no alcohol, drug, or tobacco use and an allergy to aspirin.

SOCIAL HISTORY

Fetu is a retired customer service agent who lives with his wife of 43 years, who is also retired. They live in a one-story ranch home. There are three steps to enter his home, which consists of a living room, dining room, three bedrooms, a half bathroom, and an eat-in kitchen. They have three adult children living close by with their families. Fetu identifies as Presbyterian.

REFERRAL OR PRESCRIPTION

Fetu has been transferred to the acute rehabilitation floor. He was referred for occupational therapy, physical therapy, speech therapy, and dietary services. The length of stay will be 21 days.

Occupational Therapy Initial Evaluation Findings: Rehabilitation Unit

OCCUPATIONAL PROFILE

Fetu's preadmission occupational history and experiences included being independent in all ADLs and all IADLs. His patterns of daily living most commonly included babysitting his youngest grandchild with his wife during the week. He also enjoys day trips and dining out with his wife on weekends. His interests include watching sports on television and hosting barbecues. Fetu values his independence and family life. He reported his greatest current needs are to be able to go home and not be a burden to his wife.

ADLs

Regarding self-care, Fetu was able to use a spoon and fork and drink from a cup independently, but he was dependent with cutting his food. Fetu was dependent with all dressing, bathing, grooming, and toileting. Regarding functional mobility, Fetu was able to roll independently to his right but required moderate assistance to his left. Moderate assistance was required to transition from supine and short sit in bed. Fetu was dependent on performing stand pivot transfers between the bed and commode and the bed and wheelchair. Tub transfers were not attempted. He showed noticeable signs of fatigue after transfers.

IADLs

Activities needed that provide day-to-day quality of life and relative independence were explored. Fetu was dependent in all areas of IADLs. Regarding rest and sleep, a review of the medical chart indicated that Fetu was able to sleep through the night.

MENTAL FUNCTIONS

Fetu was alert. Assessment of cognition, perception, and affect status could not be completed at the time of the evaluation because of Fetu's severe expressive aphasia.

SENSORY FUNCTIONS AND PAIN

No gross deficits were observed with visual, vestibular, taste, smell, proprioceptive and cutaneous functions. Fetu's wife reported that he was "hard of hearing." He scored pain as a 0/10 on the Wong-Baker FACES® Pain Rating Scale (Wong-Baker FACES Foundation, 2018).

CARDIOVASCULAR AND RESPIRATORY SYSTEMS FUNCTION

Assessment of cardiovascular and respiratory systems function indicated Fetu presented at a value of 4.0 on the metabolic equivalent of task.

MOVEMENT FUNCTIONS

Active range of motion (AROM), passive range of motion (PROM), and muscle strength were within normal limits (WNL) for Fetu's left upper extremity (LUE). His right upper extremity (RUE) was WNL for PROM. No AROM was present in his RUE. Left grasp strength was 41 pounds, and right grasp strength was not able to be assessed.

NEUROMUSCULAR FUNCTIONS

Fetu required moderate assistance to maintain static sitting and maximal assistance with dynamic sitting. He was dependent when standing and walking. Both the RUE and right lower extremity (RLE) were flaccid and without active movement. Deep tendon reflexes in the LUE were absent. The Fugl-Meyer Assessment for Upper Extremity (FMA–UE; Fugl-Meyer, 1975) was administered, and the scores were as follows: motor function, 2/66; sensation, 5/12; passive joint motion, 24/24; and joint pain, 24/24.

PLAN FOR DISCHARGE

Fetu will be discharged with home care services. Services will include nursing, occupational therapy, physical therapy, and speech therapy.

Questions and Activities

SAFETY OF CLIENT AND OTHERS: PRECAUTIONS AND CONTRAINDICATIONS

1. What would be the safest transfer method to transition Fetu from his bed to and from his wheelchair? Why?
2. Create a handout that identifies actions that can be taken to minimize the risk of a fall.
3. Which vital signs should be taken when working with Fetu? What are their norms? When should they be taken?
4. Fetu has been prescribed an anticoagulant. What are the precautions that need to be followed?
5. To effectively communicate with Fetu, what strategies would you use? Support your selection.
6. What common emotional reactions are associated with stroke that may affect the treatment process?
7. To maintain safety, what other factors should be considered?

OCCUPATIONS: ADLs, IADLs, EDUCATION, WORK, PLAY, SOCIAL PARTICIPATION, AND REST AND SLEEP

1. Briefly describe what the first treatment session with Fetu would be like.
2. Briefly describe how Fetu would be able to cut food.
3. Briefly describe how Fetu would be able to propel a wheelchair.
4. Identify the areas of education that would be appropriate to engage in with Fetu and explain why.
5. Would work, play, socialization, or sleep be addressed for Fetu? Why or why not?

PERFORMANCE SKILLS: MOTOR SKILLS, PROCESS SKILLS, AND SOCIAL INTERACTION SKILLS

1. Given the information provided, identify the motor, process, and social interaction skills that affect Fetu's occupational performance.
2. Which of these skills would be appropriate to address in this service delivery site? Justify your selection.
3. Which of these skills would be addressed through remediation, compensation, and education?
4. Which of these skills would be addressed through the following intervention approaches: create/promote, establish/restore, maintain, modify, and prevent?

PERFORMANCE PATTERNS: HABITS, ROUTINES, ROLES, AND RITUALS

1. Identify Fetu's useful habits, routines, roles, and rituals that support valued occupations. How can you make use of this information?
2. Identify Fetu's impoverished habits, routines, roles, and rituals that do not support valued occupations. How can you make use of this information?
3. Identify Fetu's dominating habits, routines, roles, and rituals that interfere with valued occupations. How can you make use of this information?

CLIENT FACTORS

Values, beliefs, and spirituality
How can the identified values, beliefs, and spirituality be used in this case?

Body structures
Considering the primary and secondary diagnoses, identify the related body structures.

Body functions
1. Identify how the primary and secondary diagnoses have affected the function of the identified body structures.
2. Explain the relationships between the structural and functional factors and Fetu's current level of occupational performance.

MENTAL FUNCTIONS: AFFECTIVE, COGNITIVE, AND PERCEPTUAL

1. What common affective issues related to his stroke might Fetu have to face?
2. How would these issues be addressed in occupational therapy?
3. To address these issues, what other disciplines could you refer Fetu to?
4. What common challenges related to his expressive aphasia may Fetu experience?
5. How would these challenges be addressed in occupational therapy?
6. Given the information provided, what additional mental function considerations need to be addressed?

NEUROMUSCULOSKELETAL AND MOVEMENT-RELATED FUNCTIONS

1. Given the information provided, identify neuromusculoskeletal and movement-related functions that need to be addressed. Justify your selections.

2. What negative changes can occur as a result of Fetu not being able to actively move his flaccid RUE and RLE? What can be done during his stay at the acute care facility to prevent these changes?
3. Which frames of reference can address Fetu's motor control deficits? Which one would you select? Justify your selection.
4. Compare and contrast a CVA with a brain tumor.
5. Create an exercise program for Fetu based on occupational performance.

CARDIOVASCULAR, HEMATOLOGICAL, IMMUNOLOGICAL, AND RESPIRATORY FUNCTIONS

1. Given the information provided, identify cardiovascular, hematological, immunological, and respiratory function(s) that need to be addressed. Justify your selection(s).
2. Identify the signs and symptoms of overexertion Fetu may display while engaged in his treatment sessions.

SKIN AND RELATED STRUCTURE FUNCTIONS

1. Fetu has great difficulty changing his position in bed. What are the concerns and how can these be best addressed?
2. What other skin and related structure functions should be considered?

VOICE AND SPEECH FUNCTIONS

Describe how Fetu's diagnoses may affect his voice, speech, and associated occupational performance.

ASSISTIVE TECHNOLOGIES AND DEVICES

1. What assistive technologies or adaptations might be used or made to assist Fetu while he is receiving occupational therapy services on the acute rehabilitation floor? Why?
2. What assistive technologies or adaptations might be issued before Fetu's discharge home? Why?

ETHICAL DECISION MAKING

1. You overhear Fetu's wife asking the nurse whether he will ever be able to use his arm and leg again. The nurse assures her he will be as good as new in a matter of weeks. How should this situation be best addressed?
2. During Fetu's preparation for discharge to home, you observe his wife placing five hospital towels in her shopping bag. How should this situation be best addressed?

PHARMACOLOGY

Fetu is currently taking Plavix.

1. What is the generic name?
2. Does this drug have a high alert status?
3. What is the classification of this drug?
4. What is the indication for this drug?

5. What is the action of this drug?
6. How may this drug affect client participation during a therapy session?

SOCIOCULTURAL, SOCIOECONOMIC, AND DIVERSITY FACTORS AND LIFESTYLE CHOICES

1. Given Fetu's profile, how may your own culture and beliefs affect your interaction with him?
2. Based on this self-examination, what area of cultural knowledge do you need to pursue?
3. How can this newly acquired cultural knowledge be integrated for effective outcomes?
4. How can you foster cultural interaction and awareness among your coworkers?
5. Discuss how a lack of understanding in the areas of discrimination and stigma, implicit bias, social identity, or racism may contribute to disparities in the delivery of occupational therapy services in this case.

ASSESSMENT TOOLS AND INTERPRETATION OF RESULTS

1. What is the purpose of the FMA–UE?
2. Which population is this test designed for?
3. How much time is required to administer it?
4. Provide a brief description of this assessment.
5. What is the reliability of the FMA–UE?
6. What is the validity of the FMA–UE?
7. What functional inference can be deduced from Fetu's motor function score of 2/66?
8. What additional standardized assessment can be used in this case? Why?

INTERPROFESSIONAL RELATIONSHIP AND EFFECTIVE INTRAPROFESSIONAL COLLABORATION

1. Identify the other professions that would make up the care team. Explain the focus of each.
2. Identify the roles of the occupational therapy assistant (OTA) that could be used in the occupational therapy process for this case.
3. Identify interventions that can be assigned to the OTA for this case. Justify your selections.

BILLING AND CODING

1. Identify the *International Classification of Diseases (ICD)* codes for Fetu's diagnoses.
2. For this case, identify at least two *Current Procedural Terminology (CPT®)* codes that are most appropriate. Justify your selection.

REIMBURSEMENT SYSTEMS AND DOCUMENTATION

1. Who would be the authorized individuals you could share the occupational therapy findings with? Explain why.
2. For this case, what forms and frequency of documentation will be required?
3. Which reimbursement system or systems most commonly cover occupational therapy services in this practice setting?

ADVOCACY

1. Which of the following areas of advocacy would be beneficial in this case: patient rights, matters of privacy, confidentiality, informed consent, awareness building, accessing education, and benefits/resources?
2. Create a plan to advocate for this client based on the selected areas of advocacy.

TELEHEALTH

1. How can telehealth be integrated as a component of the occupational therapy process in this case?
2. Before launching telemedicine services, what questions would be essential to ask Fetu to determine whether it is appropriate for him to engage in telemedicine services?
3. What challenges do you foresee if attempting to integrate telehealth services with this client?

Intervention Plan Formulation and Implementation

INTERVENTION PLAN FORMULATION

Create an intervention plan that includes the following:

1. List this individual's **strengths.**
2. List this individual's **barriers** in occupational performance, performance skills, and performance patterns.
3. Based on the individual's goals, health, performance, and service delivery site, **identify the barriers that will be addressed.**
4. From the barriers identified to be addressed, **formulate goals and objectives.**
5. Identify the focus of each goal and objective as either **create, promote, establish, restore, maintain, modify, or prevent.**
6. Identify the **theoretical basis, model(s) of practice, or frame(s) of reference** that will be used to address each goal and objective.
7. For each proposed goal and objective, describe clearly and precisely the **methods** that will be used. This description should include, but not be limited to, safety considerations, environmental considerations, therapeutic use of self, preparatory activities, activity selection, materials, equipment, and flow.
8. Classify the activities selected in the methods description as either **preparatory, enabling, purposeful, or occupation based.**
9. Explain how each activity can be **graded up or down,** creating the just-right challenge.
10. Provide at least two **primary sources of evidence** to support the intervention plan.

INTERVENTION PLAN IMPLEMENTATION

1. Based on your intervention plan, identify which goals and objectives require **more immediate attention.**
2. Describe your proposed **first treatment session.**
3. As the treatment session is progressing, what is **essential to be observed?**

Transition and Discontinuation

Create a plan for discharge from occupational therapy services in (hypothetical) collaboration with Fetu and members of the interprofessional team. Review the needs of Fetu, caregivers, family members, and significant others. The plan must match needs with available resources and the discharge environment.

REFERENCES

American Medical Association. (2019). *CPT® 2020 professional edition.*

Fugl-Meyer, A. R., Jääskö, L., Leyman, I., Olsson, S., & Steglind, S. (1975). The post-stroke hemiplegic patient: 1. A method for evaluation of physical performance. *Scandinavian Journal of Rehabilitation Medicine, 7,* 13–31.

Wong-Baker FACES Foundation. (2018). *Wong-Baker FACES® Pain Rating Scale.*

World Health Organization. (2019). *International statistical classification of diseases and related health problems* (11th ed.). https://icd.who.int/

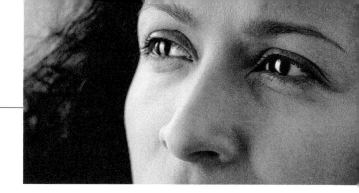

Bianca: Spinal Cord Injury, Complete C5

CLOVER HUTCHINSON, OTD, MA, OTR/L

Bianca (she, her, hers, herself)

MEDICAL HISTORY

Bianca is a 47-year-old Dominican American female who is 5' 1" and weighs 165 pounds. She was brought by emergency medical services to the emergency department after a diving accident. She presented with paralysis in all four extremities. A physical examination, X-rays, computerized tomography scan, and magnetic resonance imaging were performed. She received a diagnosis of a complete C5 spinal cord injury (SCI). She was placed on a ventilator and treated to prevent shock, and her cervical spine was immobilized. Bianca was taken to the operating room (OR), where she underwent spinal cord decompression and stabilization. From the OR, she was transferred to the neurological intensive care unit. Her medical history included breast augmentation, tummy tuck, and gluteal enhancement. Upon admission, she reported living an active life. She and her boyfriend enjoyed dining out, traveling, and dancing. She reported no caffeine, nicotine, drug, or alcohol use and has no known allergies.

SOCIAL HISTORY

Bianca lives with her boyfriend of 2 years in her boyfriend's pre–World War II two-story townhouse. There are 8 steps to the landing of the first floor and an additional 15 steps between the first and second floors. The townhouse includes a small bathroom, galley kitchen, large living room, dining room, and a single bedroom. The townhouse is located just five blocks from the salon where Bianca works. Bianca reported having a 23-year-old son who is serving in the military and has no other blood relatives in the United States. She reports being a member of the Church of Scientology.

REFERRAL OR PRESCRIPTION

Bianca was transferred to an acute rehabilitation hospital specializing in SCIs. She will receive occupational therapy; physical therapy; social work; and registered nursing, psychology, and nutritional services. Her length of stay will be 21 days.

Occupational Therapy Initial Evaluation Findings: Rehabilitation Hospital

OCCUPATIONAL PROFILE

Bianca's preadmission occupational history and experiences included being independent in all ADLs and all IADLs. Bianca has been employed as a cosmetologist for more than 20 years and has a very large clientele in the neighborhood where she lives. Her patterns of daily living most commonly included waking up at 10:00 a.m., arriving at work by 12:00 noon, and then working to 8:00 p.m. Tuesday through Saturday. She and her boyfriend frequently dined out and enjoyed going to the movies. Her interests include fashion, Latin music, and dance. She values her clients' satisfaction with her work and reported her greatest current need is to be able to walk again.

ADLs

Regarding self-care, Bianca was dependent in all areas of self-care. Regarding functional mobility, Bianca was dependent in bed mobility and transfers. During a dependent transition from supine to short sit, she reported a brief period of lightheadedness.

IADLs

Activities needed that provide day-to-day quality of life and relative independence were explored. Bianca was dependent on her ability to handle her finances, maintain her home, prepare meals, clean up, and shop. Regarding rest and sleep, Bianca reported that since her SCI she was sleeping between 3 and 4 hours per night.

MENTAL FUNCTIONS

Cognitive assessment found Bianca to be alert and oriented to person, place, time, and situation, and short- and long-term memory were intact. She was able to follow three-step commands and make her needs known. Affect appeared appropriate, except Bianca has not accepted the prognosis for her complete SCI. No gross deficits in perception were observed.

SENSORY FUNCTIONS AND PAIN

No gross deficits were observed with visual, hearing, vestibular, taste, and smell functions. Cutaneous and proprioceptive sensations below the C5 sensory level were absent. Use of the numerical rating scale (0–10) for pain indicated a score of 0 when medication is taken and 5 in the upper cervical spine without medication. The pain was described as "cramping." The Spinal Cord Independence Measure–III (Catz, 2001) was administered and resulted in a score of 20.

CARDIOVASCULAR AND RESPIRATORY SYSTEMS FUNCTION

Bianca presented with low endurance and vital capacity.

MOVEMENT FUNCTIONS

There was active bilateral movement of shoulder flexion, abduction, and extension; scapular abduction and adduction; elbow flexion; and forearm supination. There was total paralysis of the wrists, digits, trunk, and lower extremities. Passive range of motion in all extremities was within normal limits.

NEUROMUSCULAR FUNCTIONS

Bianca is dependent in sitting and standing. The muscle tone below the site of injury was flaccid, and deep tendon reflexes were absent.

PLAN FOR DISCHARGE

Bianca will be discharged to home with home care services. She will receive occupational therapy; physical therapy; and social work, registered nursing, and home health aide services.

Questions and Activities

SAFETY OF CLIENT AND OTHERS: PRECAUTIONS AND CONTRAINDICATIONS

1. Create a handout identifying the signs and symptoms of orthostatic hypotension or postural hypotension.
2. If Bianca experiences an episode of orthostatic hypotension or postural hypotension, what steps should be taken? Support your decision.
3. What are the signs and symptoms of autonomic dysreflexia to be aware of while working with Bianca?
4. If Bianca experiences an episode of autonomic dysreflexia, what immediate actions need to be taken?
5. What are the signs and symptoms of deep vein thrombosis (DVT)?
6. If Bianca develops DVT, what immediate actions need to be taken?
7. Bianca is at risk to acquire a pressure ulcer. Why? What are the most common sites where pressure ulcers form? How can occupational therapy play a role in the prevention of pressure ulcers?
8. Which vital signs should be taken when working with Bianca? What are their norms? When should they be taken?
9. Performing the manual muscle test was contraindicated at the time of the initial evaluation. Why?
10. After her SCI, Bianca now presents with a weak cough. What risks does this cough pose?
11. Identify the common psychological reactions associated with a SCI that may affect the treatment process.
12. To maintain safety, what other factors should be considered?

OCCUPATIONS: ADLs, IADLs, EDUCATION, WORK, PLAY, SOCIAL PARTICIPATION, AND REST AND SLEEP

1. Given the information provided for this case, identify the areas of occupation that will and will not be addressed. Justify your decisions.

2. Bianca's priority is to be able to make and receive calls and texts from her cell phone. What strategies can be used to accomplish this?
3. Bianca is at high risk for developing bed sores. Explain why.
4. What can be implemented to quickly allow Bianca to gain greater independence in self-feeding?
5. It was determined that a universal cuff would allow Bianca to use a spoon and fork. Identify three different cuffs. Evaluate them and select one. Justify your selection.
6. How can Bianca participate in self-grooming?

PERFORMANCE SKILLS: MOTOR SKILLS, PROCESS SKILLS, AND SOCIAL INTERACTION SKILLS

1. Given the information provided, identify the motor, process, and social interaction skills that affect Bianca's occupational performance.
2. Which of these skills would be appropriate to address within this service delivery site? Justify your selection.
3. Which of these skills would be addressed through remediation, compensation, and education?
4. Which of these skills would be addressed through the following intervention approaches: create/promote, establish/restore, maintain, modify, and prevent?

PERFORMANCE PATTERNS: HABITS, ROUTINES, ROLES, AND RITUALS

1. Identify Bianca's useful habits, routines, roles, and rituals that support valued occupations. How can you make use of this information?
2. Identify Bianca's impoverished habits, routines, roles, and rituals that do not support valued occupations. How can you make use of this information?
3. Identify Bianca's dominating habits, routines, roles, and rituals that interfere with valued occupations. How can you make use of this information?

CLIENT FACTORS

Values, beliefs, and spirituality
How can the identified values, beliefs, and spirituality be used in this case?

Body structures
Considering the primary and secondary diagnoses, identify the related body structures.

Body functions
1. Identify how the primary and secondary diagnoses have affected the function of the identified body structures.
2. Explain the relationships between the structural and functional factors and Bianca's current level of occupational performance.

MENTAL FUNCTIONS: AFFECTIVE, COGNITIVE, AND PERCEPTUAL

1. What common affective issues related to her SCI might Bianca have to face?
2. How would these issues be addressed in occupational therapy?

3. To address these issues, what other disciplines could you refer Bianca to?
4. What would be the expected stages of acceptance that Bianca would transition through? Describe the dominant characteristic of each.
5. How can each stage best be addressed?
6. Define *learned dependence,* and identify how it can be prevented.
7. Given the information provided, what additional mental function considerations need to be addressed?

NEUROMUSCULOSKELETAL AND MOVEMENT-RELATED FUNCTIONS

1. Given the information provided, identify neuromusculoskeletal and movement-related functions that need to be addressed. Justify your selections.
2. Identify the shoulder, scapula, elbow, and forearm movement that would be expected.
3. Identify the expected innervated muscles.
4. Create an exercise program for Bianca based on occupational performance.

CARDIOVASCULAR, HEMATOLOGICAL, IMMUNOLOGICAL, AND RESPIRATORY FUNCTIONS

1. Given the information provided, identify cardiovascular, hematological, immunological, and respiratory functions that need to bc addressed. Justify your selections.
2. Describe the impact of a C5 SCI on the respiratory system. Identify two scholarly sources.
3. How would the impact of her SCI on the respiratory system manifest while Bianca is engaged in her daily activities?

SKIN AND RELATED STRUCTURE FUNCTIONS

1. Which autonomic functions would be affected by Bianca's C5 SCI?
2. How would the changes in these functions affect the occupational therapy process?
3. What other skin and related structure functions should be considered?

VOICE AND SPEECH FUNCTIONS

Describe how Bianca's diagnosis may affect her voice, speech, and associated occupational performance.

ASSISTIVE TECHNOLOGIES AND DEVICES

1. What assistive technologies or adaptations might be used or made for Bianca while she is receiving occupational therapy services in the rehabilitation hospital? Why?
2. What assistive technologies or adaptations might be recommended for when she returns home? Why?

ETHICAL DECISION MAKING

1. Bianca's boyfriend confides in you that he will be breaking up with Bianca. How can this situation be best addressed?
2. Bianca's boyfriend confides in you that he will not be able to accept Bianca back into his apartment. How can this situation be best addressed?

PHARMACOLOGY

Bianca is currently receiving morphine.

1. What is the brand name?
2. Does this drug have a high alert status?
3. What is the classification of this drug?
4. What is the indication for this drug?
5. What is the action of this drug?
6. How may this drug affect client participation during a therapy session?

SOCIOCULTURAL, SOCIOECONOMIC, AND DIVERSITY FACTORS AND LIFESTYLE CHOICES

1. Given Bianca's profile, how may your own culture and beliefs affect your interaction with her?
2. Based on this self-examination, what area of cultural knowledge do you need to pursue?
3. How can this newly acquired cultural knowledge be integrated for effective outcomes?
4. How can you foster cultural interaction and awareness among your coworkers?
5. Discuss how a lack of understanding in the areas of discrimination and stigma, implicit bias, social identity, or racism may contribute to disparities in the delivery of occupational therapy services in this case.

ASSESSMENT TOOLS AND INTERPRETATION OF RESULTS

1. What is the purpose of the Spinal Cord Independence Measure III?
2. Which population is this test designed for?
3. How much time is required to administer it?
4. Provide a brief description of this assessment
5. What is the reliability of the Spinal Cord Independence Measure III?
6. What is the validity of the Spinal Cord Independence Measure III?
7. What functional inference can be deduced from Bianca's total score of 20?
8. What additional standardized assessment can be used in this case? Why?

INTERPROFESSIONAL RELATIONSHIP AND EFFECTIVE INTRAPROFESSIONAL COLLABORATION

1. Identify the other professions that would make up the care team. Explain the focus of each.
2. Identify the roles of the occupational therapy assistant (OTA) that could be used in the occupational therapy process for this case.
3. Identify interventions that can be assigned to the OTA for this case. Justify your selections.

BILLING AND CODING

1. Identify the *International Classification of Diseases (ICD)* code for Bianca's diagnosis.
2. For this case, identify at least two *Current Procedural Terminology (CPT®)* codes that are most appropriate. Justify your selection.

REIMBURSEMENT SYSTEMS AND DOCUMENTATION

1. Who would be the authorized individuals that you could share the occupational therapy findings with? Explain why.
2. For this case, what forms and frequency of documentation will be required?
3. Which reimbursement system or systems most commonly cover occupational therapy services in this practice setting?

ADVOCACY

1. Which of the following areas of advocacy would be beneficial in this case: patient rights, matters of privacy, confidentiality, informed consent, awareness building, accessing education, and/or benefits/resources?
2. Create a plan to advocate for this client based on the selected areas of advocacy.

TELEHEALTH

1. How can telehealth be integrated as a component of the occupational therapy process in this case?
2. Before launching telemedicine services, what questions would be essential to ask Bianca to determine whether it is appropriate for her to engage in telemedicine services?
3. What are the barriers, obstacles, or challenges you foresee if attempting to integrate telehealth services with this client?

Intervention Plan Formulation and Implementation

INTERVENTION PLAN FORMULATION

Create an intervention plan that includes the following:

1. List this individual's **strengths.**
2. List this individual's **barriers** in occupational performance, performance skills, and performance patterns.
3. Based on the individual's goals, health, performance, and service delivery site, **identify the barriers that will be addressed.**
4. From the barriers identified to be addressed, **formulate goals and objectives.**
5. Identify the focus of each goal and objective as either **create, promote, establish, restore, maintain, modify, or prevent.**
6. Identify the **theoretical basis, model(s) of practice, or frame(s) of reference** that will be used to address each goal and objective.
7. For each proposed goal and objective, describe clearly and precisely the **methods** that will be used. This description should include, but not be limited to, safety considerations, environmental considerations, therapeutic use of self, preparatory activities, activity selection, materials, equipment, and flow.
8. Classify the activities selected in the methods description as either **preparatory, enabling, purposeful, or occupation based.**
9. Explain how each activity can be **graded up or down,** creating the just-right challenge.
10. Provide at least two **primary sources of evidence** to support the intervention plan.

INTERVENTION PLAN IMPLEMENTATION

1. Based on your intervention plan, identify which goals and objectives require **more immediate attention.**
2. Describe your proposed **first treatment session.**
3. As the treatment session is progressing, what is **essential to be observed?**

Transition and Discontinuation

Create a plan for discharge from occupational therapy services in collaboration with Bianca and members of the interprofessional team. Review the needs of Bianca, caregivers, family members, and significant others. The plan must match needs with available resources and the discharge environment.

REFERENCES

American Medical Association. (2019). *CPT® 2020 professional edition.*

Catz, A. (2001). The Catz-Itzkovich SCIM: A revised version of the Spinal Cord Independence Measure. *Disability and Rehabilitation, 23*(6), 263–268. https://doi.org/10.1080/096382801750110919

World Health Organization. (2019). *International statistical classification of diseases and related health problems* (11th ed.). https://icd.who.int/

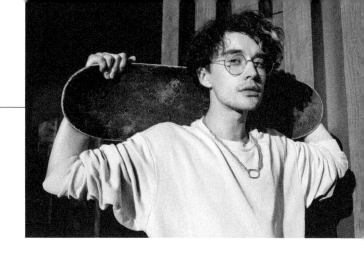

Derrick: Traumatic Brain Injury

DONALD AURIEMMA, MS ED, OTR/L

Derrick (he, him, his, himself)

MEDICAL HISTORY

Derrick is a 19-year-old Polish American male who is 6' 3" and weighs 185 pounds. He was brought to the emergency department of his regional medical center by emergency medical services after a skateboarding accident. Reports from the scene indicated that he had been drinking beer and not wearing a helmet at the time of the accident. Upon arrival, he was disoriented, complained of a headache and nausea, and was vomiting. Observable abrasions and contusions were present on his right forehead. After a physical examination, he was sent for imaging. Magnetic resonance imaging indicated a traumatic brain injury (TBI) with the presence of a large right-side hematoma that was compressing the brain. Derrick was taken immediately to the operating room for evacuation of the hematoma. Derrick's medical records indicated no significant medical history, no known allergies, and a history of alcohol and marijuana use. After surgery, he was taken to the neurological intensive care unit (NICU) for 3 days and then moved to the neurology unit for 4 days. He was then transferred to the inpatient rehabilitation unit.

SOCIAL HISTORY

Derrick is a first-year college student attending a community college; his intended major is cyber security. Derrick resides with his mother and three siblings in a three-bedroom ranch-style home. Derrick's recreational interests include skateboarding in the warmer months and snowboarding in the winter with his friends. His mother refers to him as a "daredevil." Derrick's girlfriend also enjoys skateboarding and was present at the time of the accident. They share agnostic beliefs. Derrick identifies as a pansexual.

REFERRAL OR PRESCRIPTION

After Derrick was transferred to the rehabilitation unit, he was referred for occupational therapy, physical therapy, social work, psychology, and nursing services. The length of stay will be 3 weeks.

Occupational Therapy Initial Evaluation Findings: Rehabilitation Unit

OCCUPATIONAL PROFILE

Derrick's preadmission occupational history and experiences included being independent in all ADLs and all IADLs. Derrick was in his first year at the local community college. He was employed as a part-time independent contractor in food service delivery. His patterns of daily living most commonly included waking up at 8:00 a.m. and attending classes 4 days a week. After school, he commonly worked for 2–3 hours, returned home, and then completed his school work. On weekends, he worked and spent time with his friends and girlfriend. His interests include making and posting skateboarding videos. He values living on the edge and not putting off happiness. He reported his greatest need was to return to college.

ADLs

Regarding self-care, Derrick presented as highly distractible and needed to be frequently redirected to dress, bathe, groom, and toilet. Weeping, he frequently yelled out, "Why the f*** is this so hard?" Regarding functional mobility, Derrick was able to roll, transition between supine and sit, and bridge independently. He used a straight cane and required contact guard assist and verbal cues to transfer on and off the bed, chair, and toilet equipped with a versa frame.

IADLs

Activities needed that provide day-to-day quality of life and relative independence were explored. Derrick made several unsuccessful attempts to log on to his computer, write, make a voice call, and send a text. Regarding rest and sleep, Derrick reported not being able to sleep in a "flat position" because doing so triggered severe headaches. Each night, he slept intermittently for no more than 2 hours at a time.

MENTAL FUNCTIONS

Cognitive assessment indicated that Derrick was alert and oriented to person, place, and situation, but not time. He was unable to report the correct month. While he was in the NICU, he presented with no memory of the day of his accident and the 3 days that preceded it. His long-term memory appeared grossly intact. Derrick was highly distractible and was unable to filter out common environmental stimuli during all ADLs and IADLs. Assessment of affect revealed he often cried and reported feeling anxious about missing classes. During testing, he scored a Level VII on the Ranchos Los Amigos Scale (Hagen et al., 1972). No gross perceptual deficits were noted at the time of evaluation.

SENSORY FUNCTION AND PAIN

No gross deficits were observed with hearing, taste, cutaneous, and smell functions. Blurred vision in both eyes was reported, and quick head movements resulted in reports of vertigo. Use of the numerical rating scale (0–10) indicated a score of 7 for pain in the head and cervical spine. The pain was described as "splitting."

CARDIOVASCULAR AND RESPIRATORY SYSTEM FUNCTIONS

During self-care activities, Derrick needed to stop secondary to reports of fatigue.

MOVEMENT FUNCTIONS

Passive range of motion and active range of motion in all four extremities were within defined limits (WDL). Muscle strength in both the right upper extremity (RUE) and the right lower extremity (RLE) was 5/5 using the manual muscle test. Both the left upper extremity (LUE) and the left lower extremity (LLE) was 3+/5. Coordination in the RUE appeared to be WDL, and the LUE appeared to have a mild reduction in speed and accuracy of movement. Gross grasp strength in the right hand was 79 pounds and in the left 16 pounds. Derrick presented with difficulty manipulating objects between the palm of the left hand to the tip of his left fingers.

NEUROMUSCULAR FUNCTIONS

Using clinical observation, Derrick's static and dynamic sitting balance were good, and his static and dynamic standing balance were fair. Muscle tone in the RUE and RLE was normal, and the LUE and LLE were mildly hypertonic. No primitive reflex activity was observed.

PLAN FOR DISCHARGE

Derrick will be discharged to an outpatient rehabilitation service. He will be receiving occupational and physical therapy services.

Questions and Activities

SAFETY OF CLIENT AND OTHERS: PRECAUTIONS AND CONTRAINDICATIONS

1. Identify the postsurgical precautions and contraindications that need to be followed. Justify your choices.
2. Given Derrick's impulsivity, what precautions should be followed?
3. Given Derrick's anxiety, what precautions should be followed?
4. Derrick has impaired standing balance. How will you keep him safe during upright activities?
5. Create a handout that identifies the precautions to be followed for individuals with impaired balance.
6. Identify the common psychological reactions associated with a TBI that may affect the treatment process.
7. To maintain safety, what other factors should be considered?

OCCUPATIONS: ADL, IADLs, EDUCATION, WORK, PLAY, SOCIAL PARTICIPATION, AND REST AND SLEEP

1. Given the information provided for this case, identify the areas of occupation that will and will not be addressed. Justify your decisions.
2. What strategies should be considered to allow Derrick to perform his self-care more independently?
3. What strategies should be considered to allow Derrick to use his phone and computer with less frustration?
4. What recommendations could be made to allow Derrick to experience more restful sleep?
5. What strategies should be considered to allow Derrick to transfer safely with a cane?

PERFORMANCE SKILLS: MOTOR SKILLS, PROCESS SKILLS, AND SOCIAL INTERACTION SKILLS

1. Given the information provided, identify the motor, process, and social interaction skills that affect Derrick's occupational performance.
2. Which of these skills would be appropriate to address in this service delivery site? Justify your selection.
3. Which of these skills would be addressed through remediation, compensation, and education?
4. Which of these skills would be addressed through the following intervention approaches: create/promote, establish/restore, maintain, modify, and prevent?

PERFORMANCE PATTERNS: HABITS, ROUTINES, ROLES, AND RITUALS

1. Identify Derrick's useful habits, routines, roles, and rituals that support valued occupations. How can you make use of this information?
2. Identify Derrick's impoverished habits, routines, roles, and rituals that do not support valued occupations. How can you make use of this information?
3. Identify Derrick's dominating habits, routines, roles, and rituals that interfere with valued occupations. How can you make use of this information?

CLIENT FACTORS

Values, beliefs, and spirituality
How can the identified values, beliefs, and spirituality be used in this case?

Body structures
Considering the primary and secondary diagnoses, identify the related body structures.

Body functions
1. Identify how the primary and secondary diagnoses have affected the function of the identified body structures.
2. Explain the relationships between the structural and functional factors and Derrick's current level of occupational performance.

MENTAL FUNCTIONS: AFFECTIVE, COGNITIVE, AND PERCEPTUAL

1. What common affective issues related to his TBI might Derrick have to face?
2. How would these issues be addressed in occupational therapy?

3. To address these issues, what other disciplines could you refer Derrick to?
4. What models are available to address Derrick's cognitive challenges?
5. Which models would you choose and why?
6. What activities could Derrick engage in using your selected models?
7. What models are available to address Derrick's affective challenges?
8. Which models would you choose and why?
9. What activities could Derrick engage in using your selected models?
10. Given the information provided, what additional mental function considerations need to be addressed?

NEUROMUSCULOSKELETAL AND MOVEMENT RELATED FUNCTIONS

1. Given the information provided, identify neuromusculoskeletal and movement-related functions that need to be addressed. Justify your selections.
2. What models are available to address Derrick's balance challenges?
3. Evaluate these models, select one, and justify your selection.
4. What activities could Derrick be engaged in using the selected model?
5. What models are available to address Derrick's strength challenges?
6. Evaluate these models, select one, and justify your selection.
7. What activities could Derrick be engaged in using this model?
8. Create an exercise program for Derrick based on occupational performance.

CARDIOVASCULAR, HEMATOLOGICAL, IMMUNOLOGICAL, AND RESPIRATORY FUNCTIONS

1. Given the information provided, identify cardiovascular, hematological, immunological, and respiratory functions that need to be addressed. Justify your selections.
2. Infer the reason for Derrick reporting fatigue during self-care activities.
3. What are the observable signs and reported symptoms consistent with generalized anxiety disorder in Derrick? Identify two scholarly sources.

SKIN AND RELATED STRUCTURE FUNCTIONS

1. What is an abrasion?
2. What is the common medical treatment for an abrasion?
3. What is a contusion?
4. What is the common medical treatment for a contusion?
5. What other skin and related structure functions should be considered?

VOICE AND SPEECH FUNCTIONS

Describe how Derrick's diagnosis may affect his voice, speech, and associated occupational performance.

ASSISTIVE TECHNOLOGIES AND DEVICES

1. What assistive technologies or adaptations might be used or made for Derrick while he is receiving occupational therapy services in the rehabilitation unit? Why?
2. What assistive technologies or adaptations might be recommended for when he returns home? Why?

ETHICAL DECISION MAKING

1. You reviewed the referral for services, and it was signed by a physician's assistant (PA) from the neurology unit. What is a PA, and can the referral be accepted?
2. During treatment, Derrick, in the presence of his mother, says to the therapist, "You look fat and really should go on a diet!" His mother quickly informs you that before his accident Derrick has never been rude. What might be the reason for Derrick's comment? How should it be addressed?
3. During a treatment session, Derrick's girlfriend emits a strong odor of alcohol. How should this situation be addressed?
4. During multiple treatment sessions, Derrick states that he needs to return to college so he does not fail the semester. How should this situation be addressed?

PHARMACOLOGY

Derrick is currently taking warfarin.

1. What is the brand name?
2. Does this drug have a high alert status?
3. What is the classification of this drug?
4. What is the indication for this drug?
5. What is the action of this drug?
6. How may this drug affect client participation during a therapy session?

SOCIOCULTURAL, SOCIOECONOMIC, AND DIVERSITY FACTORS AND LIFESTYLE CHOICES

1. Given Derrick's occupational profile, how may your own culture and beliefs affect your interaction with him?
2. Based on this self-examination, what areas of cultural knowledge do you need to pursue?
3. How can this newly acquired cultural knowledge be integrated for effective outcomes?
4. How can you foster cultural interaction and awareness among your coworkers?
5. Discuss how a lack of understanding in the areas of discrimination and stigma, implicit bias, social identity, or racism may contribute to disparities in the delivery of occupational therapy services in this case.

ASSESSMENT TOOLS AND INTERPRETATION OF RESULTS

1. What is the purpose of the Ranchos Los Amigos Scale?
2. Which population is this test designed for?
3. How much time is required to administer it?
4. Provide a brief description of this assessment.
5. What is the reliability of this scale?
6. What is the validity of this scale?
7. What functional inference can be deduced from Derrick's score of Level VII?
8. What additional standardized assessment can be used in this case? Why?

BILLING AND CODING

1. Identify the *International Classification of Diseases (ICD)* codes for Derrick's diagnoses.
2. For this case, identify at least two *Current Procedural Terminology (CPT®)* codes that are most appropriate. Justify your selection.

REIMBURSEMENT SYSTEMS AND DOCUMENTATION

1. Who would be the authorized individuals that you could share the occupational therapy findings with? Explain why.
2. For this case, what forms and frequency of documentation will be required?
3. Which reimbursement system or systems most commonly cover occupational therapy services in this practice setting?

TELEHEALTH

1. How can telehealth be integrated as a component of the occupational therapy process in this case?
2. Before launching telemedicine services, what questions would be essential to ask Derrick to determine whether it is appropriate for him to engage in telemedicine services?
3. What are the barriers, obstacles, or challenges you foresee if attempting to integrate telehealth services with this client?

INTERPROFESSIONAL RELATIONSHIP AND EFFECTIVE INTRAPROFESSIONAL COLLABORATION

1. Identify the other professions that would make up the care team. Explain the focus of each.
2. Identify the roles of the occupational therapy assistant (OTA) that could be used in the occupational therapy process for this case.
3. Identify interventions that can be assigned to the OTA for this case. Justify your selections.

ADVOCACY

1. Which of the following areas of advocacy would be beneficial in this case: patient rights, matters of privacy, confidentiality, informed consent, awareness building, accessing education, and benefits/resources?
2. Create a plan to advocate for this client based on the selected areas of advocacy.

Intervention Plan Formulation and Implementation

INTERVENTION PLAN FORMULATION

Create an intervention plan that includes the following:

1. List this individual's **strengths.**
2. List this individual's **barriers** in occupational performance, performance skills, and performance patterns.

3. Based on the individual's goals, health, performance, and service delivery site, **identify the barriers that will be addressed.**
4. From the barriers identified to be addressed, **formulate goals and objectives.**
5. Identify the focus of each goal and objective as either **create, promote, establish, restore, maintain, modify, or prevent.**
6. Identify the **theoretical basis, model(s) of practice, or frame(s) of reference** that will be used to address each goal and objective.
7. For each proposed goal and objective, describe clearly and precisely the **methods** that will be used. This description should include, but not be limited to, safety considerations, environmental considerations, therapeutic use of self, preparatory activities, activity selection, materials, equipment, and flow.
8. Classify the activities selected in the methods description as either **preparatory, enabling, purposeful, or occupation based.**
9. Explain how each activity can be **graded up or down,** creating the just-right challenge.
10. Provide at least two **primary sources of evidence** to support the intervention plan.

INTERVENTION PLAN IMPLEMENTATION

1. Based on your intervention plan, identify which goals and objectives require **more immediate attention.**
2. Describe your proposed **first treatment session.**
3. As the treatment session is progressing, what is **essential to be observed?**

Transition and Discontinuation

Create a plan for discharge from occupational therapy services in collaboration with Derrick and members of the interprofessional team. Review the needs of Derrick, caregivers, family members, and significant others. The plan must match needs with available resources and the discharge environment.

REFERENCES

American Medical Association. (2019). *CPT® 2020 professional edition.*

Hagen, C., Malkmus, D., & Durham, P. (1972). *Rancho Los Amigos Levels of Cognitive Functioning Scale.* Communication Disorders Service, Rancho Los Amigos Hospital.

World Health Organization. (2019). *International statistical classification of diseases and related health problems* (11th ed.). https://icd.who.int/

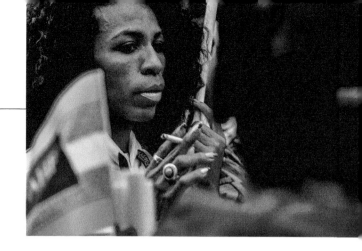

Sharon: Peripheral Vascular Disease

DONALD AURIEMMA, MS ED, OTR/L

Sharon (she, her, hers, herself)

MEDICAL HISTORY

Sharon is a 59-year-old transgender Jamaican female living in the United States. Sharon is 6' 1" and weighs 160 pounds. She was electively admitted to the hospital with gangrene on her right foot. Magnetic resonance imaging scans, X-rays, and computerized tomography scans were used to confirm the presence and spread of gangrene. Sharon underwent a right below-knee amputation (RBKA). Her medical history included peripheral vascular disease (PVD), hypertension, diabetes mellitus, and gender reassignment surgery. Upon admission, she reported smoking one to two packs of cigarettes per day and consuming 4 to 5 cups of coffee per day. She reported being sober for 10 years but reports a history of both cocaine and alcohol abuse. She is allergic to ampicillin.

SOCIAL HISTORY

Sharon is the owner of a popular florist shop with three full-time employees. She currently lives alone and reported recently breaking up with her boyfriend. She lives in a luxury three-bedroom, two-bath high rise just two blocks from her shop. Her building is new construction and is compliant with the Americans with Disabilities Act of 1990 (P. L. 101-336) regulations. She is an active member of the LBGTQIA+ community and has a broad network of friends. Her only living relatives are her mother and sister, who reside in a different state. Sharon identifies as a member of the United Church of Christ.

REFERRAL OR PRESCRIPTION

Sharon was transferred to the local rehabilitation hospital. She has been referred for occupational therapy, physical therapy, social work, psychology, and nursing services. The length of stay will be 6 days.

Occupational Therapy Initial Evaluation Findings: Rehabilitation Hospital

OCCUPATIONAL PROFILE

Sharon's preadmission occupational history and experiences included being independent in all ADLs and all IADLs. Her patterns of daily living most commonly included picking up flowers at the wholesaler between 8:00 a.m. and 9:00 a.m., picking up breakfast, and opening her shop by 10:00 a.m. Her shop hours are from 10:00 a.m. to 7:00 p.m., Tuesday through Saturday. Her interests include listening to jazz music in the evening, dining out with friends on weekends, traveling, and engaging in the arts. Sharon values her independence and the business she has created. Her reported greatest needs are to be able to return home, live independently, and get back to her florist shop as soon as possible.

ADLs

Regarding self-care, Sharon was able to feed herself independently, manage her clothes, clean herself on the toilet, dress while seated on the side of the bed when clothing was placed within her reach, and sponge bathe in bed when bathing items were made available. Tub bathing was not attempted.

Regarding functional mobility, Sharon was able to perform stand pivot transfers with contact guard assist between the bed and wheelchair, wheelchair and toilet, and wheelchair and armchair. Tub transfers were not attempted. She was able to independently propel, position, and manage components of her wheelchair. Transfers using a rolling walker were not attempted. The Amputee Mobility Predictor (AMP; Gailey et al., 2002) without prosthesis was administered, and Sharon scored a 31 (Functional Level K3).

IADLs

Activities needed that provide day-to-day quality of life and relative independence were explored. Sharon was able to manage her communications and handle finances. She was aware that currently she would not be able to maintain her home, prepare meals, or shop. Regarding rest and sleep, Sharon reported not being able to obtain restful sleep due to pain in her right residual limb.

MENTAL FUNCTIONS

Cognitive assessment found Sharon to be alert and oriented to person, place, time, and situation, and short- and long-term memory were intact. She was able to follow three-step commands and make her needs known. Assessment of affect was performed. Sharon reported feeling depressed over the loss of her leg and presented noticeably teary eyed. She does not think that she will be able to walk with a prosthesis. No gross deficits in perceptual function were observed.

SENSORY FUNCTIONS AND PAIN

No gross deficits were observed with visual, hearing, vestibular, taste, smell, and proprioceptive functions. The terminal end of her right residual limb presented with impaired touch localization and touch awareness. She reports pain at the terminal end of the residual limb. The pain was reported as a 5 using the Numerical Rating Scale (0–10). The pain was described as "tender."

CARDIOVASCULAR AND RESPIRATORY SYSTEMS FUNCTIONS

Sharon was able to perform all self-care and transfers without signs of fatigue.

MOVEMENT FUNCTIONS

Passive range of motion and active range of motion of both upper extremities (BUE) and the left lower extremity were within functional limits. Muscle strength in BUE was 4/5 using the manual muscle test (MMT). The RBKA, presented with a closed surgical wound, and has had surgical staples removed and adhesive surgical tape strips applied. The end of the residual limb was edematous, with the circumferential measurement of the right mid–calf at 17.6 inches and the left at 15.1 inches. Gross grasp strength in the right hand was 38 pounds and in the left hand was 36 pounds. No gross deficits in prehension were observed.

NEUROMUSCULAR FUNCTIONS

Static and dynamic sitting balance were normal and good, respectively. Static and dynamic standing balances were fair + and fair, respectively. Muscle tone was normal, and no deficit in reflex integration was observed.

PLAN FOR DISCHARGE

Sharon will be discharged home after completion of her 6-day stay and receive home care services. She will receive occupational therapy, physical therapy, social work, registered nursing, and home health aide services.

Questions and Activities

SAFETY OF CLIENT AND OTHERS: PRECAUTIONS AND CONTRAINDICATIONS

1. Given that Sharon has PVD, what precautions and contraindications should be considered?
2. For this case, what postsurgical precautions need to be followed?
3. Create a handout identifying precautions to be followed for individuals with impaired cutaneous sensation.
4. Identify the risks that Sharon faces when showering and bathing. How can these risks be mitigated?
5. Compare and contrast appropriate sadness over losing a limb and clinical depression.
6. Identify the common psychological reaction associated with an amputation that may affect the treatment process.
7. To maintain safety, what other factors should be considered?

OCCUPATIONS: ADLs, IADLs, EDUCATION, WORK, PLAY, SOCIAL PARTICIPATION, AND REST AND SLEEP

1. Given the information provided for this case, identify the areas of occupation that will and will not be addressed. Justify your decisions
2. What would be the recommended position(s) for Sharon during sleep?
3. What would be the recommended position of Sharon's right residual limb while she is seated in a wheelchair?
4. During patient education, what topics should be included to maximize Sharon's function and maintain her health and wellness?
5. Identify at least two strategies that can facilitate Sharon's ability to independently bathe and shower.
6. Which IADL tasks are essential to be addressed before Sharon returns home?

PERFORMANCE SKILLS: MOTOR SKILLS, PROCESS SKILLS, AND SOCIAL INTERACTION SKILLS

1. Given the information provided, identify the motor, process, and social interaction skills that affect Sharon's occupational performance.
2. Which of these skills would be appropriate to address in this service delivery site? Justify your selection.
3. Which of these skills would be addressed through remediation, compensation, and education?
4. Which of these skills would be addressed through the following intervention approaches: create/promote, establish/restore, maintain, modify, and prevent?

PERFORMANCE PATTERNS: HABITS, ROUTINES, ROLES, AND RITUALS

1. Identify Sharon's useful habits, routines, roles, and rituals that support valued occupations. How can you make use of this information?
2. Identify Sharon's impoverished habits, routines, roles, and rituals that do not support valued occupations. How can you make use of this information?
3. Identify Sharon's dominating habits, routines, roles, and rituals that interfere with valued occupations. How can you make use of this information?

CLIENT FACTORS

Values, beliefs, and spirituality
How can the identified values, beliefs, and spirituality be used in this case?

Body structures
Considering Sharon's primary and secondary diagnoses, identify the related body structures.

Body functions
1. Identify how the primary and secondary diagnoses have affected the function of the identified body structures.
2. Explain the relationships between the structural and functional factors and Sharon's current level of occupational performance.

MENTAL FUNCTIONS: AFFECTIVE, COGNITIVE, AND PERCEPTUAL

1. What common affective issues related to her amputation might Sharon have to face?
2. How would these issues be addressed in occupational therapy?
3. To address these issues, what other disciplines could you refer Sharon to?
4. Identify the stages of grief.
5. Which stage do you believe Sharon is experiencing? Support your selection.
6. How can you support Sharon through the grieving process?
7. How could the amputation affect Sharon's body image?
8. Given the information provided, what additional mental function considerations need to be addressed?

NEUROMUSCULOSKELETAL AND MOVEMENT-RELATED FUNCTIONS

1. Given the information provided, identify neuromusculoskeletal and movement-related functions that need to be addressed. Justify your selections.
2. What common techniques can be used to reduce edema in Sharon's residual limb?
3. Explain what a score of 4/5 on the MMT represents.
4. Does the muscle strength in Sharon's upper extremities need to be remediated? Justify your decision.
5. Compare and contrast phantom limb pain with residual limb pain.
6. Provide three options in addressing Sharon's residual limb pain. Explain the process you would use to select one.
7. Create an exercise program for Sharon based on occupational performance.

CARDIOVASCULAR, HEMATOLOGICAL, IMMUNOLOGICAL, AND RESPIRATORY FUNCTIONS

1. Given the information provided, identify cardiovascular, hematological, immunological, and respiratory functions that need to be addressed. Justify your selections.
2. Compare the metabolic equivalent of task (MET) value for ambulating with both lower extremities and the MET value for hopping with a single lower extremity while using a rolling walker.
3. Calculate the estimated maximal heart rate for Sharon's age. Explain how you made this determination.

SKIN AND RELATED STRUCTURE FUNCTIONS

1. What are the skin changes related to PVD?
2. Compare and contrast PVD with coronary artery disease.
3. What factors would be considered when addressing skin integrity for Sharon's residual limb?
4. What other skin and related structure functions should be considered?

VOICE AND SPEECH FUNCTIONS

Describe how Sharon's diagnosis may affect her voice, speech, and associated occupational performance.

ASSISTIVE TECHNOLOGIES AND DEVICES

1. What assistive technologies or devices might be used, adapted, or fabricated for Sharon while she is receiving occupational therapy services in the acute rehabilitation unit? Why?

2. What assistive technologies or devices might be recommended for when she returns home? Why?

ETHICAL DECISION MAKING

1. You walk past two coworkers having a private conversation. You overhear them say that according to their religion, transgender individuals are "sinners." How should this situation be best addressed?
2. You walk past Sharon's room and see her take medication out of her mouth and throw it in the garbage. How should this situation be best addressed?

PHARMACOLOGY

Sharon is currently taking cilostazol.

1. What is the brand name?
2. Does this drug have a high alert status?
3. What is the classification of this drug?
4. What is the indication for this drug?
5. What is the action of this drug?
6. How may this drug affect client participation during a therapy session?

SOCIOCULTURAL, SOCIOECONOMIC, AND DIVERSITY FACTORS AND LIFESTYLE CHOICES

1. Given Sharon's profile, how may your own culture and beliefs affect your interaction with her?
2. Based on this self-examination, what area of cultural knowledge do you need to pursue?
3. How can this newly acquired cultural knowledge be integrated for effective outcomes?
4. How can you foster cultural interaction and awareness among your coworkers?
5. Discuss how a lack of understanding in the areas of discrimination and stigma, implicit bias, social identity, or racism may contribute to disparities in the delivery of occupational therapy services in this case.

ASSESSMENT TOOLS AND INTERPRETATION OF RESULTS

1. What is the purpose of the AMP?
2. Which population is this test designed for?
3. How much time is required to administer it?
4. Provide a brief description of this assessment.
5. What is the reliability of the AMP?
6. What is the validity of the AMP?
7. What functional inference can be deduced from Sharon's score of 31?
8. What additional standardized assessment can be used in this case? Why?

INTERPROFESSIONAL RELATIONSHIP AND EFFECTIVE INTRAPROFESSIONAL COLLABORATION

1. Identify the other professions that would make up the care team. Explain the focus of each.
2. Identify the roles of the occupational therapy assistant (OTA) that could be used in the occupational therapy process for this case.

3. Identify interventions that can be assigned to the OTA for this case. Justify your selections.

BILLING AND CODING

1. Identify the *International Classification of Diseases (ICD)* codes for Sharon's diagnoses.
2. For this case, identify at least two *Current Procedural Terminology (CPT®)* codes that are most appropriate. Justify your selection.

REIMBURSEMENT SYSTEMS AND DOCUMENTATION

1. Who would be the authorized individuals that you could share the occupational therapy findings with? Explain why.
2. For this case, what forms and frequency of documentation will be required?
3. Which reimbursement system or systems most commonly cover occupational therapy services in this practice setting?

ADVOCACY

1. Which of the following areas of advocacy would be beneficial in this case: patient rights, matters of privacy, confidentiality, informed consent, awareness building, accessing education, or benefits/resources?
2. Create a plan to advocate for this client based on the selected areas of advocacy.

TELEHEALTH

1. How can telehealth be integrated as a component of the occupational therapy process in this case?
2. Before launching telemedicine services, what questions would be essential to ask Sharon to determine whether it is appropriate for her to engage in telemedicine services?
3. What are the barriers, obstacles, or challenges you foresee if attempting to integrate telehealth services with this client?

Intervention Plan Formulation and Implementation

INTERVENTION PLAN FORMULATION

Create an intervention plan that includes the following:

1. List this individual's **strengths.**
2. List this individual's **barriers** in occupational performance, performance skills, and performance patterns.
3. Based on the individual's goals, health, performance, and service delivery site, **identify the barriers that will be addressed.**
4. From the barriers identified to be addressed, **formulate goals and objectives.**
5. Identify the focus of each goal and objective as either **create, promote, establish, restore, maintain, modify, or prevent.**

6. Identify the **theoretical basis, model(s) of practice, or frame(s) of reference** that will be used to address each goal and objective.
7. For each proposed goal and objective, describe clearly and precisely the **methods** that will be used. This description should include, but not be limited to, safety considerations, environmental considerations, therapeutic use of self, preparatory activities, activity selection, materials, equipment, and flow.
8. Classify the activities selected in the methods description as either **preparatory, enabling, purposeful, or occupation based.**
9. Explain how each activity can be **graded up or down,** creating the just-right challenge.
10. Provide at least two **primary sources of evidence** to support the intervention plan.

INTERVENTION PLAN IMPLEMENTATION

1. Based on your intervention plan, identify which goals and objectives require **more immediate attention.**
2. Describe your proposed **first treatment session.**
3. As the treatment session is progressing, what is **essential to be observed?**

Transition and Discontinuation

Create a plan for discharge from occupational therapy services in collaboration with Sharon and members of the interprofessional team. Review the needs of Sharon, caregivers, family members, and significant others. The plan must match needs with available resources and the discharge environment.

REFERENCES

American Medical Association. (2019). *CPT® 2020 professional edition.*
Americans With Disabilities Act of 1990, Pub. L. 101-336, 42 U.S.C. §§ 12101–12213 (2000).
Gailey, R. S., Roach, K. E., Applegate, E. B., Cho, B., Cunniffe, B., Licht, S., . . . Nash, M. S. (2002). The Amputee Mobility Predictor: An instrument to assess determinants of the lower-limb amputee's ability to ambulate. *Archives of Physical Medicine and Tehabilitation, 83,* 613–627. https://doi.org/10.1053/apmr.2002.32309
World Health Organization. (2019). *International statistical classification of diseases and related health problems* (11th ed.). https://icd.who.int/

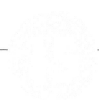

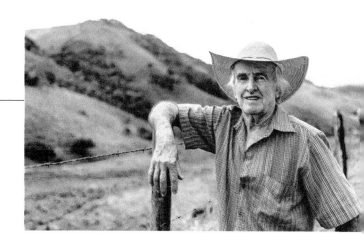

Zachary: Burn

CLOVER HUTCHINSON, OTD, MA, OTR/L

Zachary (he, him, his, himself)

MEDICAL HISTORY

Zachary is a 75-year-old Australian American male living in the United States who is 6' 0" and weighs 179 pounds. He was brought by his neighbors to the emergency department (ED) after sustaining burns while burning leaves on his property. His neighbors heard him screaming and covered him to put out the flames but did not call 911.

Physical examination findings indicated that he was alert and oriented to person, place, time, and situation but suffered full-thickness, third-degree burns to the volar aspect of his right hand, wrist, and forearm as well as the lateral aspect of his right trunk. Second-degree burns were noted to his face and left hand and forearm. Initial treatment in the ED included intravenous fluids for tissue resuscitation, tetanus prophylaxis, and wound irrigation and cooling. An electrocardiogram was normal. His vital signs were within normal range except for his blood pressure, which was 180/100 mmHg. Zachary has 27% burns to his body. This percentage of total body surface area burned was assessed using the Rule of Nines tool (Wallace, 1951). His medical history included diabetes mellitus and cataract removal in both eyes. He uses bifocals. He reports drinking 2 to 3 cups of coffee and smoking 6 to 8 cigarettes daily. He reported no drug or alcohol use and has no known allergies.

Zachary has been transferred from the ED to the burn center located 1 hour from his home. At the burn center he received a split-thickness skin graft to the volar aspect of his wrist. The donor site is his left thigh. The graft and hand were protected with a splint.

SOCIAL HISTORY

Zachary is a widower who lives with his adult children in a rural community. They reside in a large split-level cabin-style house on a vast and wooded property. There are four bedrooms, three bathrooms, and an open floor plan consisting of the kitchen, living room, and dining area. His bedroom is on the upper floor, accessible by 10 steps with a right-sided banister, and includes a full bathroom. There are 5 steps to enter the home. Zachary enjoys being surrounded by his family. Zachary identifies as an Orthodox Christian.

REFERRAL OR PRESCRIPTION

Zachary was transferred to the burn intensive care unit. He has been referred for occupational therapy, physical therapy, social work, and nursing services. The length of stay is 14 days.

Occupational Therapy Initial Evaluation: Burn Intensive Care Unit

OCCUPATIONAL PROFILE

Zachary's preadmission occupational history and experiences included being independent in all ADLs and all IADLs. He is the owner of a small propane gas company, where the day-to-day operations are handled by his children. His patterns of daily living most commonly included weekly visits to his business for updates, maintaining his yard and his small vegetable garden, preparing dinner 1 or 2 times per week, and attending church on Sundays. Zachary was able to drive to the grocery store and church. His interests include planting a variety of vegetables and sharing them with his church family. He values his independence and reports his greatest current needs are to return home and restore his prior functions, especially attending church.

ADLs

Regarding self-care, Zachary required moderate to maximum assistance to don and doff his upper body and lower body garments. He had difficulty manipulating all fasteners. He required minimal assistance with oral and facial care. After setup, he was able to feed himself with modified independence using his left nondominant hand. Toilet transfers were independent but performed with guarded movements. Toileting required minimal assistance with perineal care.

Regarding functional mobility, Zachary was able to perform bed mobility with minimal assistance, primarily requiring assistance to roll from right to left, transition to the edge of the bed, and reposition himself at the top of the bed. He ambulated independently but slowly. Zachary complains of difficulty sleeping because of pain.

IADLs

Activities needed that provide day-to-day quality of life and relative independence were explored. Zachary was not able to safely hold utensils to prepare meals or tools to perform yard work. Driving independently was unsafe at this time. Regarding rest and sleep, Zachary reported being a loud snorer and needing 10–15 minutes to gain focus after awakening in the morning.

MENTAL FUNCTIONS

Cognitive assessment found Zachary to be alert and oriented to person, place, time, and situation, and short- and long-term memory were intact. He is able to follow three-step commands and make his needs known. Affect appeared appropriate, but he expressed concerns about not being able to care for himself and is afraid of being alone at home when his children are at work. No gross deficits in perception were observed.

SENSORY FUNCTIONS

No gross deficits were observed with visual, hearing, vestibular, taste, smell, and proprioceptive functions. He reported constant pain in his right hand, forearm, and trunk, with a score of 8 on the numeric rating scale (NRS; 0–10), and in his left hand and forearm, with a score of 5–6 on the NRS. The Semmes-Weinstein Monofilament Test (Bell-Krotoski & Tomancik, 1987) revealed loss of protective sensation to the volar aspect of his right hand and diminished protective sensation to his left hand. The pain was described as "punishing."

CARDIOVASCULAR AND RESPIRATORY SYSTEMS FUNCTIONS

Assessment of sensory functions indicated no deficits in cardiovascular or respiratory functions. Zachary's blood pressure has been stabilized.

MOVEMENT FUNCTIONS

Active range of motion (AROM) and passive range of motion (PROM) were within functional limits in the left upper extremity. Muscle strength (assessed using the manual muscle test) was scored as a 4/5 for the left upper extremity. AROM and PROM to the right shoulder were limited as follows: shoulder flexion, 0–100°; shoulder abduction, 0–110°; shoulder external rotation, 0–75°; shoulder internal rotation, 0–70°; horizontal shoulder abduction, 0–95°; horizontal shoulder adduction, 0–120°; elbow flexion/extension, 30–125°; forearm supination, 0–75°; and forearm pronation, 0–85°. Wrist and digits were unable to be evaluated. Left lateral flexion of the torso was 0–15°, with left rotation of the torso at 0–20°. Edema was noted to the dorsum of the right hand, with a grade of 2 on the Pitting Edema Rating Scale (Brodovicz et al., 2009). Additionally, circumferential measurements were taken using the Figure-of Eight Method (Dewey et al., 2007): right hand, 30 cm, and left hand, 23 cm.

NEUROMUSCULAR FUNCTIONS

Zachary's static sitting balance was good (G), and dynamic sitting balance was G–. His static standing balance was G–, and dynamic standing balance was fair+. Muscle tone was within normal limits. He was guarded, secondary to pain in his trunk. Muscle tone was normal, and reflex integration was grossly intact.

PLAN FOR DISCHARGE

Zachary will be discharged to an outpatient facility and will receive occupational therapy services.

Questions and Activities

SAFETY OF CLIENT AND OTHERS: PRECAUTIONS AND CONTRAINDICATIONS

1. Generally, how long should the graft be protected?

2. Create a handout identifying the signs and symptoms of a graft failure.
3. To protect the integrity of Zachary's graft, what instructions should you provide?
4. List the signs and symptoms of an infected wound.
5. Identify the common psychological reactions associated with a severe burn that may affect the treatment process.
6. To keep Zachary and others safe, what other factors should be considered?

OCCUPATIONS: ADLs, IADLs, EDUCATION, WORK, PLAY, SOCIAL PARTICIPATION, AND REST AND SLEEP

1. Given the information provided for this case, identify the areas of occupation that will and will not be addressed. Justify your decisions.
2. What recommendations can you make to allow Zachary to experience a more restful and less painful sleep?
3. What areas of basic ADLs need to be addressed for Zachary to return home? Explain your choices.

PERFORMANCE SKILLS: MOTOR SKILLS, PROCESS SKILLS, AND SOCIAL INTERACTION SKILLS

1. Given the information provided, identify the motor, process, and social interaction skills that affect Zachary's occupational performance.
2. Which of these skills would be appropriate to address in this service delivery site? Justify your selection.
3. Which of these skills would be addressed through remediation, compensation, and education?
4. Which of these skills would be addressed through the following intervention approaches: create/promote, establish/restore, maintain, modify, and prevent?

PERFORMANCE PATTERNS: HABITS, ROUTINES, ROLES, AND RITUALS

1. Identify Zachary's useful habits, routines, roles, and rituals that support valued occupations. How can you make use of this information?
2. Identify Zachary's impoverished habits, routines, roles, and rituals that do not support valued occupations. How can you make use of this information?
3. Identify Zachary's dominating habits, routines, roles, and rituals that interfere with valued occupations. How can you make use of this information?

CLIENT FACTORS

Values, beliefs, and spirituality
How can the identified values, beliefs, and spirituality be used in this case?

Body structures
Considering Zachary's primary and secondary diagnoses, identify the related body structures.

Body functions
1. Identify how the primary and secondary diagnoses have affected the function of the identified body structures.
2. Explain the relationships between the structural and functional factors and Zachary's current level of occupational performance.

MENTAL FUNCTIONS: AFFECTIVE, COGNITIVE, AND PERCEPTUAL

1. What common affective issues related to his burns might Zachary have to face?
2. How would these issues be addressed in occupational therapy?
3. To address these issues, what other disciplines could you refer Zachary to?
4. What are the potential psychological effects of a facial burn?
5. Given the information provided, what additional mental function considerations need to be addressed?

NEUROMUSCULOSKELETAL AND MOVEMENT-RELATED FUNCTIONS

1. Given the information provided, identify neuromusculoskeletal and movement-related functions that need to be addressed. Justify your selections.
2. Identify the stages of burn rehabilitation. Explain the focus of occupational therapy for each stage.
3. What positions should Zachary's right hand be splinted in? Justify your selected positions.
4. What is a plausible rationale for why the therapist did not perform manual range-of-motion and muscle strength testing on Zachary's injured wrist and digits?
5. Explain the importance of early scar management and how it affects future movement.
6. Identify remediation activities that could be implemented to improve Zachary's range of motion.
7. Create an exercise program for Zachary based on occupational performance.

CARDIOVASCULAR, HEMATOLOGICAL, IMMUNOLOGICAL, AND RESPIRATORY FUNCTIONS

1. Given the information provided, identify cardiovascular, hematological, immunological, and respiratory functions that need to be addressed. Justify your selections.
2. Given the burn to Zachary's trunk, infer what effect it may have on respiratory function.
3. Describe the impact that severe pain has on vital signs.

SKIN AND RELATED STRUCTURE FUNCTIONS

1. Compare and contrast a split-thickness skin graft with a full-thickness skin graft.
2. Zachary has diabetes mellitus. What impact can it have on his recovery? Explain.
3. List the common signs and symptoms of a full-thickness, third-degree burn.
4. List at least three objectives for skin grafting.
5. Explain how the severity or extent of a burn is assessed.
6. Several methods are used to assess edema. Why did the therapist select the circumferential method?
7. Identify the types and mechanisms of burn injuries. Which type did Zachary sustain? What was the mechanism of injury?
8. What other skin and related structure functions should be considered?

VOICE AND SPEECH FUNCTIONS

Describe how Zachary's diagnosis may affect his voice, speech, and associated occupational performance.

ASSISTIVE TECHNOLOGIES AND DEVICES

Does Zachary need any assistive technologies or adaptations? If yes, identify which ones and explain why.

ETHICAL DECISION MAKING

1. You have been observing the nurse's treatment sessions with Zachary and you notice that the nurse is not observing universal precautions or maintaining a sterile environment during his wound care. How would you address this situation?
2. You notice a smell of smoke originating from Zachary's room. When questioned, he admits to smoking in his bathroom. What actions need to be taken?

PHARMACOLOGY

Zachary is currently being treated with silver sulfadiazine.

1. What is the brand name?
2. Does this drug have a high alert status?
3. What is the classification of this drug?
4. What is the indication for this drug?
5. What is the action of this drug?
6. How may this drug affect client participation during a therapy session?

SOCIOCULTURAL, SOCIOECONOMIC, AND DIVERSITY FACTORS AND LIFESTYLE CHOICES

1. Given Zachary's profile, how may your own culture and beliefs affect your interaction with him?
2. Based on this self-examination, what area of cultural knowledge do you need to pursue?
3. How can this newly acquired cultural knowledge be integrated for effective outcomes?
4. How can you foster cultural interaction and awareness among your coworkers?
5. Discuss how a lack of understanding in the areas of discrimination and stigma, implicit bias, social identity, or racism may contribute to disparities in the delivery of occupational therapy services in this case.

ASSESSMENT TOOLS AND INTERPRETATION OF RESULTS

1. What is the purpose of the Figure-of-Eight method and the Pitting Edema Scale (Brodovicz et al., 2009)? Briefly describe how these measurements are performed.
2. Which population are these tests designed for?
3. How much time is required to administer them?
4. Provide a brief description of each assessment.
5. What is the reliability of the Figure-of-Eight method and the Pitting Edema Scale?
6. What is the validity of the Figure-of-Eight method and the Pitting Edema Scale?
7. What other methods may be used to assess edema? Explain why?

INTERPROFESSIONAL RELATIONSHIP AND EFFECTIVE INTRAPROFESSIONAL COLLABORATION

1. Identify the roles of the occupational therapy assistant (OTA) that could be used in the occupational therapy process for this case.
2. Identify interventions that can be performed by the OTA for this case.
3. What other professionals would be part of Zachary's care and what would be their primary focus?

BILLING AND CODING

1. Identify the *International Classification of Diseases (ICD)* codes for Zachary's diagnoses.
2. For this case, identify at least two *Current Procedural Terminology (CPT®)* codes that are most appropriate. Justify your selection.

REIMBURSEMENT SYSTEMS AND DOCUMENTATION

1. Who would be the authorized individuals you could share the occupational therapy findings with? Explain why.
2. For this case, what forms and frequency of documentation will be required?
3. Which reimbursement system or systems most commonly cover occupational therapy services in this practice setting?

ADVOCACY

1. Which of the following areas of advocacy would be beneficial in this case: patient rights, matters of privacy, confidentiality, informed consent, awareness building, accessing education, or benefits/resources?
2. Create a plan to advocate for this client based on the selected areas of advocacy.

TELEHEALTH

1. How can telehealth be integrated as a component of the occupational therapy process in this case?
2. Before launching telemedicine services, what questions would be essential to ask Zachary to determine whether it is appropriate for him to engage in telemedicine services?
3. What are the barriers, obstacles, or challenges you foresee if attempting to integrate telehealth services with this client?

Intervention Plan Formulation and Implementation

INTERVENTION PLAN FORMULATION

Create an intervention plan that includes the following:

1. List this individual's **strengths.**
2. List this individual's **barriers** in occupational performance, performance skills, and performance patterns.
3. Based on the individual's goals, health, performance, and service delivery site, **identify the barriers that will be addressed.**
4. From the barriers identified to be addressed, **formulate goals and objectives.**
5. Identify the focus of each goal and objective as either **create, promote, establish, restore, maintain, modify, or prevent.**
6. Identify the **theoretical basis, model(s) of practice, or frame(s) of reference** that will be used to address each goal and objective.

7. For each proposed goal and objective, describe clearly and precisely the **methods** that will be used. This description should include, but not be limited to, safety considerations, environmental considerations, therapeutic use of self, preparatory activities, activity selection, materials, equipment, and flow.
8. Classify the activities selected in the methods description as either **preparatory, enabling, purposeful, or occupation based.**
9. Explain how each activity can be **graded up or down,** creating the just-right challenge.
10. Provide at least two **primary sources of evidence** to support the intervention plan.

INTERVENTION PLAN IMPLEMENTATION

1. Based on your intervention plan, identify which goals and objectives require **more immediate attention.**
2. Describe your proposed **first treatment session.**
3. As the treatment session is progressing, what is **essential to be observed?**

Transition and Discontinuation

Create a plan for discharge from occupational therapy services in collaboration with Zachary and members of the interprofessional team. Review the needs of Zachary, caregivers, family members, and significant others. The plan must match needs with available resources and the discharge environment.

REFERENCES

American Medical Association. (2019). *CPT® 2020 professional edition.*

Brodovicz, K. G., McNaughton, K., Uemura, N., Meininger, G., Girman, C. J., & Yale, S. H. (2009). Reliability and feasibility of methods to quantitatively assess peripheral edema. *Clinical Medicine and Research, 7,* 21–31. https://doi.org/10.3121/cmr.2009.819

Dewey, W. S., Hedman, T. L., Chapman, T. T., Wolf, S. E., & Holcomb, J. B. (2007). The reliability and concurrent validity of the Figure-of-Eight Method of measuring hand edema in patients with burns. *Journal of Burn Care and Research, 28,* 157–162. https://doi.org/10.1097/BCR.0b013e31802c9eb9

World Health Organization. (2019). *International statistical classification of diseases and related health problems* (11th ed.). https://icd.who.int/

Subacute Rehabilitation

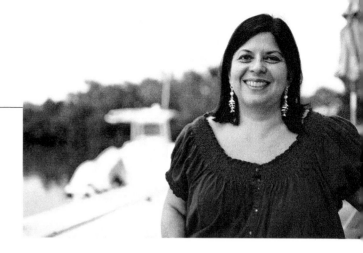

Isaura: Lupus

CLOVER HUTCHINSON, OTD, MA, OTR/L

Isaura (she, her, hers, herself)

MEDICAL HISTORY

Isaura is a 38-year-old Puerto Rican female who is 5' 4" and weighs 183 pounds. She was assisted by her friend to her rheumatologist because she was experiencing fever, extreme fatigue, painful and swollen joints, and difficulty walking. Isaura has a history of systemic lupus erythematosus (SLE). After seen by the rheumatologist, she was admitted electively to the community hospital for the acute flare-up of lupus, where she was treated with azathioprine and Plaquenil, glucocorticoids, and cytotoxic agents. Medical history includes chronic renal failure resulting in kidney transplant, diabetes mellitus, high cholesterol, and depression. Isaura reports no alcohol, drug, caffeine, or nicotine use. She has no known allergies.

SOCIAL HISTORY

Isaura reports being a lapsed Roman Catholic. She is a single mother who resides in a townhouse with her 13-year-old son and is a physical education teacher in a junior high school. She coparents with her ex-husband, who resides a mile away. Isaura recently lost her mother tragically in a motor vehicle accident. She has two sisters who live close by, and they all often spend time with each other.

REFERRAL OR PRESCRIPTION

Isaura was transferred to a subacute rehabilitation facility. She has been referred for occupational therapy, physical therapy, and social work services. The length of stay will be 10 days.

Occupational Therapy Initial Evaluation Findings: Subacute Rehabilitation

OCCUPATIONAL PROFILE

Isaura's preadmission occupational history and experiences included being independent in all ADLs and all IADLs. She has been a gym teacher for 15 years. Her patterns of daily living most commonly included waking at 6:00 a.m., dressing, eating, and taking her medications. She takes her son to school and arrives at work at 8:00 a.m. Isaura typically returns home by 4:00 p.m., prepares dinner, and oversees her son's homework. On weekends, she cares for her home, takes her son to baseball practice, and socializes with her sisters. Isaura's interests include shopping, online dating, and exploring new restaurants with her sisters. She values her coparenting relationship with her ex-husband, time spent with her son and sisters, and her stretches in remission. Her immediate goals are to return home and care for her son and to return to work.

ADLs

Regarding self-care, Isaura was able to feed, dress, groom, and toilet independently. Regarding functional mobility, Isaura was able to independently roll, bridge, scoot, and transition between supine and sit; however, she required frequent breaks because of fatigue and pain. She required minimal assistance to transfer on and off the bed, chair, and toilet using a rolling device.

IADLs

Activities needed that provide day-to-day quality of life and relative independence were explored. Isaura was able to manage her communications and finances. She believed that currently she would be unable to care for her home, prepare meals, or shop without assistance. Regarding sleep, Isaura reported being unable to obtain restful sleep, and she was sleeping no more than 2 hours at a time as a result of pain.

MENTAL FUNCTIONS

Cognitive assessment found Isaura to be alert and oriented to person, place, time, and situation, and short- and long-term memory were intact. She was able to follow three-step commands and make her needs known. Assessment of affect revealed that Isaura was feeling sad, experiencing low energy, and being easily mentally fatigued. No gross deficits in perception were observed.

SENSORY FUNCTIONS AND PAIN

No gross deficits were observed with visual, hearing, vestibular, taste, smell, proprioceptive, and cutaneous functions. Isaura reported generalized pain, with the most severe pain in her fingers, wrist, and elbows. Using the numerical rating scale (0–10), she scored her pain as a 7 and described it as "continuous and throbbing."

CARDIOVASCULAR AND RESPIRATORY SYSTEM FUNCTIONS

Isaura's overall endurance was scored as a 3–4 using the metabolic equivalent of task (MET).

MOVEMENT FUNCTIONS

Full passive range of motion and active range of motion were present in both upper extremities (BUE). The manual muscle test indicated strengths of 3+/5 in BUE. A dynamometer was used to evaluate grasp strength, which was 14 pounds in her right dominant hand and 12 pounds in her left hand. Gross grasp and pinch abilities were within functional limits in both hands.

NEUROMUSCULAR FUNCTIONS

Isaura demonstrated good static balance and dynamic sitting balance. Her static standing and dynamic balance were fair+. Standing tolerance with a walker was 5 minutes before a break was requested. Muscle tone in BUE was normal, and coordination was intact. Muscle tone in both lower extremities was normal. Reflex integration was grossly intact.

PLAN FOR DISCHARGE

Isaura will be discharged home with outpatient rehabilitation services. She will receive occupational and physical therapy.

Questions and Activities

SAFETY OF CLIENT AND OTHERS: PRECAUTIONS AND CONTRAINDICATIONS

1. Create a handout identifying precautions and contraindications for individuals diagnosed with lupus.
2. When working with an individual with lupus, the practitioner should be mindful to avoid fatigue. Explain why.
3. Given Isaura's reported pain level, what considerations should be taken when creating an intervention program?
4. Identify the common emotional reactions associated with lupus that may affect the treatment process.
5. To keep Isaura and others safe, what other factors should be considered?

OCCUPATIONS: ADLs, IADLs, EDUCATION, WORK, PLAY, SOCIAL PARTICIPATION, AND REST AND SLEEP

1. Given the information provided for this case, identify the areas of occupation that will and will not be addressed. Justify your decisions.
2. Identify the factors that affect Isaura's current level of performance.

3. How can energy conservation and work simplification concepts be incorporated into self-care, functional mobility, and IADLs?
4. What strategies can be used to facilitate restful sleep for Isaura?

PERFORMANCE SKILLS: MOTOR SKILLS, PROCESS SKILLS, AND SOCIAL INTERACTION SKILLS

1. Given the information provided, identify the motor, process, and social interaction skills that affect Isaura's occupational performance.
2. Which of these skills would be appropriate to address in this service delivery site? Justify your selection.
3. Which of these skills would be addressed through remediation, compensation, and education?
4. Which of these skills would be addressed through the following intervention approaches: create/promote, establish/restore, maintain, modify, and prevent?
5. Isaura is easily fatigued. Should this challenge be addressed through remediation or compensatory strategies, or both?
6. Isaura is experiencing pain. What physical agent modalities (PAMs) should be considered? Support your decision.
7. In addition to PAMs, what other strategies could be used to address Isaura's pain?
8. Isaura presents with 3+/5 muscle strength in BUE. Should this level of strength be addressed?
9. Given Isaura's acute flare-up of lupus, what types of exercises would be indicated, and which would be contraindicated?

PERFORMANCE PATTERNS: HABITS, ROUTINES, ROLES, AND RITUALS

1. Identify Isaura's useful habits, routines, roles, and rituals that support valued occupations. How can you make use of this information?
2. Identify Isaura's impoverished habits, routines, roles, and rituals that do not support valued occupations. How can you make use of this information?
3. Identify Isaura's dominating habits, routines, roles, and rituals that interfere with valued occupations. How can you make use of this information?

CLIENT FACTORS

Values, beliefs, and spirituality
How can the identified values, beliefs, and spirituality be used in this case?

Body structures
Considering the primary and secondary diagnoses, identify the related body structures.

Body functions
1. Identify how the primary and secondary diagnoses have affected the function of the identified body structures.
2. Explain the relationships between the structural and functional factors and Isaura's current level of occupational performance.

MENTAL FUNCTIONS: AFFECTIVE, COGNITIVE, AND PERCEPTUAL

1. Compare and contrast sadness with clinical depression.
2. Identify three depression screens that could be used to evaluate Isaura. Evaluate them, select one, and justify your decision.
3. Search the literature to determine how pain affects motivation. Provide a brief summary.
4. Given the information provided, what additional mental function considerations need to be addressed?
5. To address these issues, what other disciplines could you refer Isaura to?

NEUROMUSCULOSKELETAL AND MOVEMENT-RELATED FUNCTIONS

1. Given the information provided, identify neuromusculoskeletal and movement-related functions that need to be addressed. Justify your selections.
2. Compare and contrast muscular fatigue with cardiovascular fatigue.
3. Before Isaura's flare-up, she reported normal standing balance. What factors would you infer may be contributing to her current change in balance?
4. Create an exercise program for Isaura based on occupational performance.

CARDIOVASCULAR, HEMATOLOGICAL, IMMUNOLOGICAL, AND RESPIRATORY FUNCTIONS

1. Given the information provided, identify cardiovascular, hematological, immunological, and respiratory functions that need to be addressed. Justify your selections.
2. Identify the estimated MET value that would be required for Isaura to return to work safely as a gym teacher.
3. Describe the long-term impact of lupus on the cardiovascular system.
4. Describe the long-term impact of lupus on the respiratory system.

SKIN AND RELATED STRUCTURE FUNCTIONS

1. Compare and contrast discoid lupus erythematosus with SLE.
2. What are some initial skin changes noted in patients with lupus?
3. Explain the association between Raynaud's disease and SLE.
4. What other skin and related structure functions should be considered?

VOICE AND SPEECH FUNCTIONS

Describe how Isaura's diagnoses may affect her voice, speech, and associated occupational performance.

ASSISTIVE TECHNOLOGIES AND DEVICES

What assistive technologies or adaptations might be used or made for Isaura to use in her home while she is receiving outpatient occupational therapy services? Why?

ETHICAL DECISION MAKING

1. Isaura approaches you and confides that she finds the physical therapist "sexy" and requests that you pass on her phone number. How should this situation be addressed?
2. Isaura's roommate in the rehab facility complains to you that Isaura is up all night watching television, which prevents the roommate from obtaining restful sleep. How should this situation be addressed?

PHARMACOLOGY

Isaura is currently taking Plaquenil.

1. What is the generic name?
2. Does this drug have a high alert status?
3. What is the classification of this drug?
4. What is the indication for this drug?
5. What is the action of this drug?
6. How may this drug affect client participation during a therapy session?

SOCIOCULTURAL, SOCIOECONOMIC, AND DIVERSITY FACTORS AND LIFESTYLE CHOICES

1. Given Isaura's profile, how may your own culture and beliefs affect your interaction with her?
2. Based on this self-examination, what area of cultural knowledge do you need to pursue?
3. How can this newly acquired cultural knowledge be integrated for effective outcomes?
4. How can you foster cultural interaction and awareness among your coworkers?
5. Discuss how a lack of understanding in the areas of discrimination and stigma, implicit bias, social identity, or racism may contribute to disparities in the delivery of occupational therapy services in this case.

ASSESSMENT TOOLS AND INTERPRETATION OF RESULTS

1. What is the purpose of the MET?
2. Which population is this test designed for?
3. How much time is required to administer it?
4. Provide a brief description of this assessment.
5. What is the reliability of the MET?
6. What is the validity of the MET?
7. What functional inference can be deduced from Isaura's score of 3–4?
8. What additional standardized assessment can be used in this case? Why?

INTERPROFESSIONAL RELATIONSHIP AND EFFECTIVE INTRAPROFESSIONAL COLLABORATION

1. Identify the other professions that would make up the care team. Explain the focus of each.
2. Identify the roles of the occupational therapy assistant (OTA) that could be used in the occupational therapy process for this case.
3. Identify interventions that can be assigned to the OTA for this case. Justify your selections.

BILLING AND CODING

1. Identify the *International Classification of Diseases (ICD)* codes for Isaura's diagnoses.
2. For this case, identify at least two *Current Procedural Terminology (CPT®)* codes that are most appropriate. Justify your selection.

REIMBURSEMENT SYSTEMS AND DOCUMENTATION

1. Who would be the authorized individuals that you could share the occupational therapy findings with? Explain why.
2. For this case, what forms and frequency of documentation will be required?
3. Which reimbursement system or systems most commonly cover occupational therapy services in this practice setting?

ADVOCACY

1. Which of the following areas of advocacy would be beneficial in this case: patient rights, matters of privacy, confidentiality, informed consent, awareness building, accessing education, or benefits/resources?
2. Create a plan to advocate for this client based on the selected areas of advocacy.

TELEHEALTH

1. How can telehealth be integrated as a component of the occupational therapy process in this case?
2. Before launching telemedicine services, what questions would be essential to ask Isaura to determine whether it is appropriate for her to engage in telemedicine services?
3. What challenges do you foresee if attempting to integrate telehealth services with this client?

Intervention Plan Formulation and Implementation

INTERVENTION PLAN FORMULATION

Create an intervention plan that includes the following:

1. List this individual's **strengths.**
2. List this individual's **barriers** in occupational performance, performance skills, and performance patterns.
3. Based on the individual's goals, health, performance, and service delivery site, **identify the barriers that will be addressed.**
4. From the barriers identified to be addressed, **formulate goals and objectives.**
5. Identify the focus of each goal and objective as either **create, promote, establish, restore, maintain, modify, or prevent.**
6. Identify the **theoretical basis, model(s) of practice, or frame(s) of reference** that will be used to address each goal and objective.

7. For each proposed goal and objective, describe clearly and precisely the **methods** that will be used. This description should include, but not be limited to, safety considerations, environmental considerations, therapeutic use of self, preparatory activities, activity selection, materials, equipment, and flow.
8. Classify the activities selected in the methods description as either **preparatory, enabling, purposeful, or occupation based.**
9. Explain how each activity can be **graded up or down,** creating the just-right challenge.
10. Provide at least two **primary sources of evidence** to support the intervention plan.

INTERVENTION PLAN IMPLEMENTATION

1. Based on your intervention plan, identify which goals and objectives require **more immediate attention?**
2. Describe your proposed **first treatment session.**
3. As the treatment session is progressing, what is **essential to be observed?**

Transition and Discontinuation

Create a plan for discharge from occupational therapy services in collaboration with Isaura and members of the interprofessional team. Review the needs of Isaura, caregivers, family members, and significant others. The plan must match needs with available resources and the discharge environment.

REFERENCES

American Medical Association. (2019). *CPT® 2020 professional edition.*
World Health Organization. (2019). *International statistical classification of diseases and related health problems* (11th ed.). https://icd.who.int/

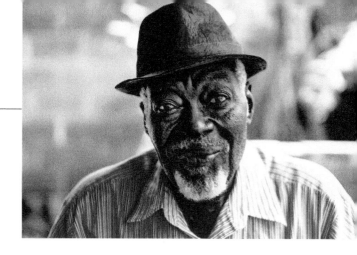

Pierre-Louis: Osteoarthritis

BEBE HANIF, MS, OTR/L

Pierre-Louis (he, him, his, himself)

MEDICAL HISTORY

Perre-Louis is an 82-year-old Haitian American male who is 6' 2" and weighs 172 pounds. He underwent an elective posterior lateral total hip replacement after a long history of right hip pain. Pierre-Louis's medical history includes osteoarthritis, diabetes mellitus, enlarged prostate gland, and glaucoma. He reported no tobacco, caffeine, or drug use. He reported social alcohol use on weekends. He has no known allergies. After surgery, he was admitted to the orthopedic floor.

SOCIAL HISTORY

Pierre-Louis's wife passed away 10 years ago. He lives alone on the first floor of a two-family house. His son lives on the second floor with his wife and two children. Pierre-Louis takes his 6-year-old twin grandchildren to school in the morning, picks them up after school, and watches them until their parents return home. His son is expecting a third child in 2 months. Many of the families on the block have lived there for more than a generation. Pierre-Louis practices Haitian Vodou.

REFERRAL OR PRESCRIPTION

Pierre-Louis was transferred to a subacute rehabilitation facility. He has been referred for occupational therapy, physical therapy, registered nursing services, and social work services. The length of stay will be 10 days.

Occupational Therapy Initial Evaluation Findings: Subacute Rehabilitation

OCCUPATIONAL PROFILE

Pierre-Louis's preadmission occupational history and experiences included being independent in all ADLs and all IADLs. Pierre-Louis is a retired chef and army veteran. His most common pattern of daily living includes waking up at 6:30 a.m., preparing his breakfast, taking the kids to school at 8:00 a.m., shopping, cleaning, picking up the kids after school, and assisting them with their homework. His interests include reading the daily newspaper, watching television, attending choir rehearsals on Friday nights, attending church on Sundays, and having dinner with his girlfriend after church. Pierre-Louis values spending time with his grandchildren and sharing time with his girlfriend. His greatest needs are to be independent and to be active in his grandchildren's lives.

ADLs

Regarding self-care, Pierre-Louis was able to feed himself independently. While seated, Pierre-Louis required supervision to don and doff upper-body clothing and maximal assistance to don and doff lower-body garments. During grooming tasks, he was able to brush his teeth and comb his hair independently. He required moderate assistance to manage clothing during toileting. Pierre-Louis scored a 60 on the Barthel Index (Mahoney & Barthel, 1965) for ADLs.

Regarding functional mobility, Pierre-Louis required moderate assistance to roll and transition from supine to sit at the edge of the bed. He reported difficulty experiencing restful sleep while supine and using an abduction wedge. He required moderate assistance and verbal cues to transfer with a walker on and off the bed, chair, raised toilet, and tub bench.

IADLs

Activities needed that provide day-to-day quality of life and relative independence were explored. Pierre-Louis was independent in telephone use and money management. He required moderate assistance for simple meal preparation and clean-up tasks. Regarding rest and sleep, Pierre-Louis reported sleeping on average 5 hours per evening and napping for 1 or 2 hours each afternoon.

MENTAL FUNCTIONS

Cognitive assessment found Pierre-Louis to be alert and oriented to person, place, time, and situation, and short- and long-term memory were intact. He was able to follow three-step commands and make his needs known. Affect appeared appropriate, and no gross deficits in perception were observed.

SENSORY FUNCTIONS AND PAIN

No gross deficits were observed with visual, hearing, vestibular, taste, smell, proprioceptive, and cutaneous functions. Using the Numerical Rating Scale (0–10), Louis-Pierre scored a 4 for pain in his right hip at rest and an 8 with movement. Pain was described as "sharp."

CARDIOVASCULAR AND RESPIRATORY SYSTEM FUNCTIONS

No deficits were noted.

MOVEMENT FUNCTIONS

Full passive range of motion and active range of motion were present in both upper extremities (BUE), and the manual muscle test indicated strength of 4/5 in BUE. Gross grasp strength in the right hand was 48 pounds and in the left hand 51 pounds. No deficits were noted in fine motor skills. Pierre-Louis had a precaution of weight bearing as tolerated (WBAT) for his right lower extremity.

NEUROMUSCULAR FUNCTIONS

Pierre-Louis demonstrated good static sitting balance and fair (F)+ dynamic sitting balance. His static standing balance was F, and his dynamic standing balance was F–. Standing tolerance with a walker was 5 minutes before a break was requested. Muscle tone in BUE was normal, and coordination was intact. Muscle tone in both lower extremities was normal. Pierre-Louis presented with limited right hip and knee extension. During functional ambulation, he was observed using a narrow base gait pattern.

PLAN FOR DISCHARGE

Pierre-Louis will be discharged home without services.

Questions and Activities

SAFETY OF CLIENT AND OTHERS: PRECAUTIONS AND CONTRAINDICATIONS

1. Create two handouts, the first identifying precautions to be followed after a posterolateral total hip arthroplasty (THA) and the second after an anterolateral total hip arthroplasty.
2. Pierre-Louis is afraid to put weight on his right leg. How would you explain WBAT?
3. What safety concerns do you anticipate?
4. The physician directed Pierre-Louis to sleep with an abduction pillow. What is it? What is its function? How long do you estimate he will need to use it?
5. Identify the common psychological reactions associated with a THA that may affect the treatment process.
6. To keep Pierre-Louis and others safe, what other factors should be considered?

OCCUPATIONS: ADLs, IADLs, EDUCATION, WORK, PLAY, SOCIAL PARTICIPATION, AND REST AND SLEEP

1. Given the information provided for this case, identify the areas of occupation that will and will not be addressed. Justify your decisions.
2. What clothing choices would you recommend for Pierre-Louis?
3. What areas of functional mobility need to be addressed for Pierre-Louis to return home? Explain.

4. What areas of basic ADLs need to be addressed to return home? Explain.
5. What equipment and strategies can be used to assist Pierre-Louis in maintaining precautions?
6. Pierre-Louis complains of difficulty cleaning himself after "doing number two." How do you address his complaint?
7. How could Pierre-Louis's lack of restful sleep be addressed?

PERFORMANCE SKILLS: MOTOR SKILLS, PROCESS SKILLS, AND SOCIAL INTERACTION SKILLS

1. Given the information provided, identify the motor, process, and social interaction skills that affect Pierre-Louis' occupational performance.
2. Which of these skills would be appropriate to address in this service delivery site? Justify your selection.
3. Which of these skills would be addressed through remediation, compensation, and education?
4. Which of these skills would be addressed through the following intervention approaches: create/promote, establish/restore, maintain, modify, and prevent?

PERFORMANCE PATTERNS: HABITS, ROUTINES, ROLES, AND RITUALS

1. Identify Pierre-Louis's useful habits, routines, roles, and rituals that support valued occupations. How can you make use of this information?
2. Identify Pierre-Louis's impoverished habits, routines, roles, and rituals that do not support valued occupations. How can you make use of this information?
3. Identify Pierre-Louis's dominating habits, routines, roles, and rituals that interfere with valued occupations. How can you make use of this information?

CLIENT FACTORS

Values, beliefs, and spirituality
How can the identified values, beliefs, and spirituality be used in this case?

Body structures
Considering Pierre-Louis's primary and secondary diagnoses, identify the related body structures.

Body functions
1. Identify how the primary and secondary diagnoses have affected the function of the identified body structures.
2. Explain the relationships between the structural and functional factors and Pierre-Louis's current level of occupational performance.

MENTAL FUNCTIONS: AFFECTIVE, COGNITIVE, AND PERCEPTUAL

1. Explain how the lack of restful sleep affects participation. Identify your sources.
2. Explain how unaddressed pain may affect participation. Identify your sources.
3. Given the information provided, what additional mental function considerations need to be addressed?

NEUROMUSCULOSKELETAL AND MOVEMENT-RELATED FUNCTIONS

1. Given the information provided, identify neuromusculoskeletal and movement-related functions that need to be addressed. Justify your selections.
2. Pierre-Louis presents with 4/5 muscle strength in all groups of BUE. Does this strength level need to be addressed? Justify your decision.
3. Pierre-Louis presents with F static standing balance and F− dynamic standing balance. How may this ability level affect his participation in daily activities?
4. Pierre-Louis's standing tolerance with a walker is 5 minutes. How may this ability level affect his participation in daily activities?
5. Compare and contrast osteoarthritis with rheumatoid arthritis.
6. Create an exercise program for Pierre-Louis based on occupational performance.

CARDIOVASCULAR, HEMATOLOGICAL, IMMUNOLOGICAL, AND RESPIRATORY FUNCTIONS

1. Given the information provided, identify cardiovascular, hematological, immunological, and respiratory functions that need to be addressed. Justify your selections.
2. Which vital signs should be taken when working with Pierre-Louis?
3. When should Pierre-Louis's vital signs be taken? Identify the norms for these vital signs. Identify two scholarly sources.

SKIN AND RELATED STRUCTURE FUNCTIONS

1. Given Pierre-Louis's age and medical condition, how long is it expected for his surgical wound to be fully healed?
2. Identify the factors that will promote or delay wound healing.
3. You notice Pierre-Louis's pants have a wet red spot just over his right hip. What could be a concern and what action would you take?
4. What other skin and related structure functions should be considered?

VOICE AND SPEECH FUNCTIONS

Describe how Pierre-Louis's diagnoses may affect his voice, speech, and associated occupational performance.

ASSISTIVE TECHNOLOGIES AND DEVICES

1. What assistive technologies or adaptations might be used or made for Pierre-Louis while he receives occupational therapy services? Support your choices.
2. What assistive technologies or adaptations might be recommended when he returns home? Support your choices.

ETHICAL DECISION MAKING

1. According to the surgeon, Pierre-Louis has a stay of 10 days in subacute rehabilitation. Given the setting and the projected length of stay, how would you prioritize his therapeutic needs?

2. Pierre-Louis speaks English with a heavy Creole accent, and at times you find it difficult to understand him. How could this situation be addressed?
3. During an occupational therapy session, Pierre-Louis's girlfriend inquired about his blood pressure. How should you address this question while maintaining compliance with the Health Insurance Portability and Accountability Act of 1996 (P. L. 104-191)?
4. Pierre-Louis's abduction pillow is missing. Identify your options, make a selection, and support your decision.

PHARMACOLOGY

Pierre-Louis is currently taking Sectral.

1. What is the generic name?
2. Does this drug have a high alert status?
3. What is the classification of this drug?
4. What is the indication for this drug?
5. What is the action of this drug?
6. How may this drug affect client participation during a therapy session?

SOCIOCULTURAL, SOCIOECONOMIC, AND DIVERSITY FACTORS AND LIFESTYLE CHOICES

1. Given Pierre-Louis's profile, how may your own culture and beliefs affect your interaction with him?
2. Based on this self-examination, what area of cultural knowledge do you need to pursue?
3. How can this newly acquired cultural knowledge be integrated for effective outcomes?
4. How can you foster cultural interaction and awareness among your coworkers?
5. Discuss how a lack of understanding in the areas of discrimination and stigma, implicit bias, social identity, or racism may contribute to disparities in the delivery of occupational therapy services in this case.

ASSESSMENT TOOLS AND INTERPRETATION OF RESULTS

1. What is the purpose of the Barthel Index?
2. Which population is this test designed for?
3. How much time is required to administer it?
4. Provide a brief description of this assessment.
5. What is the reliability of the Barthel Index?
6. What is the validity of the Barthel Index?
7. What functional inference can be deduced from Pierre-Louis's score of 60 on the Barthel Index?
8. What additional standardized assessment can be used in this case? Why?

INTERPROFESSIONAL RELATIONSHIP AND EFFECTIVE INTRAPROFESSIONAL COLLABORATION

1. Identify the other professions that would make up the care team. Explain the focus of each.
2. Identify the roles of the occupational therapy assistant (OTA) that could be used in the occupational therapy process for this case.
3. Identify interventions that can be assigned to the OTA for this case. Justify your selections.

BILLING AND CODING

1. Identify the *International Classification of Diseases (ICD)* codes for this individual's diagnoses.
2. For this case, identify at least two *Current Procedural Terminology (CPT®)* codes that are most appropriate. Justify your selection.

REIMBURSEMENT SYSTEMS AND DOCUMENTATION

1. Who would be the authorized individuals that you could share the occupational therapy findings with? Explain why.
2. For this case, what forms and frequency of documentation will be required?
3. Which reimbursement system or systems most commonly cover occupational therapy services in this practice setting?

ADVOCACY

1. Which of the following areas of advocacy would be beneficial in this case: patient rights, matters of privacy, confidentiality, informed consent, awareness building, accessing education, or benefits/resources?
2. Create a plan to advocate for this client based on the selected areas of advocacy.

TELEHEALTH

1. How can telehealth be integrated as a component of the occupational therapy process in this case?
2. Before launching telemedicine services, what questions would be essential to ask Pierre-Louis to determine whether it is appropriate for him to engage in telemedicine services?
3. What are the barriers, obstacles, or challenges you foresee if attempting to integrate telehealth services with this client?

Intervention Plan Formulation and Implementation

INTERVENTION PLAN FORMULATION

Create an intervention plan that includes the following:

1. List this individual's **strengths.**
2. List this individual's **barriers** in occupational performance, performance skills, and performance patterns.
3. Based on the individual's goals, health, performance, and service delivery site, **identify the barriers that will be addressed.**
4. From the barriers identified to be addressed, **formulate goals and objectives.**
5. Identify the focus of each goal and objective as either **create, promote, establish, restore, maintain, modify, or prevent.**
6. Identify the **theoretical basis, model(s) of practice, or frame(s) of reference** that will be used to address each goal and objective.

7. For each proposed goal and objective, describe clearly and precisely the **methods** that will be used. This description should include, but not be limited to, safety considerations, environmental considerations, therapeutic use of self, preparatory activities, activity selection, materials, equipment, and flow.
8. Classify the activities selected in the methods description as either **preparatory, enabling, purposeful, or occupation based.**
9. Explain how each activity can be **graded up or down,** creating the just-right challenge.
10. Provide at least two **primary sources of evidence** to support the intervention plan.

INTERVENTION PLAN IMPLEMENTATION

1. Based on your intervention plan, identify which goals and objectives require **more immediate attention.**
2. Describe your proposed **first treatment session.**
3. As the treatment session is progressing, what is **essential to be observed?**

Transition and Discontinuation

Create a plan for discharge from occupational therapy services in collaboration with Pierre-Louis and members of the interprofessional team. Review the needs of Pierre-Louis, caregivers, family members, and significant others. The plan must match needs with available resources and the discharge environment.

REFERENCES

American Medical Association. (2019). *CPT® 2020 professional edition.*

Health Insurance Portability and Accountability Act of 1996 (HIPAA), Pub. L. 104-191, 42 U.S.C. § 300gg, 29 U.S.C. §§ 1181–1183, and 42 U.S.C. §§ 1320d–1320d9.

Mahoney, F. I., & Barthel, D. (1965). Functional evaluation: The Barthel Index. *Maryland State Medical Journal, 14,* 56–61.

World Health Organization. (2019). *International statistical classification of diseases and related health problems* (11th ed.). https://icd.who.int/

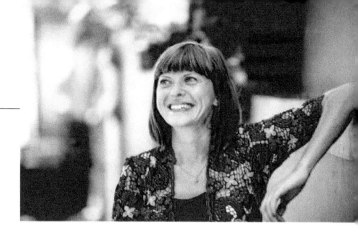

Rosalind: Multiple Sclerosis

EVA RODRIGUEZ, PhD, OTR

Rosalind (she, her, hers, herself)

MEDICAL HISTORY

Rosalind is a 51-year-old Ukrainian American female who is 5' 3" and weighs 111 pounds. She was electively admitted to her regional hospital by her neurologist for observation and assessment because she reported weakness and difficulty ambulating with her straight cane. Magnetic resonance imaging scans of the brain showed gadolinium-enhancing lesions in the cerebrum, parietal, and temporal areas. These scans also indicated lesions on thoracic vertebrae 1 and 2. Rosalind was diagnosed with an acute episode of multiple sclerosis (MS). Her medical history includes primary progressive relapsing MS (onset at age 30) and optic neuritis with a right homonymous hemianopsia visual field loss of 5° peripherally. Rosalind reported the use of dimethyltryptamine (DMT) and medical marijuana in liquid form. She reported no tobacco, drug, or caffeine use. Rosalind reported being allergic to codeine-based medications.

SOCIAL HISTORY

Rosalind is a speech–language pathologist in the local school district. She lives with her spouse, Sarah, and their three dogs in a ranch-style home in the suburbs. Sarah is a nurse practitioner with a private practice and works long hours, 3 days a week. Rosalind's family (three siblings, and their partners and children) live within walking distance of her home. Rosalind identifies as an Orthodox Christian and Sarah identifies as Jewish.

REFERRAL OR PRESCRIPTION

Rosalind was transferred to a subacute rehabilitation facility. She has been referred for occupational therapy, physical therapy, registered nursing services, speech therapy, and social work services. The length of stay will be 20 days.

Occupational Therapy Initial Evaluation Findings: Subacute Rehabilitation

OCCUPATIONAL PROFILE

Rosalind's preadmission occupational history and experiences included being independent in all ADLs and all IADLs. She has a master's degree in speech-language pathology. Her primary role at home includes caring for her dogs, which is shared with Sarah during the weekends. Her daily routine begins at 6:00 a.m. with preparing her fair-trade coffee and walking the dogs for about 20 minutes. After their walk, Rosalind prepares herself for work, which includes preparing her vegan lunch. After work, she shops for any last-minute ingredients and prepares weeknight dinners. On the weekends, Rosalind shares shopping and laundry responsibilities with her spouse. They have a cleaning service for the home twice a week. Her interests include cooking, machine quilting, and volunteering for activities related to LGBTQIA+ issues. Rosalind values her family and friends and enjoys socializing with them. She enjoys preparing large meals with her spouse for social gatherings.

ADLs

Regarding self-care, Rosalind was able to feed herself independently. She was able to don and doff loose-fitting clothing, including socks, but required short rest periods, specifically for lower body dressing. She was able to manage various clothing fasteners (zippers, buttons, snaps, hooks, laces) but with reported difficulty because of mild decreased tactile awareness. When standing in front of the bathroom sink, she required contact guard assist (CGA) while brushing her teeth, washing her face, applying makeup, and brushing her hair. During bathing, she required CGA for both upper- and lower-extremity hygiene.

Regarding functional mobility, Rosalind was able to independently roll and transition between prone and supine. She needed minimal assistance to transition to a short sit in bed. She required CGA to transition from short sit from the edge of the bed to standing with a narrow-base quad cane. Rosalind required minimal assistance and redirection to attention to tasks during transfers on and off the chair, toilet, and tub secondary to verbally over engaging with the therapist. After transfer evaluations, she expressed fatigue and required a brief rest period before the evaluation could continue.

IADLs

Activities needed that provide day-to-day quality of life and relative independence were explored. Rosalind expressed concerns about her ability to shop, prepare meals, take care of the dogs, and return to work upon discharge. Regarding rest and sleep, Rosalind reported frequently having difficulty falling asleep and being consumed with worry.

MENTAL FUNCTIONS

Cognitive assessment found Rosalind to be alert and oriented to person, place, time, and situation, and short- and long-term memory were intact. She presented with a delayed response during verbal pragmatic communication and reported "brain fog." Rosalind was distractible and impulsive and required verbal redirection and repetition of instructions. Her Mini-Mental Status Examination (Folstein et al., 2010) was scored at 22. She presented with a pseudobulbar affect. No gross perceptual deficits were noted.

SENSORY FUNCTIONS AND PAIN

No gross deficits were observed with hearing, vestibular, taste, smell, and proprioceptive functions. Cutaneous sensory testing indicated impaired tactile awareness and tactile localization in both hands. Visual testing indicated decreased peripheral visual field loss (5° right homonymous hemianopia). No pain was reported.

CARDIOVASCULAR AND RESPIRATORY SYSTEMS FUNCTIONS

No deficits were noted in these areas.

MOVEMENT FUNCTIONS

Rosalind presented within normal limits for both active range of motion and passive range of motion in all extremities. Rosalind was able to form all gross grasp patterns of the hand but had difficulty with hand manipulation skills. She presented with impaired bilateral gross grasp, with strength measured at 10 pounds on the right dominant side and 8 pounds on the nondominant side, using the Jamar dynamometer.

NEUROMUSCULAR FUNCTIONS

Rosalind was able to maintain balance against moderate resistance during both static and dynamic sitting. While standing, she presented with minimal weight shifting and difficulty crossing the midline. Deep tendon reflex testing in all four extremities yielded brisk responses.

PLAN FOR DISCHARGE

Rosalind will be discharged to home with home health services that include occupational therapy; physical therapy; speech therapy; and registered nursing, social work, and home health aide services.

Questions and Activities

SAFETY OF CLIENT AND OTHERS: PRECAUTIONS AND CONTRAINDICATIONS

1. Create a handout identifying the precautions and contraindications addressing an acute flare-up of MS.
2. Considering Rosalind's current level of balance, what precautions should be followed?
3. Compare and contrast balance and equilibrium.

4. What precautions should Rosalind follow during engagement in ADLs given her cutaneous sensory deficits?
5. Given Rosalind's cognitive status, what precautions should be followed?
6. Identify the common emotional reactions associated with MS that may affect the treatment process.
7. To keep Rosalind and others safe, what other factors should be considered?

OCCUPATIONS: ADLs, IADLs, EDUCATION, WORK, PLAY, SOCIAL PARTICIPATION, AND REST AND SLEEP

1. Given the information provided for this case, identify the areas of occupation that will and will not be addressed. Justify your decisions.
2. Rosalind has difficulty managing fasteners. What strategies would you use to address this challenge?
3. Rosalind currently requires assistance to bathe. What strategies would you use to address this situation?
4. Rosalind is currently unsafe transferring independently. What strategies would you use to address this situation?
5. During a treatment session, Rosalind states, "I would give anything to obtain a good night's sleep." How would you address this challenge?
6. Before her admission, Rosalind shopped for food by walking to her local supermarket but is aware it will not be possible when she returns home. What options would you offer her to consider?

PERFORMANCE SKILLS: MOTOR SKILLS, PROCESS SKILLS, AND SOCIAL INTERACTION

1. Given the information provided, identify the motor, process, and social interaction skills that affect Rosalind's occupational performance.
2. Which of these skills would be appropriate to address in this service delivery site? Justify your selection.
3. Which of these skills would be addressed through remediation, compensation, and education?
4. Which of these skills would be addressed through the following intervention approaches: create/promote, establish/restore, maintain, modify, and prevent?

PERFORMANCE PATTERNS: HABITS, ROUTINES, ROLES, AND RITUALS

1. Identify Rosalind's useful habits, routines, roles, and rituals that support valued occupations. How can you make use of this information?
2. Identify Rosalind's impoverished habits, routines, roles, and rituals that do not support valued occupations. How can you make use of this information?
3. Identify Rosalind's dominating habits, routines, roles, and rituals that interfere with valued occupations. How can you make use of this information?

CLIENT FACTORS

Values, beliefs, and spirituality
How can the identified values, beliefs, and spirituality be used in this case?

Body structures
Considering Rosalind's primary and secondary diagnoses, identify the related body structures.

Body Functions

1. Identify how the primary and secondary diagnoses have affected the function of the identified body structures.
2. Explain the relationships between the structural and functional factors and Rosalind's current level of occupational performance.

MENTAL FUNCTIONS: AFFECTIVE, COGNITIVE, AND PERCEPTUAL

1. Identify common cognitive changes associated with progressive MS. Identify your source.
2. Identify common affective changes associated with progressive MS. Identify your source.
3. Identify how the pseudobulbar affect may affect the occupational therapy process.
4. What measures and strategies are available to address Rosalind's impulsivity and distractibility?
5. Given the information provided, what additional mental function considerations need to be addressed?

NEUROMUSCULOSKELETAL AND MOVEMENT-RELATED FUNCTIONS

1. Given the information provided, identify neuromusculoskeletal and movement-related functions that need to be addressed. Justify your selections.
2. Identify three different assessments or scales that can be used to evaluate Rosalind's balance. Evaluate them and then select one. Justify your decision.
3. Use the selected assessment or scale to determine the rating for Rosalind's sitting and standing balance.
4. Identify the tool that was most likely used to measure Rosalind's gross grasp strength.
5. Given her current gross grasp strength, what areas of ADLs or IADLs would be most affected?
6. Compare and contrast MS with myasthenia gravis.
7. The muscle strength in all muscle groups has been estimated at 3+/5. Should Rosalind's strength be addressed through a remediation or compensation model? Defend your selection.
8. Create an exercise program for Rosalind based on occupational performance.

CARDIOVASCULAR, HEMATOLOGICAL, IMMUNOLOGICAL, AND RESPIRATORY FUNCTIONS

1. Given the information provided, identify cardiovascular, hematological, immunological, and respiratory functions that need to be addressed. Justify your selections.
2. Rosalind experiences fatigue, which is typical for individuals with MS. Is the fatigue that she is experiencing muscular or cardiovascular?
3. Are there immunological changes associated with MS? If so, identify and explain what they are.
4. Are there any cardiopulmonary changes associated with MS? If so, identify and explain what they are.

SKIN AND RELATED STRUCTURE FUNCTIONS

1. Given Rosalind's diminished cutaneous sensation, identify and describe the appropriate test or tests that could be used to assess touch localization and touch awareness.
2. What other skin and related structure functions should be considered?

VOICE AND SPEECH FUNCTIONS

Describe how Rosalind's diagnoses may affect her voice, speech, and associated occupational performance.

ASSISTIVE TECHNOLOGIES AND DEVICES

1. What assistive technologies or adaptations might be used or made for Rosalind while she is receiving occupational therapy services in subacute rehabilitation? Why?
2. What assistive technologies or adaptations might be recommended for when she returns home? Why?

ETHICAL DECISION MAKING

1. Rosalind has informed you that she intends to return to work immediately upon discharge. How could this situation be addressed?
2. How could implicit bias affect your interaction with Rosalind?

PHARMACOLOGY

Rosalind is currently taking DMT.

1. What is the brand name?
2. Does this drug have a high alert status?
3. What is the classification of this drug?
4. What is the indication for this drug?
5. What is the action of this drug?
6. How may this drug affect client participation during a therapy session?

SOCIOCULTURAL, SOCIOECONOMIC, AND DIVERSITY FACTORS AND LIFESTYLE CHOICES

1. Given Rosalind's profile, how may your own culture and beliefs affect your interaction with her?
2. Based on this self-examination, what area of cultural knowledge do you need to pursue?
3. How can this newly acquired cultural knowledge be integrated for effective outcomes?
4. How can you foster cultural interaction and awareness among your coworkers?
5. Discuss how a lack of understanding in the areas of discrimination and stigma, implicit bias, social identity, or racism may contribute to disparities in the delivery of occupational therapy services in this case.

ASSESSMENT TOOLS AND INTERPRETATION OF RESULTS

1. What is the purpose of the Jamar dynamometer?
2. Which population is this test designed for?
3. How much time is required to administer it?
4. Provide a brief description of this assessment.
5. What is the reliability of the Jamar dynamometer?
6. What is the validity of the Jamar dynamometer?
7. What functional inference can be deduced from Rosalind's measures of grasp strength?
8. What additional standardized assessment can be used in this case? Why?

INTERPROFESSIONAL RELATIONSHIP AND EFFECTIVE INTRAPROFESSIONAL COLLABORATION

1. Identify the other professions that would make up the care team. Explain the focus of each.
2. Identify the roles of the occupational therapy assistant (OTA) that could be used in the occupational therapy process for this case.
3. Identify interventions that can be assigned to the OTA for this case. Justify your selections.

BILLING AND CODING

1. Identify the *International Classification of Diseases (ICD)* codes for Rosalind's diagnoses.
2. For this case, identify at least two *Current Procedural Terminology (CPT®)* codes that are most appropriate. Justify your selection.

REIMBURSEMENT SYSTEMS AND DOCUMENTATION

1. Who would be the authorized individuals that you could share the occupational therapy findings with? Explain why.
2. For this case, what forms and frequency of documentation will be required?
3. Which reimbursement system or systems most commonly cover occupational therapy services in this practice setting?

ADVOCACY

1. Which of the following areas of advocacy would beneficial for this case: patient rights, matters of privacy, confidentiality, informed consent, awareness building, accessing education, or benefits/resources?
2. Create a plan to advocate for this client based on the selected areas of advocacy.

TELEHEALTH

1. How can telehealth be integrated as a component of the occupational therapy process in this case?
2. Before launching telemedicine services, what questions would be essential to ask Rosalind to determine whether it is appropriate for her to engage in telemedicine services?
3. What are the barriers, obstacles, or challenges you foresee if attempting to integrate telehealth services with this client?

Intervention Plan Formulation and Implementation

INTERVENTION PLAN FORMULATION

Create an intervention plan that includes the following:

1. List this individual's **strengths.**
2. List this individual's **barriers** in occupational performance, performance skills, and performance patterns.

3. Based on the individual's goals, health, performance, and service delivery site, **identify the barriers that will be addressed.**
4. From the barriers identified to be addressed, **formulate goals and objectives.**
5. Identify the focus of each goal and objective as either **create, promote, establish, restore, maintain, modify, or prevent.**
6. Identify the **theoretical basis, model(s) of practice, or frame(s) of reference** that will be used to address each goal and objective.
7. For each proposed goal and objective, describe clearly and precisely the **methods** that will be used. This description should include, but not be limited to, safety considerations, environmental considerations, therapeutic use of self, preparatory activities, activity selection, materials, equipment, and flow.
8. Classify the activities selected in the methods description as either **preparatory, enabling, purposeful, or occupation based.**
9. Explain how each activity can be **graded up or down,** creating the just-right challenge.
10. Provide at least two **primary sources of evidence** to support the intervention plan.

INTERVENTION PLAN IMPLEMENTATION

1. Based on your intervention plan, identify which goals and objectives require **more immediate attention.**
2. Describe your proposed **first treatment session.**
3. As the treatment session is progressing, what is **essential to be observed?**

Transition and Discontinuation

Create a plan for discharge from occupational therapy services in collaboration with Rosalind and members of the interprofessional team. Review the needs of Rosalind, caregivers, family members, and significant others. The plan must match needs with available resources and the discharge environment.

REFERENCES

American Medical Association. (2019). *CPT® 2020 professional edition.*
Folstein, M. F., White, T., Folstein, S. E., & Messer, M. A. (2010). *Mini-Mental State Examination (MMSE–2).* PAR.
World Health Organization. (2019). *International statistical classification of diseases and related health problems* (11th ed.). https://icd.who.int/

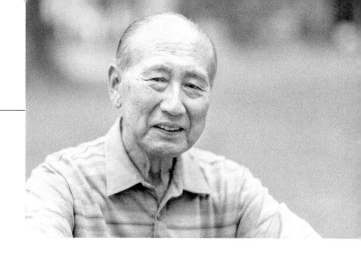

Aki: Congestive Heart Failure

FREDERICK WOLODIN, MS, OTR/L

Aki (he, him, his, himself)

MEDICAL HISTORY

Aki is a 91-year-old Japanese American male who is 6' and weighs 175 pounds. He was brought in by emergency services from subacute rehabilitation with shortness of breath, pedal edema, productive cough, and confusion. Upon arrival, Aki was alert and oriented to person and place. His blood pressure (BP) was 160/82, heart rate (HR) was 88, respiration rate (RR) was 24, and temperature was 97.5°. An X-ray of his lungs and heart revealed bilateral pleural effusion and an enlarged heart. An electrocardiogram revealed a left thickened ventricle and arrhythmia. He received a diagnosis of congestive heart failure (CHF) with an ejection fraction of 20%.

His medical history includes coronary artery disease, hypertension, atrial fibrillation, diabetes mellitus, Stage 4 chronic kidney disease, osteoarthritis after a right total hip replacement (THR) 13 years ago, and a left THR 15 years ago. He was admitted to the telemetry care unit for 3 days. Upon medical stabilization, he was sent to the stepdown unit and then to the medical floor. Aki reported no drug, alcohol, tobacco, or caffeine use. He has no known allergies.

SOCIAL HISTORY

Aki lives alone in an assisted living facility (ALF) located in a Japanese community. He has two male adult children and four grandchildren and enjoys weekly visits from his family. Aki identifies as practicing Shinto.

REFERRAL OR PRESCRIPTION

Aki was transferred to a subacute rehabilitation facility. He has been referred for occupational therapy, physical therapy, registered nursing services, and social work services. The length of stay will be 21 days.

Occupational Therapy Initial Evaluation Findings: Subacute Rehabilitation

OCCUPATIONAL PROFILE

Aki was independent with all ADLs and all IADLs. He grew up with his immigrant parents, who spoke only Japanese. He had one sister, who passed away from breast cancer at age 30. Aki worked for his father, who owned and managed a tailor shop, which Aki inherited upon his father's retirement. His mother was a homemaker. He has a bachelor's degree in liberal arts. Aki's most common pattern of daily living includes waking up at 6:00 a.m., performing his self-care, and eating breakfast. His interests include watching the local and international news from Asia. Aki was active at the ALF and was the ombudsman. He values work, education, family, and individual independence. His reported greatest needs are to return to the ALF and to be able to care for his own needs.

ADLs

Regarding self-care, Aki performed his upper-body dressing with minimal assistance sitting at the edge of the bed. He attempted to initiate lower-body dressing; however, he required total assistance for that task. Aki was able to feed himself with setup. He required moderate assistance for anterior hygiene and maximal assistance for posterior hygiene. Bathing was not assessed at this time.

Regarding functional mobility, Aki transitioned to and from supine to sit with maximal assistance and rolled side to side with moderate assistance with the use of the bed rail. He transferred to and from the bed, armchair, wheelchair, and toilet with maximum assistance with use of the rolling walker. Aki required verbal cuing 50% of the time to maintain proper hand placement.

IADLs

Activities needed that provide day-to-day quality of life and relative independence were explored. Aki required moderate assistance to manage his cell phone, medication, and finances. He was unable to prepare a simple meal and perform light housekeeping tasks. Regarding rest and sleep, Aki reported a life-long pattern of going to bed at 9:00 p.m. and awakening at 5:00 a.m. and obtaining restorative sleep.

MENTAL FUNCTIONS

Cognitive assessment found Aki to be alert and oriented to person, place, time, and situation, and long-term memory was intact. He presented with mild impairment in short-term memory. Aki demonstrated a lack of safety awareness by attempting to perform transfers unassisted. He was able to follow two- and three-step commands and make his needs known. Affect appeared appropriate, and no gross deficits in perception were observed.

SENSORY FUNCTIONS AND PAIN

No gross deficits were observed with visual, hearing, vestibular, taste, and smell functions. Light touch, deep pressure, and thermal sensation were grossly intact to both upper extremities (BUE) and were moderately impaired in the distal portions of both lower extremities (BLE). Aki reported experiencing no pain.

CARDIOVASCULAR AND RESPIRATORY SYSTEMS FUNCTION

Aki's vital signs at rest were as follows: BP, 148/70; RR, 18; HR, 82; and oxygen saturation (SpO2), 98% on room air. His vital signs after transferring from the bed to the commode using a rolling walker were as follows: BP, 160/82; RR, 26; HR, 96; and SpO2, 95% on room air. His metabolic equivalent task value was 3.0. Aki presented with pitting edema of 2+ to BLE. He was functionally classified as Class III using the New York Heart Association (NYHA) Classification of Heart Failure (Criteria Committee of the New York Heart Association, 1994).

MOVEMENT FUNCTIONS

Active range of motion and passive range of motion in BUE were within normal limits. Aki's muscle strength was estimated to be 3+/5 for BUE. His fine motor abilities were grossly intact for gross grasp formation, pinch pattern formation, and in-hand manipulation.

NEUROMUSCULAR FUNCTIONS

Aki's static and dynamic sitting balance were good. His static standing balance was fair−, and his dynamic standing balance was poor+. Standing tolerance was 2 minutes. Muscle tone was normal, and reflex integration was grossly intact.

PLAN FOR DISCHARGE

Upon discharge, Aki will return to the ALF.

Questions and Activities

SAFETY OF CLIENT AND OTHERS: PRECAUTIONS AND CONTRAINDICATIONS

1. Create a handout identifying the signs and symptoms of CHF.
2. What are the signs and symptoms of cardiac distress?
3. Identify the cardiac precautions that need to be observed while working with Aki.
4. What are the precautions to follow for a THR? Does Aki need to follow them?
5. Identify factors that would support Aki being classified as a fall risk.
6. Why did the therapist estimate Aki's muscle strength instead of performing a manual muscle test?
7. To keep Aki and others safe, what other factors should be considered?

OCCUPATIONS: ADLs, IADLs, EDUCATION, WORK, PLAY, SOCIAL PARTICIPATION, AND REST AND SLEEP

1. Given the information provided for this case, identify the areas of occupation that will and will not be addressed. Justify your decisions.
2. What articles of clothing would make Aki most comfortable during his stay at subacute rehabilitation?
3. What areas of functional mobility need to be addressed for Aki to return to the ALF? Explain.
4. What areas of basic ADLs need to be addressed for Aki to return to the ALF? Explain.
5. Aki is diagnosed with diabetes mellitus. What are the dietary considerations he should observe?
6. Aki is diagnosed with hypertension. What are the dietary considerations he should observe?
7. Which areas of IADLs need to be addressed for Aki to return to the ALF? Explain.

PERFORMANCE SKILLS: MOTOR SKILLS, PROCESS SKILLS, AND SOCIAL INTERACTION SKILLS

1. Given the information provided, identify the motor, process, and social interaction skills that affect Aki's occupational performance.
2. Which of these skills would be appropriate to address in this service delivery site?
3. Which of these skills would be addressed through remediation, compensation, and education?
4. Which of these skills would be addressed through the following intervention approaches: create/promote, establish/restore, maintain, modify, and prevent?

PERFORMANCE PATTERNS: HABITS, ROUTINES, ROLES, AND RITUALS

1. Identify Aki's useful habits, routines, roles, and rituals that support valued occupations. How can you make use of this information?
2. Identify Aki's impoverished habits, routines, roles, and rituals that do not support valued occupations. How can you make use of this information?
3. Identify Aki's dominating habits, routines, roles, and rituals that interfere with valued occupations. How can you make use of this information?

CLIENT FACTORS

Values, beliefs, and spirituality
How can the identified values, beliefs, and spirituality be used in this case?

Body structures
Considering Aki's primary and secondary diagnoses, identify the related body structures.

Body Functions
1. Identify how the primary and secondary diagnoses have affected the function of the identified body structures.
2. Explain the relationships between the structural and functional factors and Aki's current level of occupational performance.

MENTAL FUNCTIONS: AFFECTIVE, COGNITIVE, AND PERCEPTUAL

1. Identify common affective changes that may be associated with CHF. How would they be addressed in occupational therapy?

2. Identify common cognitive changes that may be associated with CHF. How would they be addressed in occupational therapy?
3. What other services would be available for Aki to address these changes?
4. Given the information provided, what additional mental function considerations need to be addressed?

NEUROMUSCULOSKELETAL AND MOVEMENT-RELATED FUNCTIONS

1. Given the information provided, identify neuromusculoskeletal and movement-related functions that need to be addressed. Justify your selections.
2. Compare and contrast right heart failure with left heart failure.
3. Identify remediation activities that could be implemented to improve Aki's muscular strength.
4. Identify remediation activities that could be implemented to improve Aki's standing balance.
5. Identify remediation activities that could be implemented to improve Aki's standing tolerance.
6. Create an exercise program for Aki based on occupational performance.

CARDIOVASCULAR, HEMATOLOGICAL, IMMUNOLOGICAL, AND RESPIRATORY FUNCTIONS

1. Given the information provided, identify cardiovascular, hematological, immunological, and respiratory functions that need to be addressed. Justify your selections.
2. Given Aki's current level of cardiac function, what strategies should be considered to optimize his participation? Justify your selection.
3. What remediation strategies should be considered to improve Aki's cardiovascular endurance? Justify your selection.

SKIN AND RELATED STRUCTURE FUNCTIONS

1. Aki presented with reduced cutaneous sensation in BLE. Identify possible contributing factors.
2. What other skin and related structure functions should be considered?

VOICE AND SPEECH FUNCTIONS

Describe how the diagnoses may affect Aki's voice, speech, and associated occupational performance.

ASSISTIVE TECHNOLOGIES AND DEVICES

Does Aki need any assistive technologies or adaptations? If yes, identify them and explain why he needs them.

ETHICAL DECISION MAKING

1. On several occasions, you observed Aki consuming a bag of potato chips. How can this situation be best addressed?
2. In the therapy gym, a colleague says to you, "Why do you give him so much of your time? He is old and is going to die soon." How should this statement be best addressed?

PHARMACOLOGY

Aki is currently taking Diucardin.

1. What is the generic name?
2. Does this drug have a high alert status?
3. What is the classification of this drug?
4. What is the indication for this drug?
5. What is the action of this drug?
6. How may this drug affect client participation during a therapy session?

SOCIOCULTURAL, SOCIOECONOMIC, AND DIVERSITY FACTORS AND LIFESTYLE CHOICES

1. Given Aki's profile, how may your own culture and beliefs affect your interaction with him?
2. Based on this self-examination, what area of cultural knowledge do you need to pursue?
3. How can this newly acquired cultural knowledge be integrated for effective outcomes?
4. How can you foster cultural interaction and awareness among your coworkers?
5. Discuss how a lack of understanding in the areas of discrimination and stigma, implicit bias, social identity, or racism may contribute to disparities in the delivery of occupational therapy services in this case.

ASSESSMENT TOOLS AND INTERPRETATION OF RESULTS

1. What is the purpose of the NYHA Classification of Heart Failure?
2. Which population is this test designed for?
3. How much time is required to administer it?
4. Provide a brief description of this assessment.
5. What is the reliability of the NYHA Classification of Heart Failure?
6. What is the validity of the NYHA Classification of Heart Failure?
7. What functional inference can be deduced from Aki's functional Class III classification?
8. What additional standardized assessment can be used in this case? Why?

INTERPROFESSIONAL RELATIONSHIP AND EFFECTIVE INTRAPROFESSIONAL COLLABORATION

1. Identify the other professions that would make up the care team. Explain the focus of each.
2. Identify the roles of the occupational therapy assistant (OTA) that could be used in the occupational therapy process for this case.
3. Identify interventions that can be assigned to the OTA for this case. Justify your selections.

BILLING AND CODING

1. Identify the *International Classification of Diseases (ICD)* codes for Aki's diagnoses.
2. For this case, identify at least two *Current Procedural Terminology (CPT®)* codes that are most appropriate. Justify your selection.

REIMBURSEMENT SYSTEMS AND DOCUMENTATION

1. Who would be the authorized individuals that you could share the occupational therapy findings with? Explain why.
2. For this case, what forms and frequency of documentation will be required?
3. Which reimbursement system or systems most commonly cover occupational therapy services in this practice setting?

ADVOCACY

1. Which of the following areas of advocacy would be beneficial in this case: patient rights, matters of privacy, confidentiality, informed consent, awareness building, accessing education, or benefits/resources?
2. Create a plan to advocate for this client based on the selected areas of advocacy.

TELEHEALTH

1. How can telehealth be integrated as a component of the occupational therapy process in this case?
2. Before launching telemedicine services, what questions would be essential to ask Aki to determine whether it is appropriate for him to engage in telemedicine services?
3. What are the barriers, obstacles, or challenges you foresee if attempting to integrate telehealth services with this client?

Intervention Plan Formulation and Implementation

INTERVENTION PLAN FORMULATION

Create an intervention plan that includes the following:

1. List this individual's **strengths.**
2. List this individual's **barriers** in occupational performance, performance skills, and performance patterns.
3. Based on the individual's goals, health, performance, and service delivery site, **identify the barriers that will be addressed.**
4. From the barriers identified to be addressed, **formulate goals and objectives.**
5. Identify the focus of each goal and objective as either **create, promote, establish, restore, maintain, modify, or prevent.**
6. Identify the **theoretical basis, model(s) of practice, or frame(s) of reference** that will be used to address each goal and objective.
7. For each proposed goal and objective, describe clearly and precisely the **methods** that will be used. This description should include, but not be limited to, safety considerations, environmental considerations, therapeutic use of self, preparatory activities, activity selection, materials, equipment, and flow.
8. Classify the activities selected in the methods description as either **preparatory, enabling, purposeful, or occupation based.**
9. Explain how each activity can be **graded up or down,** creating the just-right challenge.
10. Provide at least two **primary sources of evidence** to support the intervention plan.

INTERVENTION PLAN IMPLEMENTATION

1. Based on your intervention plan, identify which goals and objectives require **more immediate attention.**
2. Describe your proposed **first treatment session.**
3. As the treatment session is progressing, what is **essential to be observed?**

Transition and Discontinuation

Create a plan for discharge from occupational therapy services in collaboration with Aki and members of the interprofessional team. Review the needs of Aki, caregivers, family members, and significant others. The plan must match needs with available resources and the discharge environment.

REFERENCES

American Medical Association. (2019). *CPT® 2020 professional edition.*

Criteria Committee of the New York Heart Association. (1994). *Nomenclature and criteria for diagnosis of diseases of the heart and great vessels* (9th ed.). Little, Brown and Company.

World Health Organization. (2019). *International statistical classification of diseases and related health problems* (11th ed.). https://icd.who.int/

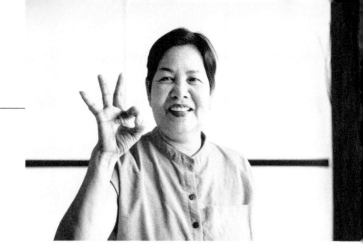

Ting: Osteoporosis

DONALD AURIEMMA, MS ED, OTR/L

Ting (she, her, hers, herself)

MEDICAL HISTORY

Ting is a 72-year-old Malaysian American female who is 5' 2" and weighs 165 pounds. She arrived at the emergency department (ED) of her local community hospital reporting a slip and fall in her bathtub. She presented with stooped posture and complained of severe back pain. After a physical examination, she was sent for X-rays and a computerized axial tomography scan. She was diagnosed with compression fractures of her second and fourth thoracic vertebrae. She was fitted with a thoracic lumbar sacral orthosis (TLSO) and prescribed pain medication.

Her medical history includes hypertension, peripheral vascular disease, osteopenia, myocardial infarction, and blindness in her left eye secondary to a motor vehicle accident. She reported no alcohol, drug, or nicotine use and has no known allergies. From the ED, she was sent to the orthopedic floor for 24 hours of observation.

SOCIAL HISTORY

Ting is a retired custodial worker. She lives alone in a modest one-bedroom, fifth-floor apartment in a building without an elevator. She has no living relatives in the United States and lost her only child in a car accident. She is a practicing Buddhist and socializes with other members of the temple after days and nights of meditation and study.

REFERRAL OR PRESCRIPTION

Ting was transferred to a subacute rehabilitation facility. She has been referred for occupational therapy, physical therapy, registered nursing services, and social work services. The length of stay will be 10 days.

Occupational Therapy Initial Evaluation Findings: Subacute Rehabilitation

OCCUPATIONAL PROFILE

Ting's preadmission occupational history and experiences included being independent in all ADLs and all IADLs. She is a retired mall custodial worker and has lived alone since the passing of her husband 10 years ago. Her patterns of daily living most commonly included having a light breakfast in the morning and spending at least 3 days at the temple engaged in meditation and study. Her interests include visiting friends and watching game shows on television. Ting values truth and understanding. She reported her greatest needs are to be able to return home, live independently, and be able to once again attend her temple.

ADLs

Regarding self-care, Ting was able to independently feed herself and dress both upper extremities (BUE), but she needed moderate assistance to don and doff her pants, shoes, and socks. She was able to independently wash BUE but required moderate assistance washing both lower extremities (BLE). She was able to manage her clothing and clean herself after toileting. Regarding functional mobility, Ting was able to independently roll side to side and required minimal assistance to transition between supine and sitting. She used a rolling walker and required minimal assistance to transfer on and off the bed, chair, toilet, and tub.

IADLs

Activities needed that provide day-to-day quality of life and relative independence were explored. Ting independently managed her communications and finances. She was aware that currently she would not be able to maintain her home, prepare meals, or shop. Regarding rest and sleep, Ting reported being unable to find a comfortable sleeping position and sleeping intermittently at night.

MENTAL FUNCTIONS

Cognitive assessment found Ting to be alert and oriented to person, place, time, and situation, and short- and long-term memory were intact. She was able to follow three-step commands and make her needs known. Her affect appeared appropriate, and Ting stated that she is "highly motivated" to start therapy. No gross deficits in perception were observed.

SENSORY FUNCTIONS AND PAIN

No gross deficits were observed with hearing, vestibular, taste, smell, proprioceptive, and cutaneous functions. Ting reported visual acuity of 20/20 in her right eye and legal blindness in her left. She was unable to detect light or movement in her left eye. Pain in the thoracic spine was reported to be an 8 using the Numerical Rating Scale (0–10). Ting reported fluctuating pain levels between 7 and 10. The pain level at the time of evaluation was reported as an 8. Pain was described as "sharp and continuous." An eye exam was administered using the Snellen Eye Chart (Hetherington, 1954), and a score of 20/400 was obtained.

CARDIOVASCULAR AND RESPIRATORY SYSTEMS FUNCTIONS

Ting experienced intermittent claudication during ambulation.

MOVEMENT FUNCTIONS

Passive range of motion and active range of motion in BUE were within defined limits. Testing muscle strength with the manual muscle test (MMT) was contraindicated at the time of evaluation. Prehension was intact for gross grasp, pinch, and in-hand manipulation skills.

NEUROMUSCULAR FUNCTIONS

Coordination, tone, and reflex integration in BUE and BLE were intact.

PLAN FOR DISCHARGE

Ting will be discharged home and receive services through a certified home health agency. Services will include occupational therapy, physical therapy, social work, nursing, and home health aide services.

Questions and Activities

SAFETY OF CLIENT AND OTHERS: PRECAUTIONS AND CONTRAINDICATIONS

1. Create a handout identifying precautions for individuals with spinal fractures.
2. What wearing schedule will Ting most likely follow with her TLSO?
3. Identify the risks of wearing a TLSO. How can these risks be mitigated?
4. The MMT was contraindicated at the initial evaluation. Why?
5. Identify the common psychological reactions associated with osteoporosis that may affect the treatment process.
6. To keep Ting and others safe, what other factors should be considered?

OCCUPATIONS: ADLs, IADLs, EDUCATION, WORK, PLAY, SOCIAL PARTICIPATION, AND REST AND SLEEP

1. Given the information provided for this case, identify the areas of occupation that will and will not be addressed. Justify your decisions.
2. What strategies can be used to allow Ting to regain independence in lower body dressing?
3. What strategies can be used to allow Ting to regain independence in lower body bathing?
4. What recommendations can you make to allow Ting to experience more restful sleep?

5. What strategies can be used to allow Ting to gain independence transitioning between supine and short sitting?
6. What areas of functional mobility need to be addressed and how?
7. Because Ting will be living alone when she returns home, identify areas of IADLs that need to be addressed. Explain how they should be addressed.

PERFORMANCE SKILLS: MOTOR SKILLS, PROCESS SKILLS, AND SOCIAL INTERACTION SKILLS

1. Given the information provided, identify the motor, process, and social interaction skills that affect Ting's occupational performance.
2. Which of these skills would be appropriate to address in this service delivery site? Justify your selection.
3. Which of these skills would be addressed through remediation, compensation, and education?
4. Which of these skills would be addressed through the following intervention approaches: create/promote, establish/restore, maintain, modify, and prevent?

PERFORMANCE PATTERNS: HABITS, ROUTINES, ROLES, AND RITUALS

1. Identify Ting's useful habits, routines, roles, and rituals that support valued occupations. How can you make use of this information?
2. Identify Ting's impoverished habits, routines, roles, and rituals that do not support valued occupations. How can you make use of this information?
3. Identify Ting's dominating habits, routines, roles, and rituals that interfere with valued occupations. How can you make use of this information?

CLIENT FACTORS

Values, beliefs, and spirituality
How can the identified values, beliefs, and spirituality be used in this case?

Body structures
Considering Ting's primary and secondary diagnoses, identify the related body structures.

Body functions

1. Identify how the primary and secondary diagnoses have affected the function of the identified body structures.
2. Explain the relationships between the structural and functional factors and Ting's current level of occupational performance.

MENTAL FUNCTIONS: AFFECTIVE, COGNITIVE, AND PERCEPTUAL

1. How may high levels of pain affect Ting's motivation over time?
2. Given the information provided, what additional mental function considerations need to be addressed?

NEUROMUSCULOSKELETAL AND MOVEMENT-RELATED FUNCTIONS

1. Given the information provided, identify neuromusculoskeletal and movement-related functions that need to be addressed. Justify your selections.
2. Compare and contrast osteoporosis with osteopenia.
3. List the common lifting restrictions for individuals with spinal fractures.
4. Which of Ting's tasks or activities may need to be modified as a result of lifting restrictions?
5. Create an exercise program for Ting based on occupational performance.

CARDIOVASCULAR, HEMATOLOGICAL, IMMUNOLOGICAL, AND RESPIRATORY FUNCTIONS

1. Given the information provided, identify cardiovascular, hematological, immunological and respiratory functions that need to be addressed.
2. Explain how severe pain affects cardiovascular, hematological, immunological, and respiratory functions.

SKIN AND RELATED STRUCTURE FUNCTIONS

1. What would be the visible signs and reported symptoms of a poorly fitted TLSO?
2. If you become aware of a poorly fitted TLSO, what steps should be taken?
3. What other skin and related structure functions should be considered?

VOICE AND SPEECH FUNCTIONS

Describe how Ting's diagnoses may affect her voice, speech, and associated occupational performance.

ASSISTIVE TECHNOLOGIES AND DEVICES

1. What assistive technologies or adaptations might be used or made for Ting while she is receiving occupational therapy services at the subacute rehabilitation center? Why?
2. What assistive technologies or adaptations might be recommended for when she returns home? Why?

ETHICAL DECISION MAKING

1. While performing a functional ambulation task, a patient with a known brain injury pinches Ting on her buttocks as he wheels his wheelchair past her. How should this action be addressed?
2. In preparation for discharge, Ting informs you that she has no food in her home. How should this situation be addressed?

PHARMACOLOGY

Ting is currently taking Oxycontin.

1. What is the generic name?
2. Does this drug have a high alert status?
3. What is the classification of this drug?
4. What is the indication for this drug?

5. What is the action of this drug?
6. How may this drug affect client participation during a therapy session?

SOCIOCULTURAL, SOCIOECONOMIC, AND DIVERSITY FACTORS AND LIFESTYLE CHOICES

1. Given Ting's profile, how may your own culture and beliefs affect your interaction with her?
2. Based on this self-examination, what areas of cultural knowledge do you need to pursue?
3. How can this newly acquired cultural knowledge be integrated for effective outcomes?
4. How can you foster cultural interaction and awareness among your coworkers?
5. Discuss how a lack of understanding in the areas of discrimination and stigma, implicit bias, social identity, or racism may contribute to disparities in the delivery of occupational therapy services in this case.

ASSESSMENT TOOLS AND INTERPRETATION OF RESULTS

1. What is the purpose of the Snellen Eye Chart?
2. Which population is this test designed for?
3. How much time is required to administer it?
4. Provide a brief description of this assessment.
5. What is the reliability of the Snellen Eye Chart?
6. What is the validity of the Snellen Eye Chart?
7. What functional inference can be deduced from Ting's score of 20/400 in her left eye?
8. What additional standardized assessment can be used in this case? Why?

INTERPROFESSIONAL RELATIONSHIP AND EFFECTIVE INTRAPROFESSIONAL COLLABORATION

1. Identify the other professions that would make up the care team. Explain the focus of each.
2. Identify the roles of the occupational therapy assistant (OTA) that could be used in the occupational therapy process for this case.
3. Identify interventions that can be assigned to the OTA for this case. Justify your selections.

BILLING AND CODING

1. Identify the *International Classification of Diseases (ICD)* codes for Ting's diagnoses.
2. For this case, identify at least two *Current Procedural Terminology (CPT®)* codes that are most appropriate. Justify your selection.

REIMBURSEMENT SYSTEMS AND DOCUMENTATION

1. Who would be the authorized individuals that you could share the occupational therapy findings with? Explain why.
2. For this case, what forms and frequency of documentation will be required?
3. Which reimbursement system or systems most commonly cover occupational therapy services in this practice setting?

ADVOCACY

1. Which of the following areas of advocacy would be beneficial in this case: patient rights, matters of privacy, confidentiality, informed consent, awareness building, accessing education, or benefits/resources?
2. Create a plan to advocate for this client based on the selected areas of advocacy.

TELEHEALTH

1. How can telehealth be integrated as a component of the occupational therapy process in this case?
2. Before launching telemedicine services, what questions would be essential to ask Ting to determine whether it is appropriate for her to engage in telemedicine services?
3. What are the barriers, obstacles, or challenges you foresee if attempting to integrate telehealth services with this client?

Intervention Plan Formulation and Implementation

INTERVENTION PLAN FORMULATION

Create an intervention plan that includes the following:

1. List this individual's **strengths.**
2. List this individual's **barriers** in occupational performance, performance skills, and performance patterns.
3. Based on the individual's goals, health, performance, and service delivery site, **identify the barriers that will be addressed.**
4. From the barriers identified to be addressed, **formulate goals and objectives.**
5. Identify the focus of each goal and objective as either **create, promote, establish, restore, maintain, modify, or prevent.**
6. Identify the **theoretical basis, model(s) of practice, or frame(s) of reference** that will be used to address each goal and objective.
7. For each proposed goal and objective, describe clearly and precisely the **methods** that will be used. This description should include, but not be limited to, safety considerations, environmental considerations, therapeutic use of self, preparatory activities, activity selection, materials, equipment, and flow.
8. Classify the activities selected in the methods description as either **preparatory, enabling, purposeful, or occupation based.**
9. Explain how each activity can be **graded up or down,** creating the just-right challenge.
10. Provide at least two **primary sources of evidence** to support the intervention plan.

INTERVENTION PLAN IMPLEMENTATION

1. Based on your intervention plan, identify which goals and objectives require **more immediate attention.**
2. Describe your proposed **first treatment session.**
3. As the treatment session is progressing, what is **essential to be observed?**

Transition and Discontinuation

Create a plan for discharge from occupational therapy services in collaboration with Ting and members of the interprofessional team. Review the needs of Ting, caregivers, family members, and significant others. The plan must match needs with available resources and the discharge environment.

REFERENCES

American Medical Association. (2019). *CPT® 2020 professional edition.*

Hetherington, R. (1954). The Snellen Chart as a test of visual acuity. *Psychologische Forschung, 24,* 349–357. https://doi.org/10.1007/BF00422033

World Health Organization. (2019). *International statistical classification of diseases and related health problems* (11th ed.). https://icd.who.int/

Skilled Nursing Facility or Long-Term Care

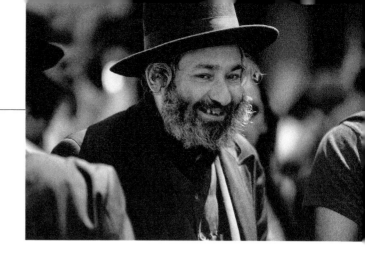

Jacob: Alzheimer's Disease

BEBE HANIF, MS, OTR/L

Jacob: (he, him, his, himself)

MEDICAL HISTORY

Jacob is a 94-year-old Israeli male living in the United States, who is 5' 11" and weighs 193 pounds. He was brought in by emergency medical services to the emergency department after a fall. He was found by the certified nursing assistant on the floor on the right side of his bed at the skilled nursing facility (SNF). A computed tomography scan of the head, X-rays, and blood tests were performed. The scan and X-ray results were negative. His blood test revealed a urinary tract infection. Medical history includes Alzheimer's disease, renal disease, diabetes mellitus, chronic obstructive pulmonary disease, and congestive heart failure. There is no reported alcohol, drug, caffeine, or tobacco use, and he has no known allergies.

SOCIAL HISTORY

Jacob has been a resident in the SNF for the past 6 years. He is a retired delicatessen owner who previously lived and worked in Brooklyn, New York. His wife passed away 15 years ago. He has a son, two grandchildren, and three great-grandchildren who visit occasionally. Jacob practices Hasidic Judaism.

REFERRAL OR PRESCRIPTION

Jacob was transferred back to the SNF for restorative care. He has been referred for occupational and physical therapy. The length of treatment will be 30 days.

Occupational Therapy Initial Evaluation Findings: Skilled Nursing Facility

OCCUPATIONAL PROFILE

Jacob's preadmission occupational history and experiences included requiring assistance in all ADLs. He is nonverbal and follows commands inconsistently. His common pattern of daily living includes being fed, cleaned, and dressed by the nursing assistant and then transferred to his wheelchair and placed in the dining room with the other residents. Daily activities in the dining room include current affairs, games, music, and movies. He is toileted after lunch and returns to bed before dinner. Jacob is not able to state his values, interests, or greatest need.

ADLs

Regarding self-care, Jacob required maximum assistance to feed himself and to dress his upper body. He was dependent with grooming, toileting, bathing, and lower body dressing. The FIM® (Uniform Data System for Medical Rehabilitation, 1997) was completed, and a total score of 51 was obtained. Regarding functional mobility, Jacob required maximum assistance to roll and transition from supine to sit at the edge of the bed. He transferred to and from all surfaces with maximum assistance.

IADLs

Activities needed that provide day-to-day quality of life and relative independence were explored. Jacob was dependent in all areas. Regarding rest and sleep, the medical record indicated that Jacob frequently falls asleep during the day, frequently awakens during the evening, and at times can become agitated.

MENTAL FUNCTIONS

Jacob is alert and oriented times 1 to self. Short- and long-term memory were both impaired. He was able to follow one-step commands but not two-step commands.

SENSORY FUNCTIONS AND PAIN

No gross deficits were observed with visual, hearing, vestibular, taste, smell, proprioceptive, and cutaneous functions. Use of the Wong-Baker FACES® Pain Rating Scale (Wong-Baker FACES Foundation, 2018) indicated a score of 4 in the right upper extremity. No description of pain was able to be obtained.

CARDIOVASCULAR AND RESPIRATORY SYSTEMS FUNCTIONS

Jacob's blood pressure was 143/92 mm Hg, oxygen saturation on room air was 93%, and heart rate was 84 beats per minute.

MOVEMENT FUNCTIONS

Limited active range of motion and passive range of motion were noted in all extremities; goniometric assessment was unable to be performed. The manual muscle test (grossly) indicated a score of 3 to 3+/5 for both upper extremities (BUE) and both lower extremities (BLE).

NEUROMUSCULAR FUNCTIONS

Jacob was able to sit at the edge of the bed with maximum assistance. Static and dynamic sitting balance were 3–/5 (F-), and static and dynamic standing balance were 2/5 (P). Muscle tone in BUE and BLE was rigid. Bradykinesia and tremors were present.

PLAN FOR DISCHARGE

Jacob will be discharged to his home at the SNF.

Questions and Activities

SAFETY OF CLIENT AND OTHERS: PRECAUTIONS AND CONTRAINDICATIONS

1. Create a handout that provides recommendations to maximize communication with Jacob.
2. What safety concerns do you anticipate because Jacob has a history of falls?
3. What safety concerns do you anticipate because Jacob presents with impaired vision and hearing?
4. To keep Jacob and others safe, what other factors should be considered?

OCCUPATIONS: ADLs, IADLs, EDUCATION, WORK, PLAY, SOCIAL PARTICIPATION, AND REST AND SLEEP

1. Given the information provided for this case, identify the areas of occupation that will and will not be addressed. Justify your decisions.
2. What clothing choices would you recommend for Jacob to avoid discomfort?
3. What equipment and strategies do you anticipate can be used to increase Jacob's safety in bed and in the wheelchair?
4. Would you address any functional mobility skills with Jacob?
5. Would you address socialization or sleep with Jacob? Why or why not?

PERFORMANCE SKILLS: MOTOR SKILLS, PROCESS SKILLS, AND SOCIAL INTERACTION SKILLS

1. Given the information provided, identify the motor, process, and social interaction skills that affect Jacob's occupational performance.
2. Which of these skills would be appropriate to address in this service delivery site? Justify your selection.
3. Which of these skills would be addressed through remediation, compensation, and education?
4. Which of these skills would be addressed through the following intervention approaches: create/promote, establish/restore, maintain, modify, and prevent?

PERFORMANCE PATTERNS: HABITS, ROUTINES, ROLES, AND RITUALS

1. Identify Jacob's useful habits, routines, roles, and rituals that support valued occupations. How can you make use of this information?
2. Identify Jacob's impoverished habits, routines, roles, and rituals that do not support valued occupations. How can you make use of this information?
3. Identify Jacob's dominating habits, routines, roles, and rituals that interfere with valued occupations. How can you make use of this information?

CLIENT FACTORS

Values, beliefs, and spirituality
How can the identified values, beliefs and spirituality be used in this case?

Body structures
Considering Jacob's primary and secondary diagnoses, identify the related body structures.

Body functions
1. Identify how the primary and secondary diagnoses have affected the function of the identified body structures.
2. Explain the relationships between the structural and functional factors and current level of occupational performance.

MENTAL FUNCTIONS: AFFECTIVE, COGNITIVE, AND PERCEPTUAL

1. Compare and contrast Alzheimer's disease with Lewy body dementia.
2. Identify three strategies that could be used to maximize effective communication with Jacob. How would you evaluate them?
3. Identify sources that could provide effective strategies to maximize Jacob's ability to use his available vision and hearing.
4. Given the information provided, what additional mental function considerations need to be addressed?

NEUROMUSCULOSKELETAL AND MOVEMENT-RELATED FUNCTIONS

1. Given the information provided, identify neuromusculoskeletal and movement-related functions that need to be addressed. Justify your selections.
2. Based on the finding "patient was able to sit at the edge of the bed with maximum assist," should Jacob's static balance be assigned a grade of poor or poor+? Provide your reference.
3. Based on the finding "patient was unable to stand/pivot for transfer bed to a wheelchair," which commercial device or devices are available to assist?
4. Create an exercise program to be provided to Jacob's care providers that is based on occupational performance.

CARDIOVASCULAR, HEMATOLOGICAL, IMMUNOLOGICAL, AND RESPIRATORY FUNCTIONS

1. Given the information provided, identify cardiovascular, hematological, immunological, and respiratory functions that need to be addressed. Justify your selections.

2. Which vital signs should be taken when working with Jacob? Identify the norms for each of these vital signs and when they should be taken.

SKIN AND RELATED STRUCTURE FUNCTIONS

1. On arrival at the occupational therapy area, you notice a swelling on Jacob's right arm. What would be a concern and what possible actions would you take?
2. What other skin and related structure functions should be considered?

VOICE AND SPEECH FUNCTIONS

Describe how Jacob's diagnoses may affect his voice, speech, and associated occupational performance.

ASSISTIVE TECHNOLOGIES AND DEVICES

What assistive technologies or adaptations might be used or made for Jacob for comfort or positioning? Why?

ETHICAL DECISION MAKING

1. Jacob becomes agitated and restless in the evenings. What strategies would you use to calm him?
2. Jacob's grandson comes to you, uses a racial slur, and demands that you place his grandfather in a restorative occupational therapy program. What is your reaction, what do you say, and how do you support your decision?

PHARMACOLOGY

Jacob is currently taking Aricept.

1. What is the generic name?
2. Does this drug have a high alert status?
3. What is the classification of this drug?
4. What is the indication for this drug?
5. What is the action of this drug?
6. How may this drug affect client participation during basic ADLs?

SOCIOCULTURAL, SOCIOECONOMIC, AND DIVERSITY FACTORS AND LIFESTYLE CHOICES

1. Given Jacob's profile, how may your own culture and beliefs affect your interaction with him?
2. Based on this self-examination, what area of cultural knowledge do you need to pursue?
3. How can this newly acquired cultural knowledge be integrated for effective outcomes?
4. How can you foster cultural interaction and awareness among your coworkers?
5. Discuss how a lack of understanding in the areas of discrimination and stigma, implicit bias, social identity, or racism may contribute to disparities in the delivery of occupational therapy services in this case.

ASSESSMENT TOOLS AND INTERPRETATION OF RESULTS

1. What is the purpose of the FIM?
2. Which population is this test designed for?
3. How much time is required to administer it?
4. Provide a brief description of this assessment.
5. What is the reliability of the FIM?
6. What is the validity of the FIM?
7. What functional inference can be deduced from Jacob's score of 51?
8. What additional standardized assessment can be used in this case? Why?

INTERPROFESSIONAL RELATIONSHIP AND EFFECTIVE INTRAPROFESSIONAL COLLABORATION

1. Identify the other professions that would make up the care team. Explain the focus of each.
2. Identify the roles of the occupational therapy assistant (OTA) that could be used in the occupational therapy process for this case.
3. Identify interventions that can be assigned to the OTA for this case. Justify your selections.

BILLING AND CODING

1. Identify the *International Classification of Diseases (ICD)* codes for Jacob's diagnoses.
2. For this case, identify at least two *Current Procedural Terminology (CPT®)* codes that are most appropriate. Justify your selection.

REIMBURSEMENT SYSTEMS AND DOCUMENTATION

1. Who would be the authorized individuals that you could share the occupational therapy findings with? Explain why.
2. For this case, what forms and frequency of documentation will be required?
3. Which reimbursement system or systems most commonly cover occupational therapy services in this practice setting?

ADVOCACY

1. Which of the following areas of advocacy would be beneficial in this case: patient rights, matters of privacy, confidentiality, informed consent, awareness building, accessing education, or benefits/ resources?
2. Create a plan to advocate for this client based on the selected areas of advocacy.

TELEHEALTH

1. How can telehealth be integrated as a component of the occupational therapy process in this case?
2. Before launching telemedicine services, what questions would be essential to ask Jacob's caregivers to determine whether it is appropriate for him to engage in telemedicine services?
3. What challenges do you foresee if attempting to integrate telehealth services with this client?

Intervention Plan Formulation and Implementation

INTERVENTION PLAN FORMULATION

Create an intervention plan that includes the following:

1. List this individual's **strengths.**
2. List this individual's **barriers** in occupational performance, performance skills, and performance patterns.
3. Based on the individual's goals, health, performance, and service delivery site, **identify the barriers that will be addressed.**
4. From the barriers identified to be addressed, **formulate goals and objectives.**
5. Identify the focus of each goal and objective as either **create, promote, establish, restore, maintain, modify, or prevent.**
6. Identify the **theoretical basis, model(s) of practice, or frame(s) of reference** that will be used to address each goal and objective.
7. For each proposed goal and objective, describe clearly and precisely the **methods** that will be used. This description should include, but not be limited to, safety considerations, environmental considerations, therapeutic use of self, preparatory activities, activity selection, materials, equipment, and flow.
8. Classify the activities selected in the methods description as either **preparatory, enabling, purposeful, or occupation based.**
9. Explain how each activity can be **graded up or down,** creating the just-right challenge.
10. Provide at least two **primary sources of evidence** to support the intervention plan.

INTERVENTION PLAN IMPLEMENTATION

1. Based on your intervention plan, identify which goals and objectives require **more immediate attention.**
2. Describe your proposed **first treatment session.**
3. As the treatment session is progressing, what is **essential to be observed?**

Transition and Discontinuation

Create a plan for discharge from occupational therapy services in collaboration with Jacob and members of the interprofessional team. Review the needs of Jacob, caregivers, family members, and significant others. The plan must match needs with available resources and the discharge environment.

REFERENCES

American Medical Association. (2019). *CPT® 2020 professional edition.*
Uniform Data System for Medical Rehabilitation. (1997). *Guide for the Uniform Data Set for Medical Rehabilitation (including the FIM® instrument), version 5.1.* Author.
Wong-Baker FACES Foundation. (2018). *Wong-Baker FACES® Pain Rating Scale.*
World Health Organization. (2019). *International statistical classification of diseases and related health problems* (11th ed.). https://icd.who.int/

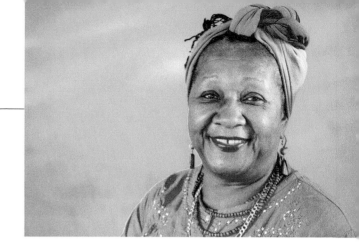

Aretha: End-Stage Renal Disease

VIKRAM PAGPATAN, OTR/L, ATP, BCP, CLA

Aretha (she, her, hers, herself)

MEDICAL HISTORY

Aretha is a 78-year-old Trinidadian American female who is 5' 9" and weighs 230 pounds. Aretha was found unresponsive in a pool of blood by her daughter, who called emergency medical services, and she was subsequently taken to her community hospital's emergency department (ED). A physical examination, X-rays, and blood tests were done. The exam revealed that Aretha's right bicep had an arteriovenous fistula and was in a deconditioned state. From the ED, she was sent to the operating room, and a surgical repair of the fistula was performed. Her medical history includes end-stage renal disease, Type 2 diabetes mellitus, generalized anxiety disorder, ovarian cancer, and osteoarthritis. Aretha has a surgical history of a complete hysterectomy and a humeral fixation after a mechanical fall. Aretha undergoes hemodialysis three times a week. She reported no alcohol, drug, tobacco, or caffeine use. She reported a wheat allergy.

SOCIAL HISTORY

Aretha is originally from Trinidad and Tobago and has resided in the Bronx, New York, for more than 20 years. Aretha has two sons who are both employed full time in the city's sanitation department as shift supervisors, and a daughter who is a school principal. Aretha has been a widow for 7 years and resides alone in a cooperative building. Her unit is a studio apartment with elevator access. Aretha has been retired for 12 years but is employed as a substitute teacher on a per diem basis for a contract agency. She owns a vehicle that is used by her neighbor to drive her to her medical and hemodialysis appointments. Aretha is a member of Jehovah's Witnesses and has weekly religious obligations at her place of worship.

REFERRAL OR PRESCRIPTION

Aretha was transferred to a skilled nursing facility (SNF) for restorative care. She has been referred for occupational therapy, physical therapy, social work, and registered nursing services. The length of stay will be 30 days.

Occupational Therapy Initial Evaluation Findings: Skilled Nursing Facility

OCCUPATIONAL PROFILE

Aretha's preadmission occupational history and experiences included being independent in all ADLs and requiring minimal assistance for homemaking tasks such as laundry, house cleaning, and food shopping. Before her hospitalization, Aretha hired a neighbor to help her with these tasks. She is also driven by her neighbor to and from the dialysis center 3 days per week. Her daily routine on the remaining 4 days included waking early, bathing, eating breakfast, and then traveling to and spending the day at the Kingdom Hall. She values her time, family, and spiritual community. Her interests include tutoring at-risk children in her community and cooking traditional Caribbean dishes. She reported her greatest needs are to return home and reestablish her previous level of independence and to be healthy enough to receive a kidney transplant.

ADLs

Regarding self-care, Aretha required contact guard assistance (CGA) for upper- and lower-body dressing as well as minimal to moderate assistance for bathing and toileting. Regarding functional mobility, Aretha was able to roll, transition between supine and short sit, and bridge independently. She requires CGA to transfer, using a wide-based quad cane on and off the chair, bed, and toilet. When standing, Aretha reports feeling dizzy and anxious. She disclosed a history of falling on three separate occasions at home when transferring out of her bathtub.

IADLs

Activities needed that provide day-to-day quality of life and relative independence were explored. Aretha was able to manage her finances, use her mobile device, and prepare meals but was unable to clean her home, shop, and do laundry. Regarding rest and sleep, Aretha reported waking up frequently during the night because of "intense throbbing" sensations in her knees.

MENTAL FUNCTIONS

Cognitive assessment found Aretha to be alert and oriented to person, place, time, and situation, and short- and long-term memory were intact. She was able to follow three-step commands and make her needs known. Her affect appeared appropriate. Aretha was found to be calm and cooperative but was in denial of her limitations. The Beck Anxiety Inventory (BAI; Beck & Steer, 1993) was administered, and a score of 25 was recorded. No gross deficits in perception were observed.

SENSORY FUNCTIONS AND PAIN

No gross deficits were observed with visual, hearing, taste, smell, and proprioceptive functions. A vestibular assessment revealed that sudden transitions resulted in dizziness. She presented with a diminished light touch in both upper extremities and reported tingling sensations in her right dominant hand, localized to digits 1–3. Aretha reported "tenderness and hypersensitivity" to touch at the fistula site. She reported pain as a 5 in both knees using the Numerical Rating Scale (0–10).

CARDIOVASCULAR AND RESPIRATORY SYSTEMS FUNCTION

Aretha's resting blood pressure is 162/93 mmHg, and her heart rate is 103 beats per minute. She experienced shortness of breath when ambulating for a distance greater than 200 feet. Her baseline oxygen saturation is 96%, and her respiration rate is 18 breaths per minute.

MOVEMENT FUNCTIONS

Aretha's active range of motion (AROM) in all extremities was within defined limits (WDL) with the exception of the right upper extremity, which had shoulder flexion of 0–110°, shoulder abduction of 0–105°, shoulder external rotation of 0–70°, shoulder internal rotation of 0–80°, and shoulder horizontal adduction of 0–95°. Muscle strength in both upper extremities was grossly 3–/5 in shoulder groups and 3+/5 in distal groups. Gross grasp strength was 11 pounds on the right and 9 pounds on the left. Fine motor abilities were intact for grasp formation, pinch formation, and in-hand manipulation.

NEUROMUSCULAR FUNCTIONS

Aretha's static and dynamic sitting balance was 4/5 (good). Her static and dynamic standing balance was 3+/5 (fair+). Her standing tolerance was 3–5 minutes. Abrupt movements resulted in dizziness. Muscle tone was found to be WDL in both upper and lower extremities. Reflex integration was grossly intact.

PLAN FOR DISCHARGE

Aretha is expected to be discharged home with home care services. Services will include occupational therapy; physical therapy; and registered nursing, social work, and home health aide services.

Questions and Activities

SAFETY OF CLIENT AND OTHERS: PRECAUTIONS AND CONTRAINDICATIONS

1. Create a handout that identifies the general precautions for an individual with a fistula.
2. Can blood pressure be taken on the right upper extremity? Why or why not?
3. What resting blood pressure threshold would make occupational therapy treatment contraindicated?
4. What resting heart rate would make occupational therapy treatment contraindicated?
5. To keep Aretha and others safe, what other factors should be considered?

OCCUPATIONS: ADLs, IADLs, EDUCATION, WORK, PLAY, SOCIAL PARTICIPATION, AND REST AND SLEEP

1. Given the information provided for this case, identify the areas of occupation that will and will not be addressed. Justify your decisions.
2. How does a fistula affect self-care activities?
3. What recommendations can you make to allow Aretha to obtain more restful sleep?
4. What strategies can be used for Aretha to gain independence during bathing?
5. What strategies can be used for Aretha to gain independence during dressing?

PERFORMANCE SKILLS: MOTOR SKILLS, PROCESS SKILLS, AND SOCIAL INTERACTION SKILLS

1. Given the information provided, identify the motor, process, and social interaction skills that affect Aretha's occupational performance.
2. Which of these skills would be appropriate to address in this service delivery site? Justify your selection.
3. Which of these skills would be addressed through remediation, compensation, and education?
4. Which of these skills would be addressed through the following intervention approaches: create/promote, establish/restore, maintain, modify, and prevent?

PERFORMANCE PATTERNS: HABITS, ROUTINES, ROLES, AND RITUALS

1. Identify Aretha's useful habits, routines, roles, and rituals that support valued occupations. How can you make use of this information?
2. Identify Aretha's impoverished habits, routines, roles, and rituals that do not support valued occupations. How can you make use of this information?
3. Identify Aretha's dominating habits, routines, roles, and rituals that interfere with valued occupations. How can you make use of this information?

CLIENT FACTORS

Values, beliefs, and spirituality
How can Aretha's values, beliefs, and spirituality be used in this case?

Body structures
Considering Aretha's primary and secondary diagnoses, identify the related body structures.

Body functions
1. Identify how the primary and secondary diagnoses have affected the function of the identified body structures.
2. Explain the relationships between the structural and functional factors and Aretha's current level of occupational performance.

MENTAL FUNCTIONS: AFFECTIVE, COGNITIVE, AND PERCEPTUAL

1. Identify a current theory or theories to address Aretha's anxiety. Briefly explain your choice.
2. Describe an approach you would use with Aretha to gain a more realistic view of her physical capabilities. Justify your proposed approach.
3. Given the information provided, what additional mental function considerations need to be addressed?

NEUROMUSCULOSKELETAL AND MOVEMENT-RELATED FUNCTIONS

1. Given the information provided, identify neuromusculoskeletal and movement-related functions that need to be addressed. Justify your selections.
2. Identify strategies that can be used to address the restoration of AROM of the right shoulder given the presence of the fistula.
3. Describe how impaired standing balance can contribute to the risk of falls. Site two sources to support your position.
4. List at least three activities that Aretha may have difficulty performing given her current standing tolerance.
5. Create an exercise program for Aretha based on occupational performance.

CARDIOVASCULAR, HEMATOLOGICAL, IMMUNOLOGICAL, AND RESPIRATORY FUNCTIONS

1. Given the information provided, identify cardiovascular, hematological, immunological, and respiratory functions that need to be addressed. Justify your selections.
2. Compare and contrast end-stage renal disease with acute renal failure.
3. Identify the metabolic equivalent of task value that you would currently assign to Aretha. Support your decision.
4. Explain how Aretha's baseline blood pressure could affect treatment.
5. Compare and contrast the signs and symptoms of vertigo with orthostatic hypotension.

SKIN AND RELATED STRUCTURE FUNCTIONS

1. What skin care should be provided in the area of the fistula?
2. Identify the possible explanation for the report of tingling sensations to digits 1–3.
3. Identify the long-term skin changes related to diabetes.
4. What other skin and related structure functions should be considered?

VOICE AND SPEECH FUNCTIONS

Describe how Aretha's diagnoses may affect her voice, speech, and associated occupational performance.

ASSISTIVE TECHNOLOGIES AND DEVICES

1. What assistive technologies or adaptations might be used or made for Aretha while she is receiving occupational therapy services in the SNF? Why?
2. What assistive technologies or adaptations might be recommended for Aretha when she returns home? Why?

ETHICAL DECISION MAKING

1. During treatment, a staff member mistakenly identifies Aretha as African American. How would you address this mistake?
2. After a treatment session, Aretha provides you with literature about her religion. What would you think or feel? What would you do?

PHARMACOLOGY

Aretha is taking erythropoietin.

1. What is the brand name?
2. Does this drug have a high alert status?
3. What is the classification of this drug?
4. What is the indication for this drug?
5. What is the action of this drug?
6. How may this drug affect client participation during a therapy session?

SOCIOCULTURAL, SOCIOECONOMIC, AND DIVERSITY FACTORS AND LIFESTYLE CHOICES

1. Given Aretha's profile, how may your own culture and beliefs affect your interaction with her?
2. Based on this self-examination, what area of cultural knowledge do you need to pursue?
3. How can this newly acquired cultural knowledge be integrated for effective outcomes?
4. How can you foster cultural interaction and awareness among your coworkers?
5. Discuss how a lack of understanding in the areas of discrimination and stigma, implicit bias, social identity, or racism may contribute to disparities in the delivery of occupational therapy services in this case.

ASSESSMENT TOOLS AND INTERPRETATION OF RESULTS

1. What is the purpose of the BAI?
2. Which population is this test designed for?
3. How much time is required to administer it?
4. Provide a brief description of this assessment.
5. What is the reliability of the BAI?
6. What is the validity of the BAI?
7. What additional standardized assessment can be used in this case? Why?

INTERPROFESSIONAL RELATIONSHIP AND EFFECTIVE INTRAPROFESSIONAL COLLABORATION

1. Identify the other professions that would make up the care team. Explain the focus of each.
2. Identify the roles of the occupational therapy assistant (OTA) that could be used in the occupational therapy process for this case.
3. Identify interventions that can be assigned to the OTA for this case. Justify your selections.

BILLING AND CODING

1. Identify the *International Classification of Diseases (ICD) codes* for Aretha's diagnoses.
2. For this case, identify at least two *Current Procedural Terminology (CPT®)* codes that are most appropriate. Justify your selection.

REIMBURSEMENT SYSTEMS AND DOCUMENTATION

1. Who would be the authorized persons you could share the occupational therapy findings with? Explain why.
2. Who would be the unauthorized persons with whom you could not share the occupational therapy findings without written permission? Explain why.
3. What forms of documentation will be required for this case?

ADVOCACY

1. Which of the following areas of advocacy would be beneficial in this case: patient rights, matters of privacy, confidentiality, informed consent, awareness building, accessing education, or benefits/resources?
2. Create a plan to advocate for this client based on the selected areas of advocacy.

TELEHEALTH

1. How can telehealth be integrated as a component of the occupational therapy process in this case?
2. Before launching telemedicine services, what questions would be essential to ask Aretha to determine whether it is appropriate for her to engage in telemedicine services?
3. What are the barriers, obstacles, or challenges you foresee if attempting to integrate telehealth services with this client?

Intervention Plan Formulation and Implementation

INTERVENTION PLAN FORMULATION

Create an intervention plan that includes the following:

1. List this individual's **strengths.**
2. List this individual's **barriers** in occupational performance, performance skills, and performance patterns.
3. Based on the individual's goals, health, performance, and service delivery site, **identify the barriers that will be addressed.**
4. From the barriers identified to be addressed, **formulate goals and objectives.**
5. Identify the focus of each goal and objective as either **create, promote, establish, restore, maintain, modify, or prevent.**
6. Identify the **theoretical basis, model(s) of practice, or frame(s) of reference** that will be used to address each goal and objective.
7. For each proposed goal and objective, describe clearly and precisely the **methods** that will be used. This description should include, but not be limited to, safety considerations, environmental considerations, therapeutic use of self, preparatory activities, activity selection, materials, equipment, and flow.
8. Classify the activities selected in the methods description as either **preparatory, enabling, purposeful, or occupation based.**
9. Explain how each activity can be **graded up or down,** creating the just-right challenge.
10. Provide at least two **primary sources of evidence** to support the intervention plan.

INTERVENTION PLAN IMPLEMENTATION

1. Based on your intervention plan, identify which goals and objectives require **more immediate attention.**
2. Describe your proposed **first treatment session.**
3. As the treatment session is progressing, what is **essential to be observed?**

Transition and Discontinuation

Create a plan for discharge from occupational therapy services in collaboration with Aretha and members of the interprofessional team. Review the needs of Aretha, caregivers, family members, and significant others. The plan must match needs with available resources and the discharge environment.

REFERENCES

American Medical Association. (2019). *CPT® 2020 professional edition.*

Beck, A. T., & Steer, R. A. (1993). *Beck Anxiety Inventory manual.* Psychological Corporation.

World Health Organization. (2019). *International statistical classification of diseases and related health problems* (11th ed.). https://icd.who.int/

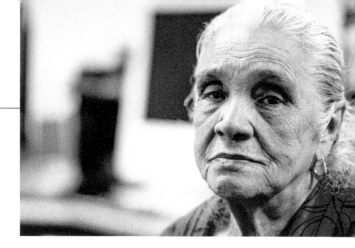

Epa: Diabetes

DONALD AURIEMMA, MS ED, OTR/L

Epa (she, her, hers, herself)

MEDICAL HISTORY

Epa is a 72-year-old Polynesian American who is 5' 4" and weighs 178 pounds. She was admitted to a skilled nursing facility (SNF) after an above-knee amputation of her right lower extremity. At age 3, she was diagnosed with juvenile-onset diabetes mellitus. Her medical history includes diabetic retinopathy, which has led to legal blindness; renal failure requiring dialysis; and left ventricular congestive heart failure. She reported no alcohol, substance, nicotine, or caffeine use. Epa reported being allergic to animal dander.

SOCIAL HISTORY

Epa has lived with her spouse, Roger, for 42 years. They own a loft together in lower Manhattan. The loft has served as both a home and working studio for both her and Roger. For the past 2 years, they have eaten all meals out and had a cleaning service for their home. Epa and Roger have a large community of friends, who mostly include photographers as well as performing and studio artists. They have traveled the world together pursuing their photographic endeavors and have been fixtures in the New York art community. Epa identifies as an animist.

REFERRAL OR PRESCRIPTION

Epa was transferred to a SNF for restorative care. She has been referred for occupational therapy, physical therapy, social work, and registered nursing services. The length of stay will be 30 days.

Occupational Therapy Initial Evaluation Findings: Skilled Nursing Facility

OCCUPATIONAL PROFILE

Epa's preadmission occupational history and experiences included requiring assistance to perform most of her ADLs and all IADLs. Epa is a renowned photographer who was forced to retire as a result of her failing vision and health. Her works are on display at both the Museum of Modern Art and the Smithsonian. For the past 10 years, Epa and Roger have hired people to care for their home. Her failing health has required Roger to assist her with most of her basic ADLs. Epa is on hemodialysis and frequently finds herself without energy. Epa values her contribution to the art world, her marriage to Roger, and notions of equality and equity. Her interests include spending quality time with Roger. She reported her greatest needs are not to be a burden on Roger, being as independent as possible, and being able to engage remotely with the members of her art community.

ADLs

Regarding self-care, Epa was able to self-feed when food and utensils were placed within her reach. With moderate assistance, she could dress and bathe her upper extremities but needed total assistance with lower extremities. She was able to brush her teeth but required moderate assistance to shave. Epa required moderate assistance to manage clothing after toileting. Regarding functional mobility, Epa was able to roll in bed independently but required maximal assistance to transition between supine and both short and long sitting positions. She required maximal assistance to perform stand pivot transfers between the bed and wheelchair and the wheelchair and commode.

IADLs

Activities needed that provide day-to-day quality of life and relative independence were explored. Epa was not able to manage her home or finances and required assistance with communication devices. The Lawton IADL Scale (Lawton & Brody, 1969) was administered, and Epa obtained a total score of 2 (i.e., 1 point for *answers phone but does not dial* and 1 point for *is responsible for taking medication in correct dosages at correct time*). Regarding rest and sleep, Epa reported sleeping only 2 hours at a time secondary to hypersensitivity in her right residual limb.

MENTAL FUNCTIONS

Cognitive assessment found Epa to be alert and oriented to person, place, time, and situation, and short- and long-term memory were intact. She was able to follow three-step commands and make her needs known. Affect appeared appropriate, but she became noticeably teary-eyed when she referred to the burden she has placed on Roger. No gross deficits in perception were observed.

SENSORY FUNCTIONS AND PAIN

No gross deficits were observed with hearing, vestibular, taste, smell, and proprioceptive functions. Epa reported a corrected visual acuity of 20/200 in both eyes. She presented with diminished light touch, deep pressure, and thermal sensation in both hands. All digits presented with a delayed capillary refill and shiny skin. No pain was reported.

CARDIOVASCULAR AND RESPIRATORY SYSTEMS FUNCTION

Epa's cardiovascular endurance was assessed at 2.5 using the metabolic equivalent of task (MET).

MOVEMENT FUNCTIONS

Passive range of motion and active range of motion were within defined limits. Muscle strength in all groups of the left upper extremity (LUE) was 3+/5. The manual muscle test (MMT) of the right upper extremity (RUE) was not performed because of the presence of an arteriovenous fistula. Assessment of fine motor abilities identified difficulty using palmar pinch and tip-to-tip pinch and manipulating small objects.

NEUROMUSCULAR FUNCTIONS

The Balance Grading Review was used to assess Epa's static and dynamic sitting balance, which were good, and her static and dynamic standing balance, which were poor. She could tolerate short sitting for up to 30 minutes before complaints of fatigue. Standing tolerance was not assessed, and muscle tone was normal. Reflex integration was grossly intact.

PLAN FOR DISCHARGE

After completion of her subacute stay, Epa will transition to become a resident at the SNF.

Questions and Activities

SAFETY OF CLIENT AND OTHERS: PRECAUTIONS AND CONTRAINDICATIONS

1. Create a handout identifying the postsurgical precautions to be followed after a lower extremity amputation.
2. Given that Epa presents with impaired cutaneous sensory loss in both hands, what precautions need to be considered?
3. Because Epa has been diagnosed with left ventricular heart failure, what precautions need to be followed?
4. Identify the precautions that should be followed for legal blindness. Cite your source and justify your selection.
5. Compare and contrast legal blindness with low vision.
6. Identify the common emotional reactions associated with an amputation that may affect the treatment process.
7. To keep Epa and others safe, what other factors should be considered?

OCCUPATIONS: ADLs, IADLs, EDUCATION, WORK, PLAY, SOCIAL PARTICIPATION, AND REST AND SLEEP

1. Given the information provided for this case, identify the areas of occupation that will and will not be addressed. Justify your decisions.
2. How is *legal blindness* defined?
3. How would you maximize Epa's residual vision during engagement in the occupational therapy process?
4. Considering Epa's MET value, which self-care task would be the least and most challenging for her?
5. Considering Epa's MET value, what areas of functional mobility should be addressed first?
6. Transfers commonly can be performed using a sliding board, sliding method, squat pivot method, stand pivot method, or an ambulation device. Which method would be the most appropriate for Epa? Explain why.
7. What recommendations can be made to facilitate more restful sleep for Epa?

PERFORMANCE SKILLS: MOTOR SKILLS, PROCESS SKILLS, AND SOCIAL INTERACTION SKILLS

1. Given the information provided, identify the motor, process, and social interaction skills that affect Epa's occupational performance.
2. Which of these skills would be appropriate to address in this service delivery site? Justify your selection.
3. Which of these skills would be addressed through remediation, compensation, and education?
4. Which of these skills would be addressed through the following intervention approaches: create/promote, establish/restore, maintain, modify, and prevent?

PERFORMANCE PATTERNS: HABITS, ROUTINES, ROLES, AND RITUALS

1. Identify Epa's useful habits, routines, roles, and rituals that support valued occupations. How can you make use of this information?
2. Identify Epa's impoverished habits, routines, roles, and rituals that do not support valued occupations. How can you make use of this information?
3. Identify Epa's dominating habits, routines, roles, and rituals that interfere with valued occupations. How can you make use of this information?

CLIENT FACTORS

Values, beliefs, and spirituality
How can the identified values, beliefs, and spirituality be used in this case?

Body structures
Considering Epa's primary and secondary diagnoses, identify the related body structures.

Body Functions
1. Identify how the primary and secondary diagnoses have affected the function of the identified body structures.
2. Explain the relationships between the structural and functional factors and Epa's current level of occupational performance.

MENTAL FUNCTIONS: AFFECTIVE, COGNITIVE, AND PERCEPTUAL

1. Search the literature and identify how amputation affects body image. Provide a brief summary of the findings.
2. Given the information provided, what additional mental function considerations need to be addressed?

NEUROMUSCULOSKELETAL AND MOVEMENT-RELATED FUNCTIONS

1. Given the information provided, identify neuromusculoskeletal and movement-related functions that need to be addressed. Justify your selections.
2. How has Epa's right above-knee amputation affected her center of gravity?
3. What considerations should be made when designing a treatment plan for an individual with a lower-extremity amputation that accounts for a shift in the center of gravity?
4. The MMT was contraindicated for Epa's RUE. Explain why.
5. Is Epa a candidate to remediate muscle strength in her LUE? Explain why.
6. Create an exercise program for Epa based on occupational performance.

CARDIOVASCULAR, HEMATOLOGICAL, IMMUNOLOGICAL, AND RESPIRATORY FUNCTIONS

1. Given the information provided, identify cardiovascular, hematological, immunological, and respiratory functions that need to be addressed. Justify your selections.
2. Compare and contrast Type 1 diabetes with Type 2 diabetes.
3. Do you believe Epa will be a candidate to receive a prosthetic leg? Justify your decision.
4. Create a handout identifying energy conservation principles.
5. Identify the type or types of monitoring required when working with a person who has ventricular heart failure.
6. Identify the signs and symptoms of hyperglycemia and hypoglycemia.
7. What must be done for a client who experiences an episode of hyperglycemia or hypoglycemia?

SKIN AND RELATED STRUCTURE FUNCTIONS

1. What is an indication of a prolonged capillary refill?
2. What might be an explanation for Epa's diminished light touch, deep pressure, and thermal sensation in both hands?
3. What other skin and related structure functions should be considered?

VOICE AND SPEECH FUNCTIONS

Describe how Epa's diagnoses may affect her voice, speech, and associated occupational performance.

ASSISTIVE TECHNOLOGIES AND DEVICES

What assistive technologies or adaptations might be used or made for Epa while she is receiving occupational therapy services? Why?

ETHICAL DECISION MAKING

1. Epa informs you that she and Roger have not engaged in any sexual intimacy for more than 3 months. She asks you how the facility would ensure their privacy if they choose to be sexually intimate. What is required to best address her question?
2. You observe that because of Epa's celebrity status, she receives a higher level of care than others. How should this situation be addressed?
3. Without prompting, during a treatment session Epa expresses her belief that God is only a creation of man's imagination. How should this situation be addressed?

PHARMACOLOGY

Epa is currently taking Humalog.

1. What is the generic name?
2. Does this drug have a high alert status?
3. What is the classification of this drug?
4. What is the indication for this drug?
5. What is the action of this drug?
6. How may this drug affect client participation during a therapy session?

SOCIOCULTURAL, SOCIOECONOMIC, AND DIVERSITY FACTORS AND LIFESTYLE CHOICES

1. Given Epa's profile, how may your own culture and beliefs affect your interaction with her?
2. Based on this self-examination, what area of cultural knowledge do you need to pursue?
3. How can this newly acquired cultural knowledge be integrated for effective outcomes?
4. Discuss how a lack of understanding in the areas of discrimination and stigma, implicit bias, social identity, or racism may contribute to disparities in the delivery of occupational therapy services in this case.

ASSESSMENT TOOLS AND INTERPRETATION OF RESULTS

1. What is the purpose of the Lawton IADL Scale?
2. Which population is this test designed for?
3. How much time is required to administer it?
4. Provide a brief description of this assessment.
5. What is the reliability of the Lawton IADL Scale?
6. What is the validity of the Lawton IADL Scale?
7. What functional inference can be deduced from Epa's score of 2 on the scale?
8. What additional standardized assessment can be used in this case? Why?

INTERPROFESSIONAL RELATIONSHIP AND EFFECTIVE INTRAPROFESSIONAL COLLABORATION

1. Identify the other professions that would make up the care team. Explain the focus of each.
2. Identify the roles of the occupational therapy assistant (OTA) that could be used in the occupational therapy process for this case.
3. Identify interventions that can be assigned to the OTA for this case. Justify your selections.

BILLING AND CODING

1. Identify the *International Classification of Diseases (ICD)* codes for Epa's diagnoses.
2. For this case, identify at least two *Current Procedural Terminology (CPT®)* codes that are most appropriate. Justify your section.

REIMBURSEMENT SYSTEMS AND DOCUMENTATION

1. Who would be the authorized individuals that you could share the occupational therapy findings with? Explain why.
2. Which reimbursement system or systems most commonly cover occupational therapy services in this practice setting?
3. For this case, what forms and frequency of documentation will be required?

ADVOCACY

1. Which of the following areas of advocacy would be beneficial in this case: patient rights, matters of privacy, confidentiality, informed consent, awareness building, accessing education, and/or benefits/ resources?
2. Create a plan to advocate for this client based on the selected areas of advocacy.

TELEHEALTH

1. How can telehealth be integrated as a component of the occupational therapy process in this case?
2. Before launching telemedicine services, what questions would be essential to ask Epa to determine whether it is appropriate for her to engage in telemedicine services?
3. What are the barriers, obstacles, or challenges you foresee if attempting to integrate telehealth services with this client?

Intervention Plan Formulation and Implementation

INTERVENTION PLAN FORMULATION

Create an intervention plan that includes the following:

1. List this individual's **strengths.**
2. List this individual's **barriers** in occupational performance, performance skills, and performance patterns.
3. Based on the individual's goals, health, performance, and service delivery site, **identify the barriers that will be addressed.**
4. From the barriers identified to be addressed, **formulate goals and objectives.**
5. Identify the focus of each goal and objective as either **create, promote, establish, restore, maintain, modify, or prevent.**
6. Identify the **theoretical basis, model(s) of practice, or frame(s) of reference** that will be used to address each goal and objective.

7. For each proposed goal and objective, describe clearly and precisely the **methods** that will be used. This description should include, but not be limited to, safety considerations, environmental considerations, therapeutic use of self, preparatory activities, activity selection, materials, equipment, and flow.
8. Classify the activities selected in the methods description as either **preparatory, enabling, purposeful, or occupation based.**
9. Explain how each activity can be **graded up or down,** creating the just-right challenge.
10. Provide at least two **primary sources of evidence** to support the intervention plan.

INTERVENTION PLAN IMPLEMENTATION

1. Based on your intervention plan, identify which goals and objectives require **more immediate attention.**
2. Describe your proposed **first treatment session.**
3. As the treatment session is progressing, what is **essential to be observed?**

Transition and Discontinuation

Create a plan for discharge from occupational therapy services in collaboration with Epa and members of the interprofessional team. Review the needs of Epa, caregivers, family members, and significant others. The plan must match needs with available resources and the discharge environment.

REFERENCES

American Medical Association. (2019). *CPT® 2020 professional edition.*

Lawton, M. P., & Brody, E. M. (1969). Assessment of older people: Self-maintaining and instrumental activities of daily living. *The Gerontologist, 9,* 179–186. https://doi.org/10.1093/geront/9.3_Part_1.179

World Health Organization. (2019). *International statistical classification of diseases and related health problems* (11th ed.). https://icd.who.int/

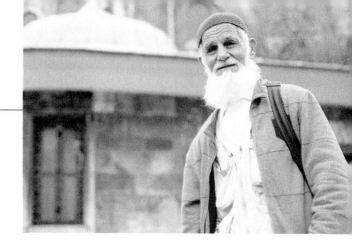

Mohammad: Chronic Obstructive Pulmonary Disease

VIKRAM PAGPATAN, OTR/L, ATP, BCP, CLA

Mohammad (he, him, his, himself)

MEDICAL HISTORY

Mohammad is a 77-year-old Iranian American male who is 6' 2" and weighs 144 pounds. He experienced an episode of respiratory distress while working a shift as a building maintenance supervisor and was rushed to a hospital emergency department by coworkers. A physical examination, X-rays, and blood tests were performed. He received a diagnosis of chronic obstructive pulmonary disease (COPD). Mohammad's medical history includes Type 2 diabetes mellitus, a right rotator cuff tear, osteoarthritis of the left knee, and major depressive disorder. Mohammad reported no alcohol or drug use but reported smoking two to three packs of cigarettes per week for 50 years. He has no known allergies. Mohammad was stabilized and transferred to a skilled nursing facility (SNF) for short-stay rehabilitation.

SOCIAL HISTORY

Mohammad practices the Islamic faith. He resides with his two wives and his four youngest children in a 12th-floor apartment that has elevator access. The apartment consists of four bedrooms, a living room, two bathrooms with a walk-in shower, and a kitchen with an electric stove. Mohammad is the primary caregiver for his eldest wife, who requires medical assistance for medication management secondary to altered mental status and early-onset dementia. Mohammad identifies as a Sunni Muslim.

REFERRAL OR PRESCRIPTION

Mohammad was transferred to a SNF for restorative care. He has been referred for occupational therapy, physical therapy, social work, and registered nursing services. The length of stay will be 14 days.

Occupational Therapy Initial Evaluation Findings: Skilled Nursing Facility

OCCUPATIONAL PROFILE

Mohammad's preadmission occupational history and experiences included being independent in all ADLs and all IADLs. He is employed as a full-time building maintenance supervisor in a condominium complex. His patterns of daily living most commonly included arriving to work at 6:00 a.m. and returning home by 6:00 p.m. Mohammad works 4 days per week, Monday through Thursday, to support his family. He is deeply concerned that if he does not return to work by the end of 30 days, he will lose his job. Mohammad is a religious Muslim and prioritizes praying at least 5 times a day. Each prayer session takes up to 10–15 minutes, so he often takes short breaks throughout the day. Mohammad values his family and ensures that he is able to spend time with his wives and children. He reported his greatest needs are to return home and care for his family.

ADLs

Regarding self-care, Mohammad was able to independently dress and bathe his upper body but required minimal to moderate assistance with the lower body. Mohammad became noticeably anxious and experienced shortness of breath (SOB) during lower body care. Regarding functional mobility, Mohammad was able to independently roll from side to side and transition from supine to sit but experienced mild SOB. During functional ambulation and transfers with the use of a rolling walker, he required supervision.

IADLs

Activities needed that provide day-to-day quality of life and relative independence were explored. Mohammad's younger wife has assumed responsibility to care for the elder wife, maintain the home, prepare meals, and shop. Mohammad was independent in financial management and use of communication devices. Regarding rest and sleep, for comfort during sleep, Mohammad required the head of the bed to be elevated.

MENTAL FUNCTIONS

Cognitive assessment found Mohammad to be alert and oriented to person, place, time, and situation, and short- and long-term memory were intact. He was able to follow three-step commands and make his needs known. Mohammad has a fair command of the English language but reported difficulty understanding technical medical terms. Assessment of affect revealed that he feels anxious during periods of SOB and does not feel completely comfortable when providers of the opposite gender physically examine him. No gross deficits in perception were observed.

SENSORY FUNCTIONS AND PAIN

No gross deficits were observed with visual, hearing, vestibular, taste, smell, proprioceptive, and cutaneous functions. Use of the Universal Pain Assessment Tool indicated a score of 6/10 for pain in his right glenohumeral joint. The pain was described as "gnawing."

CARDIOVASCULAR AND RESPIRATORY SYSTEM FUNCTIONS

Mohammad has been prescribed supplemental oxygen at 2 liters per minute through a nasal cannula while at the SNF and has been exhibiting a daily oxygen saturation of 95%. His heart rate at rest is 90 beats per minute (BPM) and exceeds 100 BPM during basic ADLs. His respiration rate at rest is 20 breaths per minute and exceeds 26 breaths per minute with basic ADLs. The Borg Rating of Perceived Exertion (RPE) Scale (Borg, 1982; Williams, 2017) was administered, and a score of 17 was obtained.

MOVEMENT FUNCTIONS

Mohammad's active range of motion (AROM) of the left upper extremity is within defined limits (WDL), and the right upper extremity is WDL except for shoulder motions. AROM measurements for his right shoulder are flexion, 0–90°; abduction, 0–95°; internal rotation, 0–60°; and external rotation, 0–40°. Muscle strength in all muscle groups in both upper extremities was 4/5 except right shoulder musculature, which was 3–/5. Fine motor abilities for grasp patterns, pinch patterns, and in hand manipulation skills were grossly intact. Standing tolerance was 5–6 minutes.

NEUROMUSCULAR FUNCTIONS

Static and dynamic sitting balance were 5/5, and static and dynamic standing balance were 4/5. Coordination, muscle tone, and reflex integration in both upper extremities were intact.

PLAN FOR DISCHARGE

Mohammad will be discharged home without service.

Questions and Activities

SAFETY OF CLIENT AND OTHERS: PRECAUTIONS AND CONTRAINDICATIONS

1. Identify precautions to follow with the use of supplemental oxygen. Cite your source and justify your selection.
2. How may the use of supplemental oxygen affect the occupational therapy process?
3. Create a handout identifying precautions to be followed by people with COPD.
4. What are the signs of respiratory distress? If these signs are observed or reported, what actions should be taken?
5. Identify the common emotional reactions associated with COPD that may affect the treatment process.
6. To keep Mohammad and others safe, what other factors should be considered?

OCCUPATIONS: ADLs, IADLs, EDUCATION, WORK, PLAY, SOCIAL PARTICIPATION, AND REST AND SLEEP

1. Given the information provided for this case, identify the areas of occupation that will and will not be addressed. Justify your decisions.

2. Identify assistive devices or compensatory strategies that will allow Mohammad to perform the ADL of bathing.
3. Identify the areas of education that would be appropriate to engage in with Mohammad and explain why.
4. Would work, leisure, socialization, or sleep be addressed? Why or why not?
5. Given Mohammad's current functional status, estimate his current metabolic equivalent of task (MET) needed and determine which MET value would be required to return to work safely.

PERFORMANCE SKILLS: MOTOR SKILLS, PROCESS SKILLS, AND SOCIAL INTERACTION SKILLS

1. Given the information provided, identify the motor, process, and social interaction skills that affect Mohammad's occupational performance.
2. Which of these skills would be appropriate to address in this service delivery site? Justify your selection.
3. Which of these skills would be addressed through remediation, compensation, and education?
4. Which of these skills would be addressed through the following intervention approaches: create/promote, establish/restore, maintain, modify, and prevent?

PERFORMANCE PATTERNS: HABITS, ROUTINES, ROLES, AND RITUALS

1. Identify Mohammad's useful habits, routines, roles, and rituals that support valued occupations. How can you make use of this information?
2. Identify Mohammad's impoverished habits, routines, roles, and rituals that do not support valued occupations. How can you make use of this information?
3. Identify Mohammad's dominating habits, routines, roles, and rituals that interfere with valued occupations. How can you make use of this information?

CLIENT FACTORS

Values, beliefs, and spirituality
How can the identified values, beliefs, and spirituality be used in this case?

Body structures
Considering Mohammad's primary and secondary diagnoses, identify the related body structures.

Body functions
1. Identify how the primary and secondary diagnoses have affected the function of the identified body structures.
2. Explain the relationships between the structural and functional factors and Mohammad's current level of occupational performance.

MENTAL FUNCTIONS: AFFECTIVE, COGNITIVE, AND PERCEPTUAL

1. What concerns related to Mohammad's medical history may affect the occupational therapy process?
2. Identify cognitive changes associated with COPD over time. Name your source or sources.

3. What other disciplines would be available to address Mohammad's reported anxiety?
4. Given the information provided, what additional mental function considerations need to be addressed?

NEUROMUSCULOSKELETAL AND MOVEMENT-RELATED FUNCTIONS

1. Given the information provided, identify neuromusculoskeletal and movement-related functions that need to be addressed. Justify your selections.
2. Describe the signs and symptoms of a rotator cuff tear.
3. Identify the motions of the shoulder and provide the AROM norm for each.
4. Which assessment methods would have been used to assess AROM?
5. Identify three physical agent modalities that are appropriate for the management of Mohammad's pain. Select one and justify your selection.
6. Create an exercise program for Mohammad based on occupational performance.

CARDIOVASCULAR, HEMATOLOGICAL, IMMUNOLOGICAL, AND RESPIRATORY FUNCTIONS

1. Given the information provided, identify cardiovascular, hematological, immunological and respiratory functions that need to be addressed. Justify your selections.
2. Describe how pain affects vital signs.
3. Compare and contrast the norm values of vital signs for a resting adult with the norm values for children?
4. Explain critical values for vital signs.

SKIN AND RELATED STRUCTURE FUNCTIONS

1. What is cyanosis and how is it related to COPD?
2. If Mohammad exhibits cyanosis, what are the appropriate steps to take?
3. What other skin and related structure functions should be considered?

VOICE AND SPEECH FUNCTIONS

Describe how Mohammad's diagnoses may affect his voice, speech, and associated occupational performance.

ASSISTIVE TECHNOLOGIES AND DEVICES

What assistive technologies and adaptations might be used or made for Mohammad while he is receiving occupational therapy services? Why?

ETHICAL DECISION MAKING

1. Mohammad frequently asks to take a break during the therapy session to pray. How would these breaks affect the occupational therapy process?
2. Mohammad informs you that he is being provided with meals that are not Halal. How would this situation be addressed?
3. You have been asked to titrate Mohammad's oxygen. Is this within the scope of practice?

PHARMACOLOGY

Mohammad is currently taking Duaklir.

1. What is the generic name?
2. Does this drug have a high alert status?
3. What is the classification of this drug?
4. What is the indication for this drug?
5. What is the action of this drug?
6. How may this drug affect client participation during a therapy session?

SOCIOCULTURAL, SOCIOECONOMIC, AND DIVERSITY FACTORS AND LIFESTYLE CHOICES

1. Given Mohammad's profile, how may your own culture and beliefs affect your interaction with him?
2. Based on this self-examination, what area of cultural knowledge do you need to pursue?
3. How can this newly acquired cultural knowledge be integrated for effective outcomes?
4. Discuss how a lack of understanding in the areas of discrimination and stigma, implicit bias, social identity, or racism may contribute to disparities in the delivery of occupational therapy services in this case.

ASSESSMENT TOOLS AND INTERPRETATION OF RESULTS

1. What is the purpose of the Borg RPE Scale?
2. Which population is this test designed for?
3. How much time is required to administer it?
4. Provide a brief description of this assessment.
5. What is the reliability of the Borg RPE Scale?
6. What is the validity of the Borg RPE Scale?
7. What additional standardized assessment can be used in this case? Why?

INTERPROFESSIONAL RELATIONSHIP AND EFFECTIVE INTRAPROFESSIONAL COLLABORATION

1. Identify the other professions that would make up the care team. Explain the focus of each.
2. Identify the roles of the occupational therapy assistant (OTA) that could be used in the occupational therapy process for this case.
3. Identify interventions that can be assigned to the OTA for this case. Justify your selections.

BILLING AND CODING

1. Identify the *International Classification of Diseases (ICD)* codes for Mohammad's diagnoses.
2. For this case, identify at least two *Current Procedural Terminology (CPT®)* codes that are most appropriate. Justify your selection.

REIMBURSEMENT SYSTEMS AND DOCUMENTATION

1. Who would be the authorized individuals that you could share the occupational therapy findings with? Explain why.
2. Which reimbursement system or systems most commonly cover occupational therapy services in this practice setting?
3. For this case, what forms and frequency of documentation will be required?

ADVOCACY

1. Which of the following areas of advocacy would be beneficial in this case: patient rights, matters of privacy, confidentiality, informed consent, awareness building, accessing education, or benefits/resources?
2. Create a plan to advocate for this client based on the selected areas of advocacy.

TELEHEALTH

1. How can telehealth be integrated as a component of the occupational therapy process in this case?
2. Before launching telemedicine services, what questions would be essential to ask Mohammad to determine whether it is appropriate for him to engage in telemedicine services?
3. What are the barriers, obstacles, or challenges you foresee if attempting to integrate telehealth services with this client?

Intervention Plan Formulation and Implementation

INTERVENTION PLAN FORMULATION

Create an intervention plan that includes the following:

1. List this individual's **strengths.**
2. List this individual's **barriers** in occupational performance, performance skills, and performance patterns.
3. Based on the individual's goals, health, performance, and service delivery site, **identify the barriers that will be addressed.**
4. From the **barriers** identified to be addressed, **formulate goals and objectives.**
5. Identify the focus of each goal and objective as either **create, promote, establish, restore, maintain, modify, or prevent.**
6. Identify the **theoretical basis, model(s) of practice, or frame(s) of reference** that will be used to address each goal and objective.
7. For each proposed goal and objective, describe clearly and precisely the **methods** that will be used. This description should include, but not be limited to, safety considerations, environmental considerations, therapeutic use of self, preparatory activities, activity selection, materials, equipment, and flow.
8. Classify the activities selected in the methods description as either **preparatory, enabling, purposeful, or occupation based.**
9. Explain how each activity can be **graded up or down,** creating the just-right challenge.
10. Provide at least two **primary sources of evidence** to support the intervention plan.

INTERVENTION PLAN IMPLEMENTATION

1. Based on your intervention plan, identify which goals and objectives require **more immediate attention.**
2. Describe your proposed **first treatment session.**
3. As the treatment session is progressing, what is **essential to be observed?**

Transition and Discontinuation

Create a plan for discharge from occupational therapy services in collaboration with Mohammad and members of the interprofessional team. Review the needs of Mohammad, caregivers, family members, and significant others. The plan must match needs with available resources and the discharge environment.

REFERENCES

American Medical Association. (2019). *CPT® 2020 professional edition.*

Borg, G. A. (1982). Psychophysical bases of perceived exertion. *Medicine and Science in Sports and Exercise, 14,* 377–381. https://doi.org/10.1249/00005768-198205000-00012

Williams, N. (2017). The Borg Rating of Perceived Exertion (RPE) Scale. *Occupational Medicine, 67,* 404–405. https://doi.org/10.1093/occmed/kqx063

World Health Organization. (2019). *International statistical classification of diseases and related health problems* (11th ed.). https://icd.who.int/

Home and Community Health

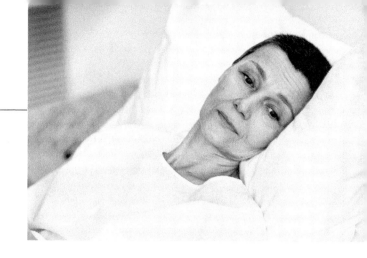

Eileen: Amyotrophic Lateral Sclerosis

DONALD AURIEMMA, MS ED, OTR/L

Eileen (she, her, hers, herself)

MEDICAL HISTORY

Eileen is a 57-year-old Irish American female who is 5' 1" and weighs 103 pounds. She was wheeled into the emergency department by her husband. She reported experiencing fever and chills for 3 days. Blood tests, urine tests, X-rays, and pulse oximetry were done. She reported receiving a diagnosis of amyotrophic lateral sclerosis (ALS) 1.5 years prior and has no other significant medical history. She reported no alcohol, tobacco, or drug use but reported consuming up to 5 cups of coffee per day. Eileen has no known allergies. She received a diagnosis of aspiration pneumonia and was transferred to a medical floor, where she received a course of intravenous antibiotics.

SOCIAL HISTORY

Eileen lives with her recently retired husband and adult son. They live in a three-bedroom ranch with two bathrooms, one of which is wheelchair accessible. Eileen recently moved into this home after her diagnosis of ALS. Eileen has a twin sister Maureen, two brothers, and another adult son serving in the U.S. Marines. She identifies as a Catholic.

REFERRAL OR PRESCRIPTION

Eileen was transferred home with home and community health care services. She has been referred for occupational therapy, physical therapy, social work, and registered nursing services. The length of stay will be 4 weeks.

Occupational Therapy Initial Evaluation Findings: Community Health Care Services

OCCUPATIONAL PROFILE

Eileen's preadmission occupational history and experiences included being dependent in all ADLs and all IADLs. Eileen has been an occupational therapist for more than 30 years. She provided home health occupational therapy services for most of her career before she retired early as a result of the progression of her illness. Eileen has a bachelor's degree in occupational therapy and had worked for several years as an adjunct faculty member.

Her most common pattern of daily living includes waking up at 7:00 a.m., being washed and fed by her husband, and then being transferred into her manual wheelchair for a stroll through their quiet suburban neighborhood. A private aide usually stays with her in the afternoons while her husband performs chores. In the early evening, she is fed, washed, and transferred into bed by her husband, where they watch television together.

Her interests include spending time with her family and close friends. She values her family, Irish heritage, strong Catholic faith, and the little time she has left. Eileen reported her greatest needs are not to be a burden to her husband and not to be placed on a ventilator or a feeding tube. She has asked her husband and close family members if they ever see her choking or struggling to breathe, to please leave the room for 15 minutes before returning.

ADLs

Regarding self-care, Eileen was dependent for all feeding, grooming, dressing, bathing, and toileting. She was observed to have frequent coughs and notable gurgling while being fed soup. The ALS Functional Rating Scale–Revised (ALSFRS–R; Cedarbaum et al., 1999) was administered, and a score of 18/48 was achieved. Regarding functional mobility, Eileen was dependent for all bed mobility, transfers, functional ambulation, and wheelchair use. Her husband physically transfers Eileen between the bed and wheelchair and power recliner.

IADLs

Activities needed that provide day-to-day quality of life and relative independence were explored. Eileen was unable to manage her cellphone, text, browse the Internet, manage money, and care for her home. Regarding rest and sleep, Eileen reported difficulty falling asleep when placed in a supine position and reported finding it very difficult to breathe.

MENTAL FUNCTIONS

Cognitive assessment found Eileen to be alert and oriented to person, place, time, and situation, and short- and long-term memory were intact. She was able to make her needs known. Affect assessment indicated that Eileen felt sad but was accepting of impending death. No gross deficits in perception were observed.

SENSORY FUNCTIONS AND PAIN

No gross deficits were observed with visual, hearing, vestibular, taste, smell, proprioceptive, and cutaneous functions. Eileen reported no pain.

CARDIOVASCULAR AND RESPIRATORY SYSTEMS FUNCTIONS

Eileen's oxygen saturation while seated in her wheelchair, erect, was 94% on room air. Her respiration rate was 24 breaths per minute.

MOVEMENT FUNCTIONS

Passive range of motion in all extremities was within defined limits. The manual muscle test indicated strengths of 2–/5 in all groups in both upper extremities and in both lower extremities. Assessment of fine motor (prehension) abilities indicated that Eileen was unable to form gross grasp and pinch patterns.

NEUROMUSCULAR FUNCTIONS

Eileen required external support to maintain a short sitting position. She was dependent in standing. Muscle tone in all extremities was hypotonic, and all deep tendon reflexes were depressed.

PLAN FOR DISCHARGE

Eileen will be discharged to the care of her husband and private aide.

Questions and Activities

SAFETY OF CLIENT AND OTHERS: PRECAUTIONS AND CONTRAINDICATIONS

1. When working with a client with ALS, what precautions and contraindications must be considered?
2. Create a handout that identifies feeding precautions for people with dysphagia.
3. Compare and contrast aspiration pneumonia with pneumonia.
4. Eileen is at high risk for developing a decubitus ulcer. Explain why. Identify the areas of her body at greatest risk. How can these ulcers be prevented?
5. Identify the common psychological reactions associated with ALS that may affect the treatment process.
6. To keep Eileen and others safe, what other factors should be considered?

OCCUPATIONS: ADLs, IADLs, EDUCATION, WORK, PLAY, SOCIAL PARTICIPATION, AND REST AND SLEEP

1. Given the information provided for this case, identify the areas of occupation that will and will not be addressed. Justify your decisions.

2. What areas of custodial care can be explored to ease the burden on her husband and private aide?
3. Eileen wishes to gain a higher level of independence with electronic communications with her friends and family. How can this goal be addressed?
4. What recommendations would allow Eileen to have more restful and safer sleep?

PERFORMANCE SKILLS: MOTOR SKILLS, PROCESS SKILLS, AND SOCIAL INTERACTION SKILLS

1. Given the information provided, identify the motor, process, and social interaction skills that affect Eileen's occupational performance.
2. Which of these skills would be appropriate to address in this service delivery site? Justify your selection.
3. Which of these skills would be addressed through remediation, compensation, and education?
4. Which of these skills would be addressed through the following intervention approaches: create/promote, establish/restore, maintain, modify, and prevent?

PERFORMANCE PATTERNS: HABITS, ROUTINES, ROLES, AND RITUALS

1. Identify Eileen's useful habits, routines, roles, and rituals that support valued occupations. How can you make use of this information?
2. Identify Eileen's impoverished habits, routines, roles, and rituals that do not support valued occupations. How can you make use of this information?
3. Identify Eileen's dominating habits, routines, roles, and rituals that interfere with valued occupations. How can you make use of this information?

CLIENT FACTORS

Values, beliefs, and spirituality
How can the identified values, beliefs, and spirituality be used in this case?

Body structures
Considering Eileen's primary and secondary diagnoses, identify the related body structures.

Body functions
1. Identify how the primary and secondary diagnoses have affected the function of the identified body structures.
2. Explain the relationships between the structural and functional factors and Eileen's current level of occupational performance.

MENTAL FUNCTIONS: AFFECTIVE, COGNITIVE, AND PERCEPTUAL

1. How does Eileen view her illness? Provide evidence to support your view.
2. Identify your thoughts and emotions that were evoked while reading this case.
3. What challenges would you face working with a person who is terminally ill?
4. Given the information provided, what additional mental function considerations need to be addressed?

NEUROMUSCULOSKELETAL AND MOVEMENT-RELATED FUNCTIONS

1. Given the information provided, identify neuromusculoskeletal and movement-related functions that need to be addressed. Justify your selections.
2. Compare and contrast ALS with Huntington's disease.
3. Eileen's muscle strength in her four extremities is 2–/5. Explain what this muscle grade is.
4. Should Eileen's reduction in muscle strength be addressed through a remediation program? Why or why not?
5. If Eileen's extremities are not passively ranged on a daily basis, it will result in accommodative shortening of the muscles. Explain the physiology of accommodative shortening.
6. How can accommodative shortening interfere with the care being provided to Eileen?
7. Create an exercise program based on occupational performance for Eileen's care providers.

CARDIOVASCULAR, HEMATOLOGICAL, IMMUNOLOGICAL, AND RESPIRATORY FUNCTIONS

1. Given the information provided, identify cardiovascular, hematological, immunological, and respiratory functions that need to be addressed. Justify your selections.
2. Identify the normal values for oxygen saturation.
3. Make an inference concerning an oxygen saturation of 94%.
4. Identify the normal range of respiration at rest.
5. Compare and contrast the signs and symptoms of respiratory distress with respiratory failure.

SKIN AND RELATED STRUCTURE FUNCTIONS

1. During your initial evaluation, you found a decubitus ulcer with partial-thickness loss of the dermis with a shallow opening in the skin. What stage does this description represent?
2. What would be your concerns?
3. What actions or actions need to be taken?
4. What other skin and related structure functions should be considered?

VOICE AND SPEECH FUNCTIONS

Describe how Eileen's diagnoses may affect her voice, speech, and occupational performance.

ASSISTIVE TECHNOLOGIES AND DEVICES

What assistive technologies and adaptations might be used or made for Eileen while she is receiving occupational therapy services at home? Why?

ETHICAL DECISION MAKING

1. Eileen has told you that if she begins to choke during your session, just leave the room; however, she does not have a do not resuscitate or do not intubate order. How should you address this situation?
2. Should occupational therapy services be delivered to a terminally ill person? Why or why not?
3. Eileen was provided with a choice between home health services or hospice care upon discharge. Compare and contrast home care with hospice care.

PHARMACOLOGY

Eileen is currently taking Radicava.

1. What is the generic name?
2. Does this drug have a high alert status?
3. What is the classification of this drug?
4. What is the indication for this drug?
5. What is the action of this drug?
6. How may this drug affect client participation during a therapy session?

SOCIOCULTURAL, SOCIOECONOMIC, AND DIVERSITY FACTORS AND LIFESTYLE CHOICES

1. How may your own culture and beliefs affect your interaction with her?
2. Based on this self-examination, what areas of cultural knowledge do you need to pursue?
3. How can this newly acquired cultural knowledge be integrated for effective outcomes?
4. Discuss how a lack of understanding in the areas of discrimination and stigma, implicit bias, social identity, or racism may contribute to disparities in the delivery of occupational therapy services in this case.

ASSESSMENT TOOLS AND INTERPRETATION OF RESULTS

1. What is the purpose of the ALSFRS-R?
2. Which population is this test designed for?
3. How much time is required to administer it?
4. Provide a brief description of this assessment.
5. What is the reliability of the ALSFRS-R?
6. What is the validity of the ALSFRS-R?
7. What functional inference can be deduced from a score of 18/48?

INTERPROFESSIONAL RELATIONSHIP AND EFFECTIVE INTRAPROFESSIONAL COLLABORATION

1. Identify the other professions that would make up the care team. Explain the focus of each.
2. Identify the roles of the occupational therapy assistant (OTA) that could be used in the occupational therapy process for this case.
3. Identify interventions that can be assigned to the OTA for this case. Justify your selections.

BILLING AND CODING

1. Identify the *International Classification of Diseases (ICD)* codes for Eileen's diagnoses.
2. For this case, identify at least two *Current Procedural Terminology (CPT®)* codes that are most appropriate. Justify your selection.

1. Who would be the authorized individuals that you could share the occupational therapy findings with? Explain why.
2. For this case, what forms and frequency of documentation will be required?
3. Which reimbursement system or systems most commonly cover occupational therapy services in this practice setting?

1. Which of the following areas of advocacy would be beneficial in this case: patient rights, matters of privacy, confidentiality, informed consent, awareness building, accessing education, or benefits/resources?
2. Create a plan to advocate for this client based on the selected areas of advocacy.

1. How can telehealth be integrated as a component of the occupational therapy process in this case?
2. Before launching telemedicine services, what questions would be essential to ask Eileen to determine whether it is appropriate for her to engage in telemedicine services?
3. What are the barriers, obstacles, or challenges you foresee if attempting to integrate telehealth services with this client?

Intervention Plan Formulation and Implementation

INTERVENTION PLAN FORMULATION

Create an intervention plan that includes the following:

1. List this individual's **strengths.**
2. List this individual's **barriers** in occupational performance, performance skills, and performance patterns.
3. Based on the individual's goals, health, performance, and service delivery site, **identify the barriers that will be addressed.**
4. From the barriers identified to be addressed, **formulate goals and objectives.**
5. Identify the focus of each goal and objective as either **create, promote, establish, restore, maintain, modify, or prevent.**
6. Identify the **theoretical basis, model(s) of practice, or frame(s) of reference** that will be used to address each goal and objective.
7. For each proposed goal and objective, describe clearly and precisely the **methods** that will be used. This description should include, but not be limited to, safety considerations, environmental considerations, therapeutic use of self, preparatory activities, activity selection, materials, equipment, and flow.
8. Classify the activities selected in the methods description as either **preparatory, enabling, purposeful, or occupation based.**
9. Explain how each activity can be **graded up or down,** creating the just-right challenge.
10. Provide at least two **primary sources of evidence** to support the intervention plan.

INTERVENTION PLAN IMPLEMENTATION

1. Based on your intervention plan, identify which goals and objectives require **more immediate attention.**
2. Describe your proposed **first treatment session.**
3. As the treatment session is progressing, what is **essential to be observed?**

Transition and Discontinuation

Create a plan for discharge from occupational therapy services in collaboration with Eileen and members of the interprofessional team. Review the needs of Eileen, caregivers, family members, and significant others. The plan must match needs with available resources and the discharge environment.

REFERENCES

American Medical Association. (2019). *CPT® 2020 professional edition.*

Cedarbaum, J. M., Stambler, N., Malta, E., Fuller, C., Hilt, D., Thurmond, B., & Nakanishi, A. (1999). The ALSFRS-R: A revised ALS functional rating scale that incorporates assessments of respiratory function. *Journal of the Neurological Sciences, 169,* 13–21. https://doi.org/10.1016/S0022-510X(99)00210-5

World Health Organization. (2019). *International statistical classification of diseases and related health problems* (11th ed.). https://icd.who.int/

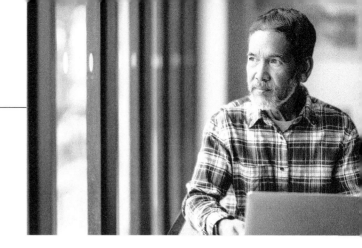

José: Alcohol Abuse

DONALD AURIEMMA, MS ED, OTR/L; CLOVER HUTCHINSON, OTD, MA, OTR/L; AND VIKRAM PAGPATAN, OTR/L, ATP, BCP, CLA

José (he, his, him, himself)

MEDICAL HISTORY

José is an 81-year-old Salvadoran American male who is 5' 6" and weighs 140 pounds. He fell in his home and was found by his son on the apartment floor with a deep laceration on his forehead. He was driven to the emergency department, where a physical examination, electrocardiogram, magnetic resonance imagining, and urine and blood tests were performed. Blood tests indicated that he was intoxicated. It was determined that José's fall was attributed to tripping over an area rug in his home that he did not see. José's medical history includes diabetes mellitus, bilateral carpal tunnel syndrome, hypertension, and poorly managed progressive primary open-angle glaucoma. He denied drug or tobacco use but reported consuming 5 to 6 bottles of beer since the death of his wife and 2 to 3 cups of coffee daily. He also revealed that he has not consistently followed his medication regimen. José has no known allergies.

SOCIAL HISTORY

José is a recent widow and lives alone in his three-bedroom, 8th-floor apartment in a city-owned building. His wife Rosa lost her battle to cancer 6 months prior. He is a retired garment worker and has one son, Edgar, who lives 5 miles from his home. Edgar and his wife are both employed and are raising their three children. José is an observer of Dominican Santeria.

REFERRAL OR PRESCRIPTION

José was transferred home with community health care services. He has been referred for occupational therapy, physical therapy, social work, registered nursing, and home health aide services. The length of stay will be 5 weeks.

Occupational Therapy Initial Evaluation Findings: Community Health Care Services

OCCUPATIONAL PROFILE

José's preadmission occupational history and experiences included being independent in all ADLs and requiring assistance with most IADLs. His most common pattern of daily living includes waking at 7 a.m., showering, and making breakfast of coffee and bread by 9:00 a.m. Since the death of Rosa, his son Edgar would see him every Saturday morning to take him shopping, clean the apartment, and help pay bills. José used to call Edgar each evening, but because José has a reduction in vision and subsequent difficulty using his phone, Edgar now calls him. José spends most days listening to Latin music and going to the senior citizens center in his building with his friend Hector. He receives meals from Meals on Wheels. José's interests include reminiscing about when he lived in El Salvador and playing bingo with Hector. He values the time and care he receives from Edgar and reported that his greatest needs are to remain sober and not disappoint his family.

ADLs

Regarding self-care, José was independent in bathing, feeding, and toileting, but he reported feeling unsatisfied with his ability to shave. Regarding functional mobility, José was able to independently roll, transition between prone and supine, and transition from supine to short sit. In the area of transfers, José was independent in sit-to-stand and toilet transfers; however, he reported feeling unsafe transferring into his tub.

IADLs

Activities needed that provide day-to-day quality of life and relative independence were explored. José reported that he no longer feels safe using the oven or the stove. He expressed frustration that he can no longer keep his home clean, pay his bills, use his phone, or search the Internet on his computer. Regarding rest and sleep, José reported sleeping between 10 and 12 hours per day.

MENTAL FUNCTIONS

Cognitive assessment found José to be alert and oriented to person, place, time, and situation, and short- and long-term memory were intact. He was able to follow three-step commands and make his needs known. Affect assessment indicated that José was frustrated and at times angry over needing help with his IADLs. No gross deficits in perception were observed.

SENSORY FUNCTIONS AND PAIN

No gross deficits were observed in hearing, vestibular, taste, smell, proprioceptive, and cutaneous functions. A gross assessment of visual acuity using a Snellen Chart revealed 20/200 corrected vision, and a Confrontation Test (Reader & Harper, 1976) to assess field of vision revealed tunnel vision. José reported no pain.

CARDIOVASCULAR AND RESPIRATORY SYSTEMS FUNCTIONS

No deficits were noted.

MOVEMENT FUNCTIONS

Passive range of motion, active range of motion, and muscular strength in all four extremities were within normal limits. Prehension assessment indicated that José was able to effectively form the hook, cylindrical, power, and spherical grasps. He was also able to effectively form lateral, tripod, scissor, palmer, and tip-to-tip pinch patterns. An awkwardness in hand manipulation skills was observed when he moved small objects between his palm and the tips of his fingers.

NEUROMUSCULAR FUNCTIONS

Both static and dynamic standing and sitting balance were normal. Muscle tone in all four extremities was normal. Reflex integration was grossly intact.

PLAN FOR DISCHARGE

José will be discharged into his own care and remain in his home.

Questions and Activities

SAFETY OF CLIENT AND OTHERS: PRECAUTIONS AND CONTRAINDICATIONS

1. Create a handout that identifies precautions that must be followed by people with progressive primary open-angle glaucoma.
2. Given José's laceration, what precautions must be considered?
3. Identify the risks associated with impaired cutaneous light touch and temperature sense in all digits. Cite your source and justify your selection.
4. Identify the common emotional reactions associated with advancing glaucoma that may affect the treatment process.
5. To keep José and others safe, what other factors should be considered?

OCCUPATIONS: ADLs, IADLs, EDUCATION, WORK, PLAY, SOCIAL PARTICIPATION, AND REST AND SLEEP

1. Given the information provided for this case, identify the areas of occupation that will and will not be addressed. Justify your decisions.
2. How can José feel safer and become more independent in preparing meals using his stove and oven?
3. How can José clean his home more independently?
4. How can José become more independent in making calls on his phone?
5. How can José become more independent using his computer to search the Internet?

PERFORMANCE SKILLS: MOTOR SKILLS, PROCESS SKILLS, AND SOCIAL INTERACTION SKILLS

1. Given the information provided, identify the motor, process, and social interaction skills that affect José's occupational performance.
2. Which of these skills would be appropriate to address in this service delivery site? Justify your selection.
3. Which of these skills would be addressed through remediation, compensation, and education?
4. Which of these skills would be addressed through the following intervention approaches: create/promote, establish/restore, maintain, modify, and prevent?

PERFORMANCE PATTERNS: HABITS, ROUTINES, ROLES, AND RITUALS

1. Identify José's useful habits, routines, roles, and rituals that support valued occupations. How can you make use of this information?
2. Identify José's impoverished habits, routines, roles, and rituals that do not support valued occupations. How can you make use of this information?
3. Identify José's dominating habits, routines, roles, and rituals that interfere with valued occupations. How can you make use of this information?

CLIENT FACTORS

Values, beliefs, and spirituality
How can the identified values, beliefs, and spirituality be used in this case?

Body structures
Considering José's primary and secondary diagnoses, identify the related body structures.

Body Functions
1. Identify how the primary and secondary diagnoses have affected the function of the identified body structures.
2. Explain the relationships between the structural and functional factors and José's current level of occupational performance.

MENTAL FUNCTIONS: AFFECTIVE, COGNITIVE, AND PERCEPTUAL

1. What strategies should be used if José becomes frustrated or angry during a therapy session?
2. Should a referral to another discipline be considered to help explore José's feelings? If so, which discipline?
3. Given the information provided, what additional mental function considerations need to be addressed?

NEUROMUSCULOSKELETAL AND MOVEMENT-RELATED FUNCTIONS

1. Given the information provided, identify neuromusculoskeletal and movement-related functions that need to be addressed. Justify your selections.
2. Compare and contrast essential tremor with symptomatic palatal tremor.
3. Given José's history of a fall, what measures can be taken to allow him to move about his home in a safer manner?

CARDIOVASCULAR, HEMATOLOGICAL, IMMUNOLOGICAL, AND RESPIRATORY FUNCTIONS

1. Given the information provided, identify cardiovascular, hematological, immunological, and respiratory functions that need to be addressed. Justify your selections.
2. Explain the physiological impact that anger and frustration have on heart rate, respiration rate, and intraocular pressure. Cite your sources and justify your selections.

SKIN AND RELATED STRUCTURE FUNCTIONS

1. What is the most probable explanation for the impaired cutaneous light touch and temperature sense in José's digits? How can these conditions affect his occupational performance?
2. Identify risks that are associated with impaired cutaneous light touch and temperature senses.
3. What preventive measures can be taken to mitigate these risks?
4. What other skin and related structure functions should be considered?

VOICE AND SPEECH FUNCTIONS

Describe how José's diagnoses may affect his voice, speech, and associated occupational performance.

ASSISTIVE TECHNOLOGIES AND DEVICES

What assistive technologies and adaptations might be used or made for José while he is receiving occupational therapy services at home? Why?

ETHICAL DECISION MAKING

1. Upon reviewing the referral or prescription for occupational therapy services, you see it is not signed by a doctor of medicine, or MD, but rather by a DO. What does DO stand for? Can occupational therapy services be referred or prescribed by a DO?
2. José reports to you that he is not taking his medication because of a lack of funds. How should this situation be addressed?
3. During your second visit, you observe that José's right wrist is swollen. When asked about it, José tells you that he tripped and fell the previous evening. He requests that you do not report it. How should this situation be addressed?
4. When you enter José's apartment, you notice a strong odor of marijuana. He informs you that he smokes it to reduce "eye pain." How should this situation be addressed?

PHARMACOLOGY

José is currently taking Timolol eye drops.

1. What is the brand name?
2. Does this drug have a high alert status?
3. What is the classification of this drug?
4. What is the indication for this drug?
5. What is the action of this drug?

6. How may this drug affect client participation during a therapy session?

SOCIOCULTURAL, SOCIOECONOMIC, AND DIVERSITY FACTORS AND LIFESTYLE CHOICES

1. Given José's profile, how may your own culture and beliefs affect your interaction with him?
2. Based on this self-examination, what area of cultural knowledge do you need to pursue?
3. How can this newly acquired cultural knowledge be integrated for effective outcomes?
4. How can you foster cultural interaction and awareness among your coworkers?
5. Discuss how a lack of understanding in the areas of discrimination and stigma, implicit bias, social identity, or racism may contribute to disparities in the delivery of occupational therapy services in this case.

ASSESSMENT TOOLS AND INTERPRETATION OF RESULTS

1. What is the purpose of the Confrontation Test?
2. Which population is this test designed for?
3. How much time is required to administer it?
4. Provide a brief description of this assessment.
5. What is the reliability of the Confrontation Test?
6. What is the validity of the Confrontation Test?
7. What functional inference can be deduced from José's score of corrected vision of 20/200?
8. What additional standardized assessment can be used in this case? Why?

INTERPROFESSIONAL RELATIONSHIP AND EFFECTIVE INTRAPROFESSIONAL COLLABORATION

1. Identify the other professions that would make up the care team. Explain the focus of each.
2. Identify the roles of the occupational therapy assistant (OTA) that could be used in the occupational therapy process for this case.
3. Identify interventions that can be assigned to the OTA for this case. Justify your selections.

BILLING AND CODING

1. Identify the *International Classification of Diseases (ICD)* codes for José's diagnoses.
2. For this case, identify at least two *Current Procedural Terminology (CPT®)* codes that are most appropriate. Justify your selection.

REIMBURSEMENT SYSTEMS AND DOCUMENTATION

1. Who would be the authorized individuals that you could share the occupational therapy findings with? Explain why.
2. For this case, what forms and frequency of documentation will be required?
3. Which reimbursement system or systems most commonly cover occupational therapy services in this practice setting?

ADVOCACY

1. Which of the following areas of advocacy would be beneficial in this case: patient rights, matters of privacy, confidentiality, informed consent, awareness building, accessing education, or benefits/resources?
2. Create a plan to advocate for this client based on the selected areas of advocacy.

TELEHEALTH

1. How can telehealth be integrated as a component of the occupational therapy process in this case?
2. Before launching telemedicine services, what questions would be essential to ask José to determine whether it is appropriate for him to engage in telemedicine services?
3. What are the barriers, obstacles, or challenges you foresee if attempting to integrate telehealth services with this client?

Intervention Plan Formulation and Implementation

INTERVENTION PLAN FORMULATION

Create an intervention plan that includes the following:

1. List this individual's **strengths.**
2. List this individual's **barriers** in occupational performance, performance skills, and performance patterns.
3. Based on the individual's goals, health, performance, and service delivery site, **identify the barriers that will be addressed.**
4. From the barriers identified to be addressed, **formulate goals and objectives.**
5. Identify the focus of each goal and objective as either **create, promote, establish, restore, maintain, modify, or prevent.**
6. Identify the **theoretical basis, model(s) of practice, or frame(s) of reference** that will be used to address each goal and objective.
7. For each proposed goal and objective, describe clearly and precisely the **methods** that will be used. This description should include, but not be limited to, safety considerations, environmental considerations, therapeutic use of self, preparatory activities, activity selection, materials, equipment, and flow.
8. Classify the activities selected in the methods description as either **preparatory, enabling, purposeful, or occupation based.**
9. Explain how each activity can be **graded up or down,** creating the just-right challenge.
10. Provide at least two **primary sources of evidence** to support the intervention plan.

INTERVENTION PLAN IMPLEMENTATION

1. Based on your intervention plan, identify which goals and objectives require **more immediate attention.**
2. Describe your proposed **first treatment session.**
3. As the treatment session is progressing, what is **essential to be observed?**

Transition and Discontinuation

Create a plan for discharge from occupational therapy services in collaboration with José and members of the interprofessional team. Review the needs of José, caregivers, family members, and significant others. The plan must match needs with available resources and the discharge environment.

REFERENCES

American Medical Association. (2019). *CPT® 2020 professional edition.*

Reader, A. L., & Harper, D. G. (1976). Confrontation visual-field testing. *JAMA, 236,* 250–250. https://doi.org/10.1001/jama.1976.03270030010002

World Health Organization. (2019). *International statistical classification of diseases and related health problems* (11th ed.). https://icd.who.int/

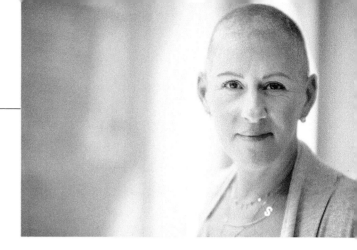

Katrina: Huntington's Disease

VIKRAM PAGPATAN, OTR/L, ATP, BCP, CLA

Katrina (she, her, hers, herself)

MEDICAL HISTORY

Katrina is a 38-year-old Georgian American female who is 5' 7" and weighs 129 pounds. Katrina was taken to the emergency department (ED) by her daughter after falling and experiencing pain in her right wrist and digits. After a physical examination and X-rays, she received a diagnosis of a right distal ulnar-radial fracture. The fracture was manually reduced and externally fixated with a plaster cast. Katrina's medical history includes Huntington's disease (HD), posttraumatic stress disorder from spousal abuse, hypertension, major depressive disorder, and aspiration pneumonia. Katrina reported no alcohol, drug, tobacco, or caffeine use. She has no known allergies. From the ED, she was transferred to a medical floor for observation and discharge planning.

SOCIAL HISTORY

Katrina recently separated from her husband and has relocated with her two high school–aged daughters to live with her 60-year-old mother. Katrina is presently on short-term disability from her telemarketing managerial position at a well-known firm. Katrina has moved into her mother's first-floor living space with two bedrooms and one bathroom. Katrina's daughters share a bedroom with their family golden retriever. Her social support has narrowed to a single lifelong friend on whom she relies heavily for moral support. Katrina was born into the Russian Orthodox church but reports not being active since being formally diagnosed with HD.

REFERRAL OR PRESCRIPTION

Katrina was transferred home with community health care services. She has been referred for occupational therapy, physical therapy, social work, home health, speech, and registered nursing services. Home services are prescribed for 6 weeks.

Occupational Therapy Initial Evaluation Findings: Community Health Care Services

OCCUPATIONAL PROFILE

Katrina's preadmission occupational history and experiences included needing assistance with bathing, dressing, and toileting from her mother and children. Additionally, she relied on them to shop, manage the home and medications, and care for their pet. Katrina had been employed for the past 10 years at the telemarketing firm, where she had been promoted to a senior-level position before she began short-term disability. She currently reports a need to apply for long-term disability. Her patterns of daily living most commonly included waking up at 5:00 a.m. and receiving assistance for bathing and self-care from a family member. She was then assisted to her home office, where she worked remotely. While Katrina worked, her mother left for work and her daughters went to school. Upon returning from school, her daughters would feed and walk the dog and prepare dinner. Katrina's interests include online shopping and researching online forums for the treatment of HD. She values her daughters and their education. She reported her greatest needs are to increase her independence and to reduce the burden on her daughters.

ADLs

Regarding self-care, Katrina was able to manage loose-fitting, pull-over garments but required total assistance for managing fasteners. In the area of feeding, Katrina required food and utensils to be set up. During toileting, she needed moderate assistance to manage lower-body garments and hygiene. For sleep and rest, Katrina reported experiencing insomnia and unrelenting fatigue. Regarding functional mobility, Katrina was able to roll and transition between supine to short sitting independently; however, she required either contact guard assistance or minimal assistance when transferring without a device. She required the same level of assistance moving within her home.

IADLs

Activities needed that provide day-to-day quality of life and relative independence were explored. Katrina reported that she recently was no longer able to effectively use her voice to manage her computer and phone. During the past several years, Katrina has relied on her daughters to care for their dog, manage her appointments, and maintain the home. She has been unable to drive since experiencing symptoms after her formal diagnosis. Katrina also relied on her daughters for shopping and meal preparation. Regarding rest and sleep, Katrina reported a history of insomnia, difficulty falling asleep, frequent nocturnal awakening, and often experienced daytime sleepiness.

MENTAL FUNCTIONS

Cognitive assessment found Katrina to be alert and oriented to person, place, time, and situation, and long-term memory was intact. Her short-term memory was impaired. She presented with difficulty in concentrating, planning, and sustaining attention. Assessment of affect found that Katrina appeared angry and irritable toward the end of the evaluation. Katrina reported contemplating thoughts of suicide in the past but denied an active plan. No gross deficits in perceptual function were observed.

SENSORY FUNCTIONS AND PAIN

No gross deficits were observed with visual, hearing, vestibular, taste, smell, proprioceptive, and cutaneous functions. Katrina reported pain in her right wrist as a 5 on the Numerical Rating Scale (0–10). She described the pain as "throbbing and constant."

CARDIOVASCULAR AND RESPIRATORY SYSTEMS FUNCTIONS

Katrina's resting vital signs were blood pressure of 156/90 mm Hg, heart rate of 92 beats per minute, respiration rate of 22 breaths per minute, and temperature of 97.6°.

MOVEMENT FUNCTIONS

Katrina presented with choreiform movements of all extremities, torso, and head. An assessment of active range of motion through observation revealed no gross deficits in all extremities. Her dominant right wrist was immobilized in a fiberglass cast and unable to be assessed. Her right hand presented as edematous and was only able to form 75% of a gross grasp. An assessment of muscle strength was unable to be performed, but she was able to mobilize all extremities against gravity.

NEUROMUSCULAR FUNCTIONS

Katrina's static and dynamic sitting balance were fair (F)+, and her standing static and dynamic were F–. She presented with involuntary bilateral ocular movements, impaired coordination, slow repetitive movements, and abnormal posturing. She reported experiencing frequent painful muscle spasms, difficulty swallowing, and difficulty effectively verbally communicating. The Johns Hopkins Fall Risk Assessment Tool (JHFRAT; Poe et al., 2005) was administered, and a score of 12 was obtained.

PLAN FOR DISCHARGE

Upon discharge, Katrina will remain at home with long-term-care services.

Questions and Activities

SAFETY OF CLIENT AND OTHERS: PRECAUTIONS AND CONTRAINDICATIONS

1. Create a handout that identifies precautions for people at high risk for aspiration pneumonia.
2. Is Katrina a fall risk? Identify three tools to assess fall risk. Evaluate them and determine which would be most appropriate in this case.
3. Identify precautions to consider when working with people at high risk for a fall.

4. Katrina exhibits involuntary movements. What precautions need to be followed during the performance of ADLs?
5. Katrina has shared thoughts of suicide. How should this information be addressed?
6. Katrina is wearing a cast. Identify the risks related to wearing a cast. Explain how these risks can be mitigated.
7. Identify the common psychological reactions associated with HD that may affect the treatment process.
8. To keep Katrina and others safe, what other factors should be considered?

OCCUPATIONS: ADLs, IADLs, EDUCATION, WORK, PLAY, SOCIAL PARTICIPATION, AND REST AND SLEEP

1. Given the information provided for this case, identify the areas of occupation that will and will not be addressed. Justify your decisions.
2. What positional strategies would you recommend for self-feeding for Katrina?
3. Compare and contrast occupational therapy with speech-language pathology regarding the scope of practice for each for self-feeding.
4. Identify the forms of caregiver education that would be necessary for reducing Katrina's risk of falls during functional mobility tasks.
5. How can Katrina maximize her engagement in self-care given her progressive condition?

PERFORMANCE SKILLS: MOTOR SKILLS, PROCESS SKILLS, AND SOCIAL INTERACTION SKILLS

1. Given the information provided, identify the motor, process, and social interaction skills that affect Katrina's occupational performance.
2. Which of these skills would be appropriate to address in this service delivery site? Justify your selection.
3. Which of these skills would be addressed through remediation, compensation, and education?
4. Which of these skills would be addressed through the following intervention approaches: create/promote, establish/restore, maintain, modify, and prevent. How can you make use of this information?

PERFORMANCE PATTERNS: HABITS, ROUTINES, ROLES, AND RITUALS

1. Identify Katrina's useful habits, routines, roles, and rituals that support valued occupations. How can you make use of this information?
2. Identify Katrina's impoverished habits, routines, roles, and rituals that do not support valued occupations. How can you make use of this information?
3. Identify Katrina's dominating habits, routines, roles and rituals that interfere with her valued occupations. How can you make use of this information?

CLIENT FACTORS

Values, beliefs, and spirituality
How can the identified values, beliefs, and spirituality be used in this case?

Body structures
Considering Katrina's primary and secondary diagnoses, identify the related body structures.

Body functions

1. Identify how the primary and secondary diagnoses have affected the function of the identified body structures.
2. Explain the relationships between the structural and functional factors and Katrina's current level of occupational performance.

MENTAL FUNCTIONS: AFFECTIVE, COGNITIVE, AND PERCEPTUAL

1. How can major depressive disorder exacerbate the symptoms of HD?
2. Katrina was observed to be angry and irritable during the end of the evaluation. How could this observation affect the delivery of treatment?
3. Katrina exhibited impairment of her short-term memory. How will this impairment affect your choice of instruction during treatment?
4. Given that Katrina has difficulty sustaining attention, how would you organize the environment to minimizc distractions?
5. Given the information provided, what additional mental function considerations need to be addressed?

NEUROMUSCULOSKELETAL AND MOVEMENT-RELATED FUNCTIONS

1. Given the information provided, identify neuromusculoskeletal and movement-related functions that need to be addressed. Justify your selections.
2. Compare and contrast choreiform with athetoid movements.
3. People with HD commonly experience significant weight loss. Explain why.
4. What recommendations can be made to minimize the risk of falls in the home?
5. Create an exercise program based on occupational performance for Katrina.

CARDIOVASCULAR, HEMATOLOGICAL, IMMUNOLOGICAL, AND RESPIRATORY FUNCTIONS

1. Given the information provided, identify cardiovascular, hematological, immunological, and respiratory functions that need to be addressed. Justify your selections.
2. Do you foresee accurately obtaining Katrina's vital signs? Explain why or why not.
3. Identify the signs and symptoms of aspiration.
4. Compare and contrast aspiration pneumonia with viral pneumonia.

SKIN AND RELATED STRUCTURE FUNCTIONS

1. What are the signs and symptoms of an improperly fitted cast?
2. How can skin integrity be compromised by involuntary movement?

VOICE AND SPEECH FUNCTIONS

Describe how Katrina's diagnoses may affect her voice, speech, and associated occupational performance.

ASSISTIVE TECHNOLOGIES AND DEVICES

What assistive technologies or adaptations might be used or made for Katrina while she is receiving occupational therapy services at home? Why?

ETHICAL DECISION MAKING

1. Katrina has recently stated, "Life is not worth living." How should this statement be addressed?
2. During treatment sessions, Katrina frequently asks you for marital advice. How should you respond?
3. As you left Katrina's home after a treatment session, her mother approached you. She shared feeling overwhelmed and emotionally drained. How should this situation best be addressed?

PHARMACOLOGY

Katrina is currently taking Celexa.

1. What is the generic name?
2. Does this drug have a high alert status?
3. What is the classification of this drug?
4. What is the indication for this drug?
5. What is the action of this drug?
6. How may this drug affect client participation during a therapy session?

SOCIOCULTURAL, SOCIOECONOMIC, AND DIVERSITY FACTORS AND LIFESTYLE CHOICES

1. Given Katrina's profile, how may your own culture and beliefs affect your interaction with her?
2. Based on this self-examination, what area of cultural knowledge do you need to pursue?
3. How can this newly acquired cultural knowledge be integrated for effective outcomes?
4. How can you foster cultural interaction and awareness among your coworkers?
5. Discuss how a lack of understanding in the areas of discrimination and stigma, implicit bias, social identity, or racism may contribute to disparities in the delivery of occupational therapy services in this case.

ASSESSMENT TOOLS AND INTERPRETATION OF RESULTS

1. What is the purpose of the JHFRAT?
2. Which population is this test designed for?
3. How much time is required to administer it?
4. Provide a brief description of this assessment.
5. What is the reliability of the JHFRAT?
6. What is the validity of the JHFRAT?
7. What functional inference can be deduced from Katrina's score of 12?
8. What additional standardized assessment can be used in this case? Why?

INTERPROFESSIONAL RELATIONSHIP AND EFFECTIVE INTRAPROFESSIONAL COLLABORATION

1. Identify the other professions that would make up the care team. Explain the focus of each.
2. Identify the roles of the occupational therapy assistant (OTA) that could be used in the occupational therapy process for this case.
3. Identify interventions that can be assigned to the OTA for this case. Justify your selections.

BILLING AND CODING

1. Identify the *International Classification of Diseases (ICD)* codes for Katrina's diagnoses.
2. For this case, identify at least two *Current Procedural Terminology (CPT®)* codes that are most appropriate. Justify your selection.

REIMBURSEMENT SYSTEMS AND DOCUMENTATION

1. Who would be the authorized individuals that you could share the occupational therapy findings with? Explain why.
2. For this case, what forms and frequency of documentation will be required?
3. Which reimbursement system or systems most commonly cover occupational therapy services in this practice setting?

ADVOCACY

1. Which of the following areas of advocacy would be beneficial in this case: patient rights, matters of privacy, confidentiality, informed consent, awareness building, accessing education, or benefits/resources?
2. Create a plan to advocate for this client based on the selected areas of advocacy.

TELEHEALTH

1. How can telehealth be integrated as a component of the occupational therapy process in this case?
2. Before launching telemedicine services, what questions would be essential to ask Katrina to determine whether it is appropriate for her to engage in telemedicine services?
3. What are the barriers, obstacles, or challenges you foresee if attempting to integrate telehealth services with this client?

Intervention Plan Formulation and Implementation

INTERVENTION PLAN FORMULATION

Create an intervention plan that includes the following:

1. List this individual's **strengths.**
2. List this individual's **barriers** in occupational performance, performance skills, and performance patterns.

3. Based on the individual's goals, health, performance, and service delivery site, **identify the barriers that will be addressed.**
4. From the barriers identified to be addressed, **formulate goals and objectives.**
5. Identify the focus of each goal and objective as either **create, promote, establish, restore, maintain, modify, or prevent.**
6. Identify the **theoretical basis, model(s) of practice, or frame(s) of reference** that will be used to address each goal and objective.
7. For each proposed goal and objective, describe clearly and precisely the **methods** that will be used. This description should include, but not be limited to, safety considerations, environmental considerations, therapeutic use of self, preparatory activities, activity selection, materials, equipment, and flow.
8. Classify the activities selected in the methods description as either **preparatory, enabling, purposeful, or occupation based.**
9. Explain how each activity can be **graded up or down,** creating the just-right challenge.
10. Provide at least two **primary sources of evidence** to support the intervention plan.

INTERVENTION PLAN IMPLEMENTATION

1. Based on your intervention plan, identify which goals and objectives require **more immediate attention.**
2. Describe your proposed **first treatment session.**
3. As the treatment session is progressing, what is **essential to be observed?**

Transition and Discontinuation

Create a plan for discharge from occupational therapy services in collaboration with Katrina and members of the interprofessional team. Review the needs of Katrina, caregivers, family members, and significant others. The plan must match needs with available resources and the discharge environment.

REFERENCES

American Medical Association. (2019). *CPT® 2020 professional edition.*

Poe, S. S., Cvach, M. M., Gartrell, D. G., Radzik, B. R., & Joy, T. L. (2005). An evidence-based approach to fall risk assessment, prevention, and management: Lessons learned. *Journal of Nursing Care Quality, 20,* 107–116. https://doi.org/10.1097/00001786-200504000-00004

World Health Organization. (2019). *International statistical classification of diseases and related health problems* (11th ed.). https://icd.who.int/

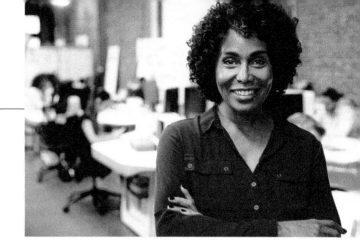

Ivy: SARS-CoV-2 (COVID-19)

CLOVER HUTCHINSON, OTD, MA, OTR/L

Ivy (she, her, hers, herself)

MEDICAL HISTORY

Ivy is a 66-year-old Nigerian American female who is 5' 2" and weighs 195 pounds. She was brought into the emergency department (ED) by her family after a complaint of persistent coughing and difficulty breathing. While in the ED, she was placed on oxygen through a nasal cannula. She had an oral temperature of 102.6° and reported a loss of smell and taste. Ivy was given a reverse transcription real-time polymerase chain reaction test, which confirmed that she was positive for the 2019 novel coronavirus (COVID-19). A high-resolution computed tomography scan was performed and revealed acute and organizing diffuse alveolar damage. Her medical history included obesity, chronic asthma, and osteoarthritis in both knees. She reported no alcohol, drug, tobacco, or caffeine use. No allergies were reported. Ivy was transferred to the general medical service ward, where she was treated for 22 days.

SOCIAL HISTORY

Ivy is employed as an office manager and disclosed that she plans to retire in 1 year. She lives with her spouse, Tricia, of 10 years in a seventh-floor apartment. Tricia has been retired for 2 years. Tricia has a son, who visits often with his two children, ages 10 and 13. All members of the family have been COVID-19 tested and reported being negative. Ivy identifies as a member of the Baptist faith.

REFERRAL OR PRESCRIPTION

Ivy was transferred home with community health care services. She has been referred for occupational therapy, physical therapy, social work, and registered nursing services. Home health services are prescribed for 4 weeks.

Occupational Therapy Initial Evaluation Findings: Community Health Care Services

OCCUPATIONAL PROFILE

Ivy's preadmission occupational history and experiences included being independent in all ADLs and all IADLs. Her patterns of daily living most commonly included waking up at 5:00 a.m., taking the train, and arriving at work by 8:00 a.m. At home, she enjoyed cooking and did most of the grocery shopping and meal preparation. Tricia performed most of the house cleaning and paid the bills. Ivy enjoyed walking with Tricia at least 3 times per week in the neighborhood park. On the weekends, they enjoyed going to the movies or local comedy shows. Ivy's interests include cooking meals from different cultures, and she values her marriage and spending time with Tricia's grandchildren. She reported her greatest need is to return to work at full capacity.

ADLs

Regarding self-care, Ivy was able to dress while sitting at the edge of the bed but required assistance with setup and frequent rest breaks. Ivy was independent in toileting and could feed herself while taking incremental breaks. She reported needing assistance from Tricia to sponge bathe. Regarding functional mobility, Ivy was able to roll from supine to her right and left side as well as transition between supine and sit and bridge in a slow effort-filled manner. She was able to transition from short sitting to stand and perform transfers with an adult rolling walker with minimal assistance.

IADLs

Activities needed that provide day-to-day quality of life and relative independence were explored. At the time of the evaluation, shopping, meal preparation, and care of the home were being performed by Tricia. Ivy reported feeling uncomfortable with technology used for financial management, such as online banking and bill paying. Ivy required assistance to manage the oxygen concentrator. Regarding rest and sleep, Ivy reported that since her diagnosis she had been experiencing insomnia, excessive sleepiness, restless leg syndrome, and nightmares.

MENTAL FUNCTIONS

Cognitive assessment found Ivy to be alert and oriented to person, place, time, and situation, and long-term memory was intact. She reported having difficulty with short-term memory for 1–2 years before admission. She was able to follow three-step commands and make her needs known. Affect appeared appropriate, but she expressed regret that she declined COVID-19 vaccination. No gross deficits in perception were observed.

SENSORY FUNCTIONS

No gross deficits were observed with hearing, vestibular, smell, proprioceptive, and cutaneous functions. Ivy reported diminished taste and smell. Visual, tactile, and auditory functions were grossly intact. The Numerical Rating Scale (0–10) revealed a pain score of 5 in both knees and a 6 for a Stage 2 decubitus ulcer located over her coccyx. The pain was described as "excruciating."

CARDIOVASCULAR AND RESPIRATORY SYSTEMS FUNCTIONS

Ivy frequently complained of fatigue and shortness of breath. Her oxygen saturation at rest was 91% and with supplemental oxygen was 96%. The Borg Rating of Perceived Exertion Scale (Mathias et al., 1986) was completed by Ivy, and she reported a score of 11 during dressing while seated and 14 during tub transfers.

MOVEMENT FUNCTIONS

Passive range of motion and active range of motion in all four extremities were within normal limits. Muscle strength in both upper extremities (BUE) and both lower extremities was 3+/5. Coordination for BUE was within defined limits. Fine motor abilities were intact for gross grasp, fine pinch, and in-hand manipulation.

NEUROMUSCULAR FUNCTIONS

Ivy's static and dynamic sitting balance were good. Her static standing balance was fair (F)+, and her dynamic standing balance was F. Ivy's muscle tone in all four extremities was normal, and reflex integration was grossly intact. The Timed Up and Go (TUG) Test (Podsiadlo & Richardson, 1991) was administered, and Ivy completed it in 17 minutes.

PLAN FOR DISCHARGE

Upon discharge, Ivy will transition to outpatient rehabilitation services. She will receive occupational and physical therapy.

Questions and Activities

SAFETY OF CLIENT AND OTHERS: PRECAUTIONS AND CONTRAINDICATIONS

1. According to current Centers for Disease Control and Prevention guidelines, what precautions must be followed when working with a person with active acute symptoms of COVID-19?
2. Create a handout identifying the early signs and symptoms of a COVID-19 infection.
3. Ivy is currently using supplemental oxygen. How is the optimal flow rate determined? What precautions must be followed?
4. Identify the signs and symptoms of respiratory distress.
5. Identify the common emotional reactions associated with a COVID-19 infection that may affect the treatment process.
6. To keep Ivy and others safe, what other factors should be considered?

OCCUPATIONS: ADLs, IADLs, EDUCATION, WORK, PLAY, SOCIAL PARTICIPATION, AND REST AND SLEEP

1. Given the information provided for this case, identify the areas of occupation that will and will not be addressed. Justify your decisions.
2. Ivy wishes to bathe in the tub. What recommendations would you make?
3. Ivy wants to know when it would be safe to resume sexual relations with her partner. How should you proceed?
4. How would you incorporate energy conservation or work simplification concepts for this case?

PERFORMANCE SKILLS: MOTOR SKILLS, PROCESS SKILLS, AND SOCIAL INTERACTION SKILLS

1. Given the information provided, identify the motor, process, and social interaction skills that affect Ivy's occupational performance.
2. Which of these skills would be appropriate to address in this service delivery site? Justify your selection.
3. Which of these skills would be addressed through remediation, compensation, and education?
4. Which of these skills would be addressed through the following intervention approaches: create/promote, establish/restore, maintain, modify, and prevent?

PERFORMANCE PATTERNS: HABITS, ROUTINES, ROLES, AND RITUALS

1. Identify Ivy's useful habits, routines, roles, and rituals that support valued occupations. How can you make use of this information?
2. Identify Ivy's impoverished habits, routines, roles, and rituals that do not support valued occupations. How can you make use of this information?
3. Identify Ivy's dominating habits, routines, roles, and rituals that interfere with valued occupations. How can you make use of this information?

CLIENT FACTORS

Values, beliefs, and spirituality
How can the identified values, beliefs, and spirituality be used in this case?

Body structures
Considering Ivy's primary and secondary diagnoses, identify the related body structures.

Body functions
1. Identify how the primary and secondary diagnoses have affected the function of the identified body structures.
2. Explain the relationships between the structural and functional factors and Ivy's current level of occupational performance.

MENTAL FUNCTIONS: AFFECTIVE, COGNITIVE, AND PERCEPTUAL

1. Ivy reports feeling frustrated with her slow recovery. How should her frustration be addressed?
2. Identify mental health concerns that have been associated with people who have been infected with COVID-19. Identify your sources.

3. At each session, Ivy pressures you to provide an estimated time frame for when she can return to work. How should this situation be addressed?
4. Given the information provided, what additional mental function considerations need to be addressed?

NEUROMUSCULOSKELETAL AND MOVEMENT-RELATED FUNCTIONS

1. Given the information provided, identify neuromusculoskeletal and movement-related functions that need to be addressed. Justify your selections.
2. Compare and contrast muscular fatigue with cardiovascular fatigue.
3. Identify three fall risk assessment tools that would be appropriate for the home care practice setting. Evaluate them and select one. Defend your selection.
4. Create a list of recommendations to minimize risk of falls within the home.
5. Create an exercise program based on occupational performance for Ivy.

CARDIOVASCULAR, HEMATOLOGICAL, IMMUNOLOGICAL, AND RESPIRATORY FUNCTIONS

1. Given the information provided, identify cardiovascular, hematological, immunological, and respiratory functions that need to be addressed. Justify your selections.
2. Identify the expected range of oxygen saturation levels for an adult population. Reference your source.
3. People with respiratory diseases commonly experience shortness of breath after the consumption of large meals. Explain why.
4. Compare and contrast supplemental oxygen with ventilator support.
5. Compare and contrast asthma with bronchitis.

SKIN AND RELATED STRUCTURE FUNCTIONS

1. What are the signs and symptoms of cyanosis?
2. What actions must be taken when signs or symptoms of cyanosis are observed?
3. What considerations should be made given the presence of the Stage 2 decubitus ulcer over Ivy's coccyx?
4. What other skin and related structure functions should be considered?

VOICE AND SPEECH FUNCTIONS

Describe how Ivy's diagnoses may affect her voice, speech, and associated occupational performance.

ASSISTIVE TECHNOLOGIES AND DEVICES

What assistive technologies or adaptations might be used or made for Ivy while she is receiving occupational therapy services at home? Why?

ETHICAL DECISION MAKING

1. Ivy reports that before your arrival, she had a fall. What are the appropriate steps that must be taken?
2. During a treatment session, you observe Ivy's partner Tricia spanking her grandchild. How should this situation be addressed?

PHARMACOLOGY

Ivy is currently taking albuterol.

1. What is the brand name?
2. Does this drug have a high alert status?
3. What is the classification of this drug?
4. What is the indication for this drug?
5. What is the action of this drug?
6. How may this drug affect client participation during a therapy session?

SOCIOCULTURAL, SOCIOECONOMIC, AND DIVERSITY FACTORS AND LIFESTYLE CHOICES

1. Given Ivy's profile, how may your own culture and beliefs affect your interaction with her?
2. Based on this self-examination, what area of cultural knowledge do you need to pursue?
3. How can this newly acquired cultural knowledge be integrated for effective outcomes?
4. How can you foster cultural interaction and awareness among your coworkers?
5. Discuss how a lack of understanding in the areas of discrimination and stigma, implicit bias, social identity, or racism may contribute to disparities in the delivery of occupational therapy services in this case.

ASSESSMENT TOOLS AND INTERPRETATION OF RESULTS

1. What is the purpose of the TUG Test?
2. Which population is this test designed for?
3. How much time is required to administer it?
4. Provide a brief description of this assessment.
5. What is the reliability of the TUG Test?
6. What is the validity of the TUG Test?
7. What functional inference can be deduced from Katrina's performance time of 17 minutes?
8. What additional standardized assessment can be used in this case? Why?

INTERPROFESSIONAL RELATIONSHIP AND EFFECTIVE INTRAPROFESSIONAL COLLABORATION

1. Identify the other professions that would make up the care team. Explain the focus of each.
2. Identify the roles of the occupational therapy assistant (OTA) that could be used in the occupational therapy process for this case.
3. Identify interventions that can be assigned to the OTA for this case. Justify your selections.

BILLING AND CODING

1. Identify the *International Classification of Diseases (ICD)* codes for Ivy's diagnoses.
2. For this case, identify at least two *Current Procedural Terminology (CPT®)* codes that are most appropriate. Justify your selection.

REIMBURSEMENT SYSTEMS AND DOCUMENTATION

1. Who would be the authorized individuals that you could share the occupational therapy findings with? Explain why.
2. For this case, what forms and frequency of documentation will be required?
3. Which reimbursement system or systems most commonly cover occupational therapy services in this practice setting?

ADVOCACY

1. Which of the following areas of advocacy would be beneficial in this case: patient rights, matters of privacy, confidentiality, informed consent, awareness building, accessing education, or benefits/ resources?
2. Create a plan to advocate for this client based on the selected areas of advocacy.

TELEHEALTH

1. How can telehealth be integrated as a component of the occupational therapy process in this case?
2. Before launching telemedicine services, what questions would be essential to ask Ivy to determine whether it is appropriate for her to engage in telemedicine services?
3. What are the barriers, obstacles, or challenges you foresee if attempting to integrate telehealth services with this client?

Intervention Plan Formulation and Implementation

INTERVENTION PLAN FORMULATION

Create an intervention plan that includes the following:

1. List this individual's **strengths.**
2. List this individual's **barriers** in occupational performance, performance skills, and performance patterns.
3. Based on the individual's goals, health, performance, and service delivery site, **identify the barriers that will be addressed.**
4. From the barriers identified to be addressed, **formulate goals and objectives.**
5. Identify the focus of each goal and objective as either **create, promote, establish, restore, maintain, modify, or prevent.**
6. Identify the **theoretical basis, model(s) of practice, or frame(s) of reference** that will be used to address each goal and objective.
7. For each proposed goal and objective, describe clearly and precisely the **methods** that will be used. This description should include, but not be limited to, safety considerations, environmental considerations, therapeutic use of self, preparatory activities, activity selection, materials, equipment, and flow.
8. Classify the activities selected in the methods description as either **preparatory, enabling, purposeful, or occupation based.**
9. Explain how each activity can be **graded up or down,** creating the just-right challenge.
10. Provide at least two **primary sources of evidence** to support the intervention plan.

INTERVENTION PLAN IMPLEMENTATION

1. Based on your intervention plan, identify which goals and objectives require **more immediate attention.**
2. Describe your proposed **first treatment session.**
3. As the treatment session is progressing, what is **essential to be observed?**

Transition and Discontinuation

Create a plan for discharge from occupational therapy services in collaboration with Ivy and members of the interprofessional team. Review the needs of Ivy, caregivers, family members, and significant others. The plan must match needs with available resources and the discharge environment.

REFERENCES

American Medical Association. (2019). *CPT® 2020 professional edition.*

Mathias, S., Nayak, U. S., & Isaacs, B. (1986). Balance in elderly patients: The "Get-Up and Go" Test. *Archives of Physical Medicine and Rehabilitation, 67,* 387–389.

World Health Organization. (2019). *International statistical classification of diseases and related health problems* (11th ed.). https://icd.who.int/

Inpatient Behavioral Health Hospital or Unit

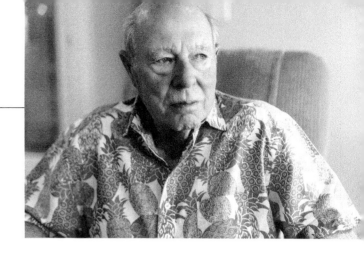

Zoran: Depression

DONALD AURIEMMA, MS ED, OTR/L

Zoran (he, him, his, himself)

MEDICAL HISTORY

Zoran is a 63-year-old German American male who is 5' 9" and weighs 210 pounds. He was taken to the emergency department by emergency medical services after a suicide attempt. Upon arrival, he presented with a self-inflicted laceration of his right distal anterior forearm at his wrist. He was rushed into surgery and had a repair of tendons of flexor digitorum profundus, flexor digitorum superficialis, flexor digitorum, flexor carpi radialis longus, flexor carpi radialis longus, and flexor carpi radialis brevis, as well as the radial artery and radial nerve. In the recovery room, he was seen by psychiatry and diagnosed with major depressive disorder (MDD). His medical history included hypertension, high cholesterol, and surgical repair of a hernia. He reported no drug, tobacco, or caffeine use, but he reported heavy alcohol use after his wife's passing. Zoran also has a history of sleep apnea but does not use any sleep aids. He has no known allergies or behavioral health history. From the surgical recovery room, he was involuntarily transferred to the inpatient behavioral health unit.

SOCIAL HISTORY

Zoran is a bus driver who owns and lives in a two-story, two-family brownstone. He planned to work until age 66 years, so he could collect maximum Social Security benefits. He and his spouse, Edna, both became infected with the 2019 novel coronavirus. Zoran survived and Edna did not. Zoran blames himself for his wife's death. He stated, "I brought that [expletive] virus home." He has one child, an engineer who lives in California. Zoran reported enjoying visits to his weekend home in the mountains and spending time with friends and family. Zoran is an observer of the Yazidi religion.

REFERRAL OR PRESCRIPTION

Zoran was transferred to an inpatient behavioral health unit. He has been referred for occupational therapy, physical therapy, social work, psychology, and registered nursing services. He will also be seen by a second occupational therapist who is a certified hand therapist from the Department of Physical Medicine and Rehabilitation. The length of stay will be 4 weeks.

Occupational Therapy Initial Evaluation Findings: Inpatient Behavioral Health Unit

OCCUPATIONAL PROFILE

Zoran's preadmission occupational history and experiences included being independent in all ADLs and IADLs. His patterns of daily living most commonly included waking on weekdays at 6:00 a.m., making himself breakfast, and working the 7:00 a.m. to 3:00 p.m. shift. He has been driving the same route for more than 25 years. He usually returns home by 4:00 p.m. and then cooks dinner. Edna usually returned home at 6:00 p.m. from work, and then they ate together. Most evenings were spent sitting in the yard, watching television, or doing household chores. Each Friday night, they would load up their car and head to their mountain home for the weekend. Zoran's interests include fishing, and he values spending time with those he cares about and being surrounded by nature. He stated, "I am a creature of habit. Routines make me comfortable." Zoran reported his greatest need is to get out of the "psych hospital."

ADLs

Regarding self-care, when Zoran was seen for the initial evaluation, he was sedated. His hair was uncombed; his breath reeked; and he wore a stained sweatshirt, pants, and sneakers. The pants and sneakers did not have laces. It was reported by the nurse that Zoran had declined being washed up and eating since his arrival. His right hand was placed in a thermoplastic dorsal block splint. Regarding functional mobility, Zoran was observed rolling and transitioning from supine to short sit independently. He required close supervision to transfer between bed and chair.

IADLs

Activities needed that provide day-to-day quality of life and relative independence were explored. Information pertaining to this area was unable to be gathered at the time of the initial evaluation. Regarding rest and sleep, the medical chart indicated that since Zoran's arrival, he had been frequently found in bed asleep during unstructured times on the unit. Medical records indicate a history of sleep apnea.

MENTAL FUNCTIONS

Cognitive assessment found Zoran to be alert and oriented to person, place, time, and situation, and short- and long-term memory were intact. He was able to follow three-step commands and make his needs known. Assessment of Zoran's affect revealed flat affect and answering questions slowly using short responses. His eyes remained fixed to the ground, and he seldom made eye contact. The following statement was repeated three times, "All this is just a big waste of time. I just want to die." No gross deficits in perceptual function were observed. The Beck Depression Inventory–II (BDI–II; Beck et al., 1996) was administered, and a score of 22 was obtained.

SENSORY FUNCTIONS AND PAIN

No gross deficits were observed with visual, hearing, vestibular, taste, smell, and proprioceptive functions. Zoran was evaluated using the Numerical Rating Scale (0–10) and reported that the pain in his right hand was a 7. The pain was described as "unbearable." He also reported that his right hand felt "numb." No gross cutaneous sensory testing was performed at the time of initial evaluation.

CARDIOVASCULAR AND RESPIRATORY SYSTEM FUNCTIONS

Zoran's vital signs were as follows: heart rate at 61 beats per minute, respiration rate at 12 breaths per minute, and blood pressure at 96/60 mm Hg.

MOVEMENT FUNCTIONS

Passive range of motion and active range of motion in all extremities were within normal limits. The right wrist and digits were not assessed. Zoran is right-hand dominant and held his right upper extremity in a guarded position.

NEUROMUSCULAR FUNCTIONS

While seated Zoran slouched in his chair, and while standing he required close supervision to transfer and ambulate. Static and dynamic sitting balance were estimated to be Fair (F)+ and static and dynamic standing balance were F–. Muscle tone was normal, and reflex integration appeared intact.

PLAN FOR DISCHARGE

Zoran will be discharged to the care of a community-based psychiatrist, psychologist, and occupational therapist.

Questions and Activities

SAFETY OF CLIENT AND OTHERS: PRECAUTIONS AND CONTRAINDICATIONS

1. Given Zoran was placed on suicide watch, what precautions must be followed?
2. Create a handout that identifies the precautions and contraindications that must be followed regarding the surgical repairs made to Zoran's right wrist.
3. Identify three up-to-date, reliable, and valid sources to obtain precautions for working with clients with MDD. Evaluate them, select the strongest source, and justify your selection.
4. Identify the common emotional reactions associated with an unsuccessful suicide attempt that may affect the treatment process.
5. To keep Zoran and others safe, what other factors should be considered?

OCCUPATIONS: ADLs, IADLs, EDUCATION, WORK, PLAY, SOCIAL PARTICIPATION, AND REST AND SLEEP

1. Given the information provided for this case, identify the areas of occupation that will and will not be addressed. Justify your decisions.
2. This case presents the unusual circumstance of two occupational therapists working with the same client in the same institution. Create a list that identifies the roles and responsibilities of each occupational therapist.
3. Zoran is right-hand dominant. What areas of basic ADLs do you believe Zoran will have difficulty performing as a result of his right hand being immobilized and his pain level of 7 in that extremity?
4. In the context of delivering occupational therapy services on a behavioral health unit, will your interaction and intervention with Zoran be delivered in a group format, individually, or a combination of both?
5. Which of Zoran's problems may be addressed in a group format?
6. What makes a group run by an occupational therapist distinctly different from one run by a social worker, recreational therapist, or psychologist?
7. Which of Zoran's problems may be addressed in an individual session?

PERFORMANCE SKILLS: MOTOR SKILLS, PROCESS SKILLS, AND SOCIAL INTERACTION SKILLS

1. Given the information provided, identify the motor, process, and social interaction skills that affect Zoran's occupational performance.
2. Which of these skills would be appropriate to address in this service delivery site? Justify your selection.
3. Which of these skills would be addressed through remediation, compensation, and education?
4. Which of these skills would be addressed through the following intervention approaches: create/promote, establish/restore, maintain, modify, and prevent?

PERFORMANCE PATTERNS: HABITS, ROUTINES, ROLES, AND RITUALS

1. Identify Zoran's useful habits, routines, roles, and rituals that support valued occupations. How can you make use of this information?
2. Identify Zoran's impoverished habits, routines, roles, and rituals that do not support valued occupations. How can you make use of this information?
3. Identify Zoran's dominating habits, routines, roles, and rituals that interfere with valued occupations. How can you make use of this information?

CLIENT FACTORS

Values, beliefs, and spirituality
How can the identified values, beliefs, and spirituality be used in this case?

Body structures
Considering Zoran's primary and secondary diagnoses, identify the related body structures.

Body functions
1. Identify how the primary and secondary diagnoses have affected the function of the identified body structures.

2. Explain the relationships between the structural and functional factors and Zoran's current level of occupational performance.

MENTAL FUNCTIONS: AFFECTIVE, COGNITIVE, AND PERCEPTUAL

1. Compare and contrast the rate of suicide attempts between males and females.
2. Create a handout identifying the signs and symptoms of MDD.
3. Explain the chemical changes that occur in the brain as a result of MDD.
4. Identify and select a model(s) or frame(s) of reference you would use to treat Zoran. Support your selection(s).
5. Given the information provided, what other mental function considerations need to be addressed?

NEUROMUSCULOSKELETAL AND MOVEMENT-RELATED FUNCTIONS

1. Given the information provided, identify neuromusculoskeletal and movement-related functions that need to be addressed. Justify your selections.
2. What forms of nonverbal communication would indicate that Zoran's condition is improving?
3. What forms of nonverbal communication would indicate that Zoran's condition is worsening?
4. Create an exercise program for Zoran based on occupational performance.

CARDIOVASCULAR, HEMATOLOGICAL, IMMUNOLOGICAL, AND RESPIRATORY FUNCTIONS

1. Given the information provided, identify cardiovascular, hematological, immunological, and respiratory functions that need to be addressed. Justify your selections.
2. Provide your insights on Zoran's vital sign measurements.
3. When Zoran transitions from sitting to standing, he usually closes his eyes and braces his body. Given his resting blood pressure, what would be your concern?

SKIN AND RELATED STRUCTURE FUNCTIONS

You observe the tips of Zoran's right fingers protruding from the applied splint. What physical signs and reported symptoms would suggest a poorly fitted device?

VOICE AND SPEECH FUNCTIONS

Describe how Zoran's diagnoses may affect his voice, speech, and associated occupational performance.

ASSISTIVE TECHNOLOGIES AND DEVICES

1. What assistive technologies or adaptations might be used or made for Zoran while he is receiving occupational therapy services on the behavioral health unit? Why?
2. What assistive technologies or adaptations might be recommended for when he returns home? Why?

ETHICAL DECISION MAKING

1. You observe Zoran trying to remove his applied splint. How should this situation be addressed?
2. Zoran asked you if you could leave him one of the plastic knives from the occupational therapy area. How should this request be addressed?
3. One of the residents on the ward informs you that they find you attractive. How should this situation be addressed?
4. Explain the concept of transference.
5. You glance into a patient room, and you observe two patients engaging in sexual intercourse. How should this situation be addressed?

PHARMACOLOGY

Zoran is currently taking Lexapro.

1. What is the generic name?
2. Does this drug have a high alert status?
3. What is the classification of this drug?
4. What is the indication for this drug?
5. What is the action of this drug?
6. How may this drug affect client participation during a therapy session?

SOCIOCULTURAL, SOCIOECONOMIC, AND DIVERSITY FACTORS AND LIFESTYLE CHOICES

1. Given Zoran's profile, how may your own culture and beliefs affect your interaction with him?
2. Based on this self-examination, what area of cultural knowledge do you need to pursue?
3. How can this newly acquired cultural knowledge be integrated for effective outcomes?
4. How can you foster cultural interaction and awareness among your coworkers?
5. Discuss how a lack of understanding in the areas of discrimination and stigma, implicit bias, social identity, or racism may contribute to disparities in the delivery of occupational therapy services in this case.

ASSESSMENT TOOLS AND INTERPRETATION OF RESULTS

1. What is the purpose of the BDI–II?
2. Which population is this test designed for?
3. How much time is required to administer it?
4. Provide a brief description of this assessment.
5. What is the reliability of the BDI–II?
6. What is the validity of the BDI–II?
7. What functional inference can be deduced from a score of 22?
8. What additional standardized assessment can be used in this case? Why?

INTERPROFESSIONAL RELATIONSHIP AND EFFECTIVE INTRAPROFESSIONAL COLLABORATION

1. Identify the other professions that would make up the care team. Explain the focus of each.

2. Identify the roles of the occupational therapy assistant (OTA) that could be used in the occupational therapy process for this case.
3. Identify interventions that can be assigned to the OTA for this case. Justify your selections.

BILLING AND CODING

1. Identify the *International Classification of Diseases (ICD)* codes for Zoran's diagnoses.
2. For this case, identify at least two *Current Procedural Terminology (CPT®)* codes that are most appropriate. Justify your selection.

REIMBURSEMENT SYSTEMS AND DOCUMENTATION

1. Who would be the authorized individuals that you could share the occupational therapy findings with? Explain why.
2. For this case, what forms and frequency of documentation will be required?
3. Which reimbursement system or systems most commonly cover occupational therapy services in this practice setting?

ADVOCACY

1. Which of the following areas of advocacy would be beneficial in this case: patient rights, matters of privacy, confidentiality, informed consent, awareness building, accessing education, or benefits/resources?
2. Create a plan to advocate for this client based on the selected areas of advocacy.

TELEHEALTH

1. How can telehealth be integrated as a component of the occupational therapy process in this case?
2. Before launching telemedicine services, what questions would be essential to ask Zoran to determine whether it is appropriate for him to engage in telemedicine services?
3. What are the barriers, obstacles, or challenges you foresee if attempting to integrate telehealth services with this client?

Intervention Plan Formulation and Implementation

INTERVENTION PLAN FORMULATION

Create an intervention plan that includes the following:

1. List this individual's **strengths.**
2. List this individual's **barriers** in occupational performance, performance skills, and performance patterns.
3. Based on the individual's goals, health, performance, and service delivery site, **identify the barriers that will be addressed.**
4. From the barriers identified to be addressed, **formulate goals and objectives.**

5. Identify the focus of each goal and objective as either **create, promote, establish, restore, maintain, modify, or prevent.**
6. Identify the **theoretical basis, model(s) of practice, or frame(s) of reference** that will be used to address each goal and objective.
7. For each proposed goal and objective, describe clearly and precisely the **methods** that will be used. This description should include, but not be limited to, safety considerations, environmental considerations, therapeutic use of self, preparatory activities, activity selection, materials, equipment, and flow.
8. Classify the activities selected in the methods description as either **preparatory, enabling, purposeful, or occupation based.**
9. Explain how each activity can be **graded up or down,** creating the just-right challenge.
10. Provide at least two **primary sources of evidence** to support the intervention plan.

INTERVENTION PLAN IMPLEMENTATION

1. Based on your intervention plan, identify which goals and objectives require **more immediate attention.**
2. Describe your proposed **first treatment session.**
3. As the treatment session is progressing, what is **essential to be observed?**

Transition and Discontinuation

Create a plan for discharge from occupational therapy services in collaboration with Zoran and members of the interprofessional team. Review the needs of Zoran, caregivers, family members, and significant others. The plan must match needs with available resources and the discharge environment.

REFERENCES

American Medical Association. (2019). *CPT® 2020 professional edition.*
Beck, A. T., Steer, R. A., & Brown, G. K. (1996). *Manual for the Beck Depression Inventory–II.* Psychological Corp.
World Health Organization. (2019). *International statistical classification of diseases and related health problems* (11th ed.). https://icd.who.int/

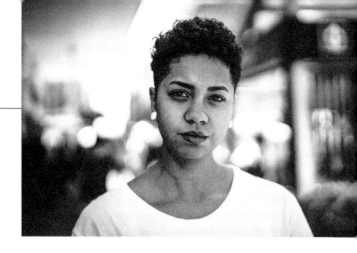

Gabriela: Bipolar Disorder

VIKRAM PAGPATAN, OTR/L, ATP, BCP, CLA

Gabriela (she, her, hers, herself)

MEDICAL HISTORY

Gabriela is a 22-year-old female Honduran citizen residing in the United States. She is 5' 4" and weighs 119 pounds. Her concerned coworkers took her to the emergency department after she experienced a manic breakdown at her workplace. Gabriela's colleagues reported that she was hyperactive for a period of 2 days, laughing uncontrollably and "appearing very off from her usual self." She was evaluated by a psychiatrist, who recommended an inpatient stay in the behavioral health unit, which Gabriela agreed to. Gabriela's medical history includes treatment for posttraumatic stress disorder (PTSD), bipolar disorder type I (BPD), and chronic sciatica. She reported no drug and tobacco use but occasional use of alcohol during social occasions and stated that she is an avid coffee drinker. Gabriela has no known allergies.

SOCIAL HISTORY

Gabriela enlisted in the U.S. Army when she was 20 after completing her associate's degree in psychology from a local institution. She served 6 years, and since her discharge from the army, she has been employed full time as an administrative assistant at a community college. She is also pursuing a bachelor's degree in psychology. She resides with her boyfriend Jason and their two dogs in a two-bedroom apartment. He is employed full time as an armed guard transport officer. Jason is currently taking online courses to complete his bachelor's degree. All of Gabriela's family lives in Honduras. Gabriela identifies as Catholic.

REFERRAL OR PRESCRIPTION

Gabriela was transferred to the inpatient behavioral health unit of her regional Veterans Administration (VA) hospital. She has been referred for occupational therapy, physical therapy, social work, psychology, and registered nursing services. The length of stay will be 4 weeks.

Occupational Therapy Initial Evaluation Findings: Inpatient Behavioral Health Unit

OCCUPATIONAL PROFILE

Gabriela's preadmission occupational history and experiences included being independent in all ADLs and all IADLs. Her patterns of daily living most commonly included leaving for work at 7:00 a.m. and returning home by 6:00 p.m. She usually eats dinner that Jason prepares, then together they take the dogs for a walk. Gabriela's interests include dining out and weekend excursions. She values time spent with Jason, pursuing her bachelor's degree, and becoming a U.S. citizen. Her greatest current needs are to restore her health and return to the activities she enjoys doing the most.

ADLs

Regarding self-care, Gabriela was independent in feeding, grooming, toileting, and bathing. She reported being up for 2–3 days at a time without bathing or sleeping. Regarding functional mobility, no gross deficits in bed mobility, transfers, or functional ambulation were observed.

IADLs

Activities needed that provide day-to-day quality of life and relative independence were explored. Gabriella's boyfriend had taken full responsibility for shopping, home management, finances, and cooking. She reported that during her manic periods she texts excessively and spends a lot of time on the Internet purchasing items that she does not need. Regarding rest and sleep, Gabriella reported insomnia and not being able to obtain a night of restful sleep.

MENTAL FUNCTIONS

Cognitive assessment found Gabriela to be alert and oriented to person, place, time, and situation, and short- and long-term memory were intact. Gabriela exhibited delays in insight and awareness, sequencing, and problem solving. She stated that she was "unable to focus for long periods of time" and that "little things" easily frustrated her. Assessment of affect was performed. Gabriela reported frequently crying over emotional topics of conversation with her colleagues and boyfriend and often finding it difficult to remember important activities such as taking her medications. Gabriela was evaluated using the Global Assessment of Functioning (GAF; Aas, 2011) and received a score of 38. No gross deficits in perceptual function were observed.

SENSORY FUNCTIONS AND PAIN

No gross deficits were observed with visual, hearing, vestibular, taste, smell, proprioceptive, and cutaneous functions. Use of the Numerical Rating Scale (0–10) indicated a score of 5 for pain in Gabriela's lower back and of 2 after taking medication for the pain. The pain was described as "jolting."

CARDIOVASCULAR AND RESPIRATORY SYSTEM FUNCTIONS

Assessment of cardiovascular and respiratory system functions indicated no deficits.

MOVEMENT FUNCTIONS

Active range of motion and passive range of motion were intact for both upper extremities and both lower extremities. Fine motor abilities were intact for gross grasp, pinch, and in-hand manipulation.

NEUROMUSCULAR FUNCTIONS

Sitting and standing were within defined limits. Muscle tone was normal, and reflex integration was grossly intact.

PLAN FOR DISCHARGE

Gabriela will be discharged home with follow-up psychiatric and psychological services at a VA satellite site.

Questions and Activities

SAFETY OF CLIENT AND OTHERS: PRECAUTIONS AND CONTRAINDICATIONS

1. Identify three up-to-date, reliable, and valid sources to obtain precautions for working with clients with mania. Evaluate them, select the strongest source, and justify your selection.
2. Create an informational handout that identifies common triggers that are associated with PTSD.
3. What activities and positions should be encouraged, and which should be avoided as a result of Gabriela's history of sciatica?
4. Identify the common emotional reactions associated with inpatient hospitalization that may affect the treatment process.
5. To keep Gabriela and others safe, what other factors should be considered?

OCCUPATIONS: ADLs, IADLs, EDUCATION, WORK, PLAY, SOCIAL PARTICIPATION, AND REST AND SLEEP

1. Given the information provided for this case, identify the areas of occupation that will and will not be addressed. Justify your decisions.
2. Prioritize the areas of occupation you have identified. Support your choices.
3. Select the top two areas of occupation from your list and provide strategies to address them.

PERFORMANCE SKILLS: MOTOR SKILLS, PROCESS SKILLS, AND SOCIAL INTERACTION SKILLS

1. Given the information provided, identify the motor, process, and social interaction skills that affect Gabriela's occupational performance.

2. Which of these skills would be appropriate to address in this service delivery site? Justify your selection.
3. Which of these skills would be addressed through remediation, compensation, and education?
4. Which of these skills would be addressed through the following intervention approaches: create/promote, establish/restore, maintain, modify, and prevent?

PERFORMANCE PATTERNS: HABITS, ROUTINES, ROLES, AND RITUALS

1. Identify Gabriela's useful habits, routines, roles, and rituals that support valued occupations. How can you make use of this information?
2. Identify Gabriela's impoverished habits, routines, roles, and rituals that do not support valued occupations. How can you make use of this information?
3. Identify Gabriela's dominating habits, routines, roles, and rituals that interfere with valued occupations. How can you make use of this information?

CLIENT FACTORS

Values, beliefs, and spirituality
How can the identified values, beliefs, and spirituality be used in this case?

Body structures
Considering Gabriela's primary and secondary diagnoses, identify the related body structures.

Body functions
1. Identify how the primary and secondary diagnoses have affected the function of the identified body structures.
2. Explain the relationships between the structural and functional factors and Gabriela's current level of occupational performance.

MENTAL FUNCTIONS: AFFECTIVE, COGNITIVE, AND PERCEPTUAL

1. Compare and contrast the affective signs and symptoms of BPD with those of PTSD.
2. Compare and contrast the cognitive and perceptual signs and symptoms of BPD with those of PTSD.
3. While working with Gabriela, what environmental considerations should be made? Justify your selection.
4. While working with Gabriela, how would you effectively use the therapeutic use of self?
5. Given the information provided, what additional mental function considerations need to be addressed?

NEUROMUSCULOSKELETAL AND MOVEMENT-RELATED FUNCTIONS

1. Given the information provided, identify neuromusculoskeletal and movement-related functions that need to be addressed. Justify your selections.
2. Should Gabriela's sciatica be addressed in the behavioral health unit?

CARDIOVASCULAR, HEMATOLOGICAL, IMMUNOLOGICAL, AND RESPIRATORY FUNCTIONS

1. Given the information provided, identify cardiovascular, hematological, immunological, and respiratory functions that need to be addressed. Justify your selections.
2. How may vital signs be affected when a person is experiencing a manic episode?
3. Explain how the "fight or flight" response is associated with PTSD.

SKIN AND RELATED STRUCTURE FUNCTIONS

What are some sympathetic skin changes that may occur during a manic or PTSD episode?

VOICE AND SPEECH FUNCTIONS

Describe how Gabriela's diagnoses may affect her voice, speech, and associated occupational performance.

ASSISTIVE TECHNOLOGIES AND DEVICES

1. What assistive technologies or adaptations might be used or made for Gabriela while she is receiving occupational therapy services on the behavioral health unit? Why?
2. What assistive technologies or adaptations might be recommended for when she returns home? Why?

ETHICAL DECISION MAKING

1. Gabriela reports that another patient on the unit has been making sexual advances toward her. How would you address this situation?
2. Gabriela confides in you that she is attracted to her psychiatrist. How would you address this disclosure?
3. Gabriella projects intimate and emotional feelings toward her health care providers. What phenomenon could this represent?

PHARMACOLOGY

Gabriela is currently taking Latuda.

1. What is the generic name?
2. Does this drug have a high alert status?
3. What is the classification of this drug?
4. What is the indication for this drug?
5. What is the action of this drug?
6. How may this drug affect client participation during a therapy session?

SOCIOCULTURAL, SOCIOECONOMIC, AND DIVERSITY FACTORS AND LIFESTYLE CHOICES

1. Given Gabriela's profile, how may your own culture and beliefs affect your interaction with her?
2. Based on this self-examination, what area of cultural knowledge do you need to pursue?

3. How can this newly acquired cultural knowledge be integrated for effective outcomes?
4. How can you foster cultural interaction and awareness among your coworkers?
5. Discuss how a lack of understanding in the areas of discrimination and stigma, implicit bias, social identity, or racism may contribute to disparities in the delivery of occupational therapy services in this case.

ASSESSMENT TOOLS AND INTERPRETATION OF RESULTS

1. What is the purpose of the GAF?
2. Which population is this test designed for?
3. How much time is required to administer it?
4. Provide a brief description of this assessment.
5. What is the reliability of the GAF?
6. What is the validity of the GAF?
7. What functional inference can be deduced from Gabriela's score of 38?
8. What additional standardized assessment can be used in this case? Why?

INTERPROFESSIONAL RELATIONSHIP AND EFFECTIVE INTRAPROFESSIONAL COLLABORATION

1. Identify the other professions that would make up the care team. Explain the focus of each.
2. Identify the roles of the occupational therapy assistant (OTA) that could be used in the occupational therapy process for this case.
3. Identify interventions that can be assigned to the OTA for this case. Justify your selections.

BILLING AND CODING

1. Identify the *International Classification of Diseases (ICD)* codes for this Gabriela's diagnoses.
2. For this case, identify at least two *Current Procedural Terminology (CPT®)* codes that are most appropriate. Justify your selection.

REIMBURSEMENT SYSTEMS AND DOCUMENTATION

1. Who would be the authorized individuals that you could share the occupational therapy findings with? Explain why.
2. For this case, what forms and frequency of documentation will be required?
3. Which reimbursement system or systems most commonly cover occupational therapy services in this practice setting?

ADVOCACY

1. Which of the following areas of advocacy would be beneficial in this case: patient rights, matters of privacy, confidentiality, informed consent, awareness building, accessing education, or benefits/resources?
2. Create a plan to advocate for this client based on the selected areas of advocacy.

TELEHEALTH

1. How can telehealth be integrated as a component of the occupational therapy process in this case?
2. Before launching telemedicine services, what questions would be essential to ask Gabriela to determine whether it is appropriate for her to engage in telemedicine services?
3. What are the barriers, obstacles, or challenges you foresee if attempting to integrate telehealth services with this client?

Intervention Plan Formulation and Implementation

INTERVENTION PLAN FORMULATION

Create an intervention plan that includes the following:

1. List this individual's **strengths.**
2. List this individual's **barriers** in occupational performance, performance skills, and performance patterns.
3. Based on the individual's goals, health, performance, and service delivery site, **identify the barriers that will be addressed.**
4. From the barriers identified to be addressed, **formulate goals and objectives.**
5. Identify the focus of each goal and objective as either **create, promote, establish, restore, maintain, modify, or prevent.**
6. Identify the **theoretical basis, model(s) of practice, or frame(s) of reference** that will be used to address each goal and objective.
7. For each proposed goal and objective, describe clearly and precisely the **methods** that will be used. This description should include, but not be limited to, safety considerations, environmental considerations, therapeutic use of self, preparatory activities, activity selection, materials, equipment, and flow.
8. Classify the activities selected in the methods description as either **preparatory, enabling, purposeful, or occupation based.**
9. Explain how each activity can be **graded up or down,** creating the just-right challenge.
10. Provide at least two **primary sources of evidence** to support the intervention plan.

INTERVENTION PLAN IMPLEMENTATION

1. Based on your intervention plan, identify which goals and objectives require **more immediate attention.**
2. Describe your proposed **first treatment session.**
3. As the treatment session is progressing, what is **essential to be observed?**

Transition and Discontinuation

Create a plan for discharge from occupational therapy services in collaboration with Gabriela and members of the interprofessional team. Review the needs of Gabriela, caregivers, family members, and significant others. The plan must match needs with available resources and the discharge environment.

REFERENCES

Aas, I. H. (2011). Guidelines for rating Global Assessment of Functioning (GAF). *Annals of General Psychiatry, 10,* 1–11.

American Medical Association. (2019). *CPT® 2020 professional edition.*

World Health Organization. (2019). *International statistical classification of diseases and related health problems* (11th ed.). https://icd.who.int/

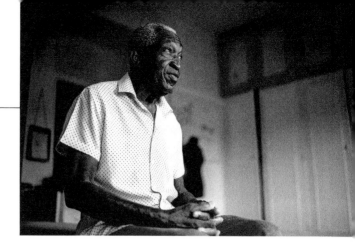

Samuel: Schizophrenia

MARY DEVADAS, MS, OTR/L, DBA, AND KERRON BLUNTE, MS, OTR/L, CLT

Samuel (he, him, his, himself)

MEDICAL HISTORY

Samuel is a 62-year-old Black male who is 6' 1" and weighs 185 pounds. He was brought into the emergency department (ED) by emergency medical services and accompanied by his wife, Ellen. Ellen stated that her husband has been off his medication for 1–2 weeks, has not slept for the past 3 days, and was hearing voices and speaking to people who did not exist. The voices were telling him he should kill himself. In the ED, Samuel had blood drawn, received magnetic resonance imaging (MRI) of his head, and was assessed by both a neurologist and a psychiatrist. He received a diagnosis of an acute psychotic episode secondary to schizophrenia. MRI imaging indicated an atypical corpus callosum and cortical atrophy. Both a sedative and an antipsychotic were administered in the ED. Samuel has a medical history of schizophrenia, hypertension, diabetes mellitus, and tardive dyskinesia. Samuel has had four admissions to an inpatient behavioral health unit since he was first diagnosed with schizophrenia; he was initially diagnosed with undifferentiated schizophrenia because of a lack of positive symptoms His wife reported that there is no caffeine, nicotine, alcohol, or substance use. He has no known allergies. Samuel was referred from the ED to an inpatient psychiatric unit because of his positive symptoms.

SOCIAL HISTORY

Samuel has been married to Ellen for 35 years. They live in a fifth-floor condo in downtown Brooklyn. They are the parents of two adult children and have four grandchildren. Samuel is a prominent self-employed artist, and his studio is in his home. Samuel enjoys traveling with his wife, spending time with his children and grandchildren, and teaching art at his community center as a volunteer. Samuel identifies as a born-again Christian.

REFERRAL OR PRESCRIPTION

Samuel was transferred to an inpatient behavioral health unit. He has been referred for occupational therapy, social work, psychology, and registered nursing services. The length of stay will be 10 days.

Occupational Therapy Initial Evaluation Findings: Inpatient Behavioral Health Unit

OCCUPATIONAL PROFILE

Samuel's preadmission occupational history and experiences included being independent in all ADLs and IADLs. He is a mixed-media artist best known for his oil paintings, pottery, and sculptures. Samuel stated that, over the years, his ability to create a detailed oil painting has declined because of tremors; however, he still enjoys other aspects of his work. His most common pattern of daily living includes waking up at 8:00 a.m., cooking and sharing breakfast with his wife, and then working in his home studio. He teaches 3 evenings per week at the community center. Other interests include traveling, cooking, gardening, spending time with his family, and socializing with friends. He values creating, sharing, and teaching art. His immediate goals are to return home and resume his typical pattern of living.

ADLs

Regarding self-care, Samuel was independent in feeding and toileting. He was unshaven and poorly groomed, and it was reported that he had not bathed in 5 days. His wife reported that Samuel had not slept for 3 days before his ED visit. Regarding functional mobility, he had no gross deficits in bed mobility but required supervision during transfers and functional ambulation since receiving the sedative in the ED. The Barthel Index (Mahoney & Barthel, 1965) for ADLs was used to assess Samuel's ADL functioning and functional mobility.

IADLs

Samuel was assessed using the Kohlman Evaluation of Living Skills (KELS; Thomson & Robnett, 2016) tool and received a total score of 6.

MENTAL FUNCTIONS

Samuel exhibited disorganized thinking and speech, having difficulty staying on topic. He was oriented to person and location but not time and situation. He acknowledged he was hearing voices. His emotions shifted between calm, anger, and agitation.

SENSORY FUNCTIONS AND PAIN

Assessment of sensory functioning indicated that his vision, hearing, cutaneous, olfactory, and proprioception were grossly intact. No pain was reported.

CARDIOVASCULAR AND RESPIRATORY SYSTEM FUNCTIONS

No deficits in cardiovascular and respiratory system functions were observed. Vital signs during the initial evaluation were blood pressure at 155/80 mm Hg, respiration rate at 16 breaths per minute, and heart rate at 61 beats per minute.

MOVEMENT FUNCTIONS

Samuel presented with lip smacking and mild uncontrollable movements of his left hand. Range of motion and muscle strength in all four extremities appeared to be within functional limits.

NEUROMUSCULAR FUNCTIONS

Muscle tone and reflex integration appeared intact. Samuel's static and dynamic sitting balance were 4/5, and his static and dynamic standing balance were 3+/5 according to a clinical assessment of balance.

PLAN FOR DISCHARGE

Samuel will be discharged to the care of a community-based psychiatrist, psychologist, and occupational therapist.

Questions and Activities

SAFETY OF CLIENT AND OTHERS: PRECAUTIONS AND CONTRAINDICATIONS

1. Identify precautions and contraindications when working with clients who are agitated.
2. Identify three up-to-date, reliable, and valid sources to obtain precautions for working with clients experiencing psychosis. Evaluate them, select the strongest source, and justify your selection.
3. Create a handout that identifies the precautions and contraindications that must be followed when interacting with a client who is experiencing psychosis.
4. To keep Samuel and others safe, what other factors should be considered?

OCCUPATIONS: ADLs, IADLs, EDUCATION, WORK, PLAY, SOCIAL PARTICIPATION, AND REST AND SLEEP

1. Given the information provided for this case, identify the areas of occupation that will and will not be addressed. Justify your decisions.
2. In the context of delivering occupational therapy services on a behavioral health unit, will your interaction and intervention with Samuel be delivered in a group format, individually, or a combination of both?
3. Which of Samuel's problems may be addressed in a group format?
4. Identify the names and goals of patient intervention groups offered at your local inpatient behavioral health facility.

5. What makes a group run by an occupational therapist distinctly different from one run by a social worker, recreational therapist, or psychologist?
6. Which of Samuel's problems may be addressed in an individual session?
7. Would work or sleep be addressed? Support your decision.

PERFORMANCE SKILLS: MOTOR SKILLS, PROCESS SKILLS, AND SOCIAL INTERACTION SKILLS

1. Given the information provided, identify the motor, process, and social interaction skills that affect Samuel's occupational performance.
2. Which of these skills would be appropriate to address in this service delivery site? Justify your selection.
3. Which of these skills would be addressed through remediation, compensation, and education?
4. Which of these skills would be addressed through the following intervention approaches: create/promote, establish/restore, maintain, modify, and prevent?

PERFORMANCE PATTERNS: HABITS, ROUTINES, ROLES, AND RITUALS

1. Identify Samuel's useful habits, routines, roles, and rituals that support valued occupations. How can you make use of this information?
2. Identify Samuel's impoverished habits, routines, roles, and rituals that do not support valued occupations. How can you make use of this information?
3. Identify Samuel's dominating habits, routines, roles, and rituals that interfere with valued occupations. How can you make use of this information?

CLIENT FACTORS

Values, beliefs, and spirituality
How can the identified values, beliefs, and spirituality be used in this case?

Body structures
Considering Samuel's primary and secondary diagnoses, identify the related body structures.

Body functions
1. Identify how the primary and secondary diagnoses have affected the function of the identified body structures.
2. Explain the relationships between the structural and functional factors and Samuel's current level of occupational performance.

MENTAL FUNCTIONS: AFFECTIVE, COGNITIVE, AND PERCEPTUAL

1. Compare and contrast disorganized type schizophrenia with paranoid type schizophrenia.
2. Create a handout identifying the signs and symptoms of psychosis.
3. Search the literature for the etiology of schizophrenia. Briefly summarize your findings and cite your sources.
4. Given the information provided, what additional mental function considerations need to be addressed?

NEUROMUSCULOSKELETAL AND MOVEMENT-RELATED FUNCTIONS

1. Given the information provided, identify neuromusculoskeletal and movement-related functions that need to be addressed. Justify your selections.
2. What forms of nonverbal communication would indicate that Samuel's condition is improving?
3. What forms of nonverbal communication would indicate that Samuel's condition is worsening?

CARDIOVASCULAR, HEMATOLOGICAL, IMMUNOLOGICAL, AND RESPIRATORY FUNCTIONS

1. Given the information provided, identify cardiovascular, hematological, immunological, and respiratory functions that need to be addressed. Justify your selections.
2. Given Samuel's history of hypertension, what must be considered in relation to hematological, immunological, or respiratory functions?

SKIN AND RELATED STRUCTURE FUNCTIONS

What should Samuel consider regarding his skin when he engages in gardening outdoors? Explain why.

VOICE AND SPEECH FUNCTIONS

Describe how Samuel's diagnoses may affect his voice, speech, and associated occupational performance.

ASSISTIVE TECHNOLOGIES AND DEVICES

1. What assistive technologies or adaptations might be used or made for Samuel while he is receiving occupational therapy services on the behavioral health unit? Why?
2. What assistive technologies or adaptations might be recommended for when he returns home? Why?

ETHICAL DECISION MAKING

1. Samuel's friend Janice, from the community center, has called the occupational therapist to inquire about Samuel's status. Janice stated that she is very concerned about Samuel and heard he is in the hospital. Identify your options to maintain compliance with the Health Insurance Portability and Accountability Act of 1996 (P. L. 104-191) when communicating with Janice. Support your options.
2. Samuel shares with you that he hates taking his antipsychotic medication. He states that it makes him sleepy, numbs his emotions, and contributes to obsessive thoughts. How does this information make you feel, what thoughts does it stimulate, and what action may be required?

PHARMACOLOGY

Samuel is currently taking Risperdal.

1. What is the generic name?
2. Does this drug have a high alert status?
3. What is the classification of this drug?
4. What is the indication for this drug?

5. What is the action of this drug?
6. How may this drug affect client participation during a therapy session?

SOCIOCULTURAL, SOCIOECONOMIC, AND DIVERSITY FACTORS AND LIFESTYLE CHOICES

1. Given Samuel's profile, how may your own culture and beliefs affect your interaction with him?
2. Based on this self-examination, what area of cultural knowledge do you need to pursue?
3. How can this newly acquired cultural knowledge be integrated for effective outcomes?
4. How can you foster cultural interaction and awareness among your coworkers?
5. Discuss how a lack of understanding in the areas of discrimination and stigma, implicit bias, social identity, or racism may contribute to disparities in the delivery of occupational therapy services in this case.

ASSESSMENT TOOLS AND INTERPRETATION OF RESULTS

1. What is the purpose of the KELS?
2. Which population is this test designed for?
3. How much time is required to administer it?
4. Provide a brief description of this assessment.
5. What is the reliability of the KELS?
6. What is the validity of the KELS?
7. What functional inference can be deduced from Samuel's total score of 6?
8. What additional standardized assessment can be used in this case? Why?

INTERPROFESSIONAL RELATIONSHIP AND EFFECTIVE INTRAPROFESSIONAL COLLABORATION

1. Identify the other professions that would make up the care team. Explain the focus of each.
2. Identify the roles of the occupational therapy assistant (OTA) that could be used in the occupational therapy process for this case.
3. Identify interventions that can be assigned to the OTA for this case. Justify your selections.

BILLING AND CODING

1. Identify the *International Classification of Diseases (ICD)* codes for Samuel's diagnoses.
2. For this case, identify at least two *Current Procedural Terminology (CPT®)* codes that are most appropriate. Justify your selection.

REIMBURSEMENT SYSTEMS AND DOCUMENTATION

1. Who would be the authorized individuals that you could share the occupational therapy findings with? Explain why.
2. For this case, what forms and frequency of documentation will be required?
3. Which reimbursement system or systems most commonly cover occupational therapy services in this practice setting?

ADVOCACY

1. Which of the following areas of advocacy would be beneficial in this case: patient rights, matters of privacy, confidentiality, informed consent, awareness building, accessing education, or benefits/resources?
2. Create a plan to advocate for this client based on the selected areas of advocacy.

TELEHEALTH

1. How can telehealth be integrated as a component of the occupational therapy process in this case?
2. Before launching telemedicine services, what questions would be essential to ask Samuel to determine whether it is appropriate for him to engage in telemedicine services?
3. What are the barriers, obstacles, or challenges you foresee if attempting to integrate telehealth services with this client?

Intervention Plan Formulation and Implementation

INTERVENTION PLAN FORMULATION

Create an intervention plan that includes the following:

1. List this individual's **strengths.**
2. List this individual's **barriers** in occupational performance, performance skills, and performance patterns.
3. Based on the individual's goals, health, performance, and service delivery site, **identify the barriers that will be addressed.**
4. From the barriers identified to be addressed, **formulate goals and objectives.**
5. Identify the focus of each goal and objective as either **create, promote, establish, restore, maintain, modify, or prevent.**
6. Identify the **theoretical basis, model(s) of practice, or frame(s) of reference** that will be used to address each goal and objective.
7. For each proposed goal and objective, describe clearly and precisely the **methods** that will be used. This description should include, but not be limited to, safety considerations, environmental considerations, therapeutic use of self, preparatory activities, activity selection, materials, equipment, and flow.
8. Classify the activities selected in the methods description as either **preparatory, enabling, purposeful, or occupation based.**
9. Explain how each activity can be **graded up or down,** creating the just-right challenge.
10. Provide at least two **primary sources of evidence** to support the intervention plan.

INTERVENTION PLAN IMPLEMENTATION

1. Based on your intervention plan, identify which goals and objectives require **more immediate attention.**
2. Describe your proposed **first treatment session.**
3. As the treatment session is progressing, what is **essential to be observed?**

Transition and Discontinuation

Create a plan for discharge from occupational therapy services in collaboration with Samuel and members of the interprofessional team. Review the needs of Samuel, caregivers, family members, and significant others. The plan must match needs with available resources and the discharge environment.

REFERENCES

American Medical Association. (2019). *CPT® 2020 professional edition.*

Health Insurance Portability and Accountability Act of 1996 (HIPAA), Pub. L. 104-191, 42 U.S.C. § 300gg, 29 U.S.C. §§ 1181–1183, and 42 U.S.C. §§ 1320d–1320d9.

Mahoney, F. I., & Barthel, D. (1965). Functional evaluation: The Barthel Index. *Maryland State Medical Journal, 14,* 56–61.

Thomson, L. K., & Robnett, R. H. (2016). *KELS: Kohlman Evaluation of Living Skills* (4th ed). AOTA Press.

World Health Organization. (2019). *International statistical classification of diseases and related health problems* (11th ed.). https://icd.who.int/

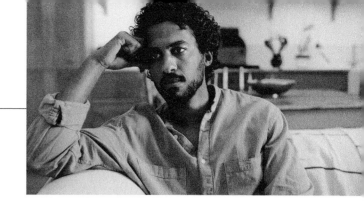

Emmanuel: Posttraumatic Stress Disorder

DONALD AURIEMMA, MS ED, OTR/L; CLOVER HUTCHINSON, OTD, MA, OTR/L;
AND VIKRAM PAGPATAN, OTR/L, ATP, BCP, CLA

Emmanuel (he, him, his, himself)

MEDICAL HISTORY

Emmanuel is a 31-year-old Moroccan American male who is 6' 2" and weighs 173 pounds. He was admitted to the behavioral health inpatient unit of the Veterans Administration (VA) hospital with a diagnosis of posttraumatic stress disorder (PTSD) after a visit to his psychiatrist. Emmanuel reported that he had assaulted his wife and had convinced her not to report it. He complained of being anxious, having difficulty sleeping, and experiencing vivid nightmares of being in combat. He expressed that he was "out of control" and feared that he would hurt himself or his family. Emmanuel's medical history includes PTSD, anxiety, depression, alcohol abuse disorder, and suicide attempts. Emmanuel reported drinking 1–2 liters of bourbon per week but reported no drug, tobacco, or caffeine use. He has no known allergies.

SOCIAL HISTORY

Emmanuel is a veteran who was discharged medically with a diagnosis of PTSD after serving 10 years in the U.S. Marine Corps. Since his discharge, he has not been able to work and is supported by his military disability income. Emmanuel has been married to his wife Alia for 6 years. Alia is an elementary school teacher, and together they have a 5-year-old daughter and reside in a two-bedroom townhouse. Socially, Emmanuel engages in activities only with Alia's friends and family. The family identifies as Shia Muslim.

REFERRAL OR PRESCRIPTION

Emmanuel was transferred to an inpatient behavioral health unit. He has been referred for occupational therapy, physical therapy, social work, psychology, and registered nursing services. The length of stay will be 30 days.

Occupational Therapy Initial Evaluation Findings: Inpatient Behavioral Health Unit

OCCUPATIONAL PROFILE

Emmanuel's preadmission occupational history and experiences included being independent in all ADLs and all IADLs. His patterns of daily living most commonly included waking at noon, doing chores around the house, and walking to pick up his daughter from school. Emmanuel joined the Marines several years after graduating high school. Since being discharged from the military, he spends most of his time at home and inconsistently attends a veterans support group that was recommended by his psychiatrist. He sometimes prepares dinner and helps his daughter with her homework. Emmanuel's interests include watching sci-fi movies and playing video games. He values spending time with his daughter and wife. Emmanuel's goal is to be a better husband and father.

ADLs

Regarding self-care, Emmanuel was independent in feeding, dressing, grooming, toileting, and bathing. Regarding functional mobility, no deficits in bed mobility, transfers, or functional ambulation were observed.

IADLs

Activities needed that provide day-to-day quality of life and relative independence were explored. Before admission, Emmanuel was responsible for paying household bills, but because he missed payments, his wife has taken over this task. He also reported that he is no longer able to participate in grocery shopping because he experiences feelings of anxiety in large and crowded spaces. Regarding rest and sleep, Emmanuel reported a history of waking up frequently during the night, having difficulty falling back to sleep, and waking up earlier than he intended. He frequently sleeps on the living room couch because he disturbs his wife's sleep by moving about, talking, and yelling while asleep.

MENTAL FUNCTIONS

Cognitive assessment found Emmanuel to be alert and oriented to person, place, time, and situation, and short- and long-term memory were intact. He reported difficulty attending and being easily angered. Assessment of affect was performed. Emmanuel expressed extreme remorse for assaulting his wife. Emmanuel was evaluated using the Suicide Assessment Five-Step Evaluation and Triage (SAFE–T; U.S. Department of Health and Human Services, 2009) assessment and scored in the moderate range. No gross deficits in perception were observed.

SENSORY FUNCTIONS AND PAIN

No gross deficits were observed with visual, hearing, vestibular, taste, smell, proprioceptive, and cutaneous functions. Use of the Numerical Rating Scale (0–10) indicated a score of 0, or no pain.

CARDIOVASCULAR AND RESPIRATORY SYSTEM FUNCTIONS

Assessment of cardiovascular and respiratory system functions indicated no deficits.

MOVEMENT FUNCTIONS

Active range of motion and passive range of motion were intact in both upper extremities and both lower extremities. Fine motor abilities were intact for grasp, pinch, and in-hand manipulation. Movements were well coordinated.

NEUROMUSCULAR FUNCTIONS

Sitting and standing balance were within defined limits. Muscle tone was normal, and reflex integration was intact.

PLAN FOR DISCHARGE

Emmanuel will be discharged home with follow-up psychiatric and psychological services at a VA satellite site.

Questions and Activities

SAFETY OF CLIENT AND OTHERS: PRECAUTIONS AND CONTRAINDICATIONS

1. What specific considerations should be made regarding Emmanuel's history of suicide attempts?
2. Create a handout identifying the behavioral changes associated with nonrestorative sleep.
3. Identify three up-to-date, reliable, and valid sources to obtain precautions for working with clients experiencing PTSD. Evaluate them, select the strongest source, and justify your selection.
4. Identify the common emotional reactions associated with the perpetration of spousal abuse that may affect the treatment process.
5. To keep Emmanuel and others safe, what other factors should be considered?

OCCUPATIONS: ADLs, IADLs, EDUCATION, WORK, PLAY, SOCIAL PARTICIPATION, AND REST AND SLEEP

1. Given the information provided for this case, identify the areas of occupation that will and will not be addressed. Justify your decisions.
2. Identify areas of occupation that Emmanuel needs to address.
3. Provide strategies for Emmanuel to obtain more restful sleep.
4. After discharge, Emmanuel wishes to participate in grocery shopping. Identify three methods that can help him accomplish this goal.
5. Provide strategies to support Emmanuel's engagement in the recommended VA support groups.
6. Emmanuel expressed a desire to once again take on the responsibility of managing household finances along with his wife. How can this goal be best addressed?

PERFORMANCE SKILLS: MOTOR SKILLS, PROCESS SKILLS, AND SOCIAL INTERACTION SKILLS

1. Given the information provided, identify the motor, process, and social interaction skills that affect Emmanuel's occupational performance.
2. Which of these skills would be appropriate to address in this service delivery site? Justify your selection.
3. Which of these skills would be addressed through remediation, compensation, and education?
4. Which of these skills would be addressed through the following intervention approaches: create/promote, establish/restore, maintain, modify, and prevent?

PERFORMANCE PATTERNS: HABITS, ROUTINES, ROLES, AND RITUALS

1. Identify Emmanuel's useful habits, routines, roles, and rituals that support valued occupations. How can you make use of this information?
2. Identify Emmanuel's impoverished habits, routines, roles, and rituals that do not support valued occupations. How can you make use of this information?
3. Identify Emmanuel's dominating habits, routines, roles, and rituals that interfere with valued occupations. How can you make use of this information?

CLIENT FACTORS

Values, beliefs, and spirituality
How can the identified values, beliefs, and spirituality be used in this case?

Body structures
Considering Emmanuel's primary and secondary diagnoses, identify the related body structures.

Body functions
1. Identify how the primary and secondary diagnoses have affected the function of the identified body structures.
2. Explain the relationships between the structural and functional factors and Emmanuel's current level of occupational performance.

MENTAL FUNCTIONS: AFFECTIVE, COGNITIVE, AND PERCEPTUAL

1. Compare and contrast the affective signs and symptoms of PTSD with those of intermittent explosive disorder.
2. Emmanuel reports being easy to anger. What environmental considerations should be made? Support your selection.
3. Identify compensatory strategies that can be used to address Emmanuel's deficit in attention.
4. Emmanuel expressed extreme remorse for assaulting his wife. How should remorse be addressed within practice?
5. Given the information provided, what additional mental function considerations need to be addressed?

NEUROMUSCULOSKELETAL AND MOVEMENT-RELATED FUNCTIONS

1. Given the information provided, identify neuromusculoskeletal and movement-related functions that need to be addressed. Justify your selections.
2. Identify nonverbal indicators of anger.

CARDIOVASCULAR, HEMATOLOGICAL, IMMUNOLOGICAL, AND RESPIRATORY FUNCTIONS

1. Given the information provided, identify cardiovascular, hematological, immunological, and respiratory functions that need to be addressed. Justify your selections.
2. Explain the relationship between the fight-or-flight response and PTSD.
3. Describe the long-term effects of alcohol abuse on these system functions.

SKIN AND RELATED STRUCTURE FUNCTIONS

What sympathetic skin changes may occur during an anxiety episode and a PTSD episode?

VOICE AND SPEECH FUNCTIONS

Describe how Emmanuel's diagnoses may affect his voice, speech, and associated occupational performance.

ASSISTIVE TECHNOLOGIES AND DEVICES

1. What assistive technologies or adaptations might be used or made for Emmanuel while he is receiving occupational therapy services in the inpatient behavioral health unit? Why?
2. What assistive technologies or adaptations might be recommended for when he returns home? Why?

ETHICAL DECISION MAKING

1. Emmanuel reported that his roommate snores loudly and stated, "I can't take him anymore." How should this situation be addressed?
2. Do you have either a legal or an ethical responsibility to report that Emmanuel had assaulted his wife?
3. Walking by Emmanuel's room, you overhear him pressuring his wife to bring in alcohol. How should this situation be addressed?

PHARMACOLOGY

Emmanuel is currently taking Zoloft.

1. What is the generic name?
2. Does this drug have a high alert status?
3. What is the classification of this drug?
4. What is the indication for this drug?
5. What is the action of this drug?
6. How may this drug affect client participation during a therapy session?

SOCIOCULTURAL, SOCIOECONOMIC, AND DIVERSITY FACTORS AND LIFESTYLE CHOICES

1. Given Emmanuel's profile, how may your own culture and beliefs affect your interaction with him?
2. Based on this self-examination, what area of cultural knowledge do you need to pursue?
3. How can this newly acquired cultural knowledge be integrated for effective outcomes?
4. How can you foster cultural interaction and awareness among your coworkers?
5. Discuss how a lack of understanding in the areas of discrimination and stigma, implicit bias, social identity, or racism may contribute to disparities in the delivery of occupational therapy services in this case.

ASSESSMENT TOOLS AND INTERPRETATION OF RESULTS

1. What is the purpose of the SAFE–T assessment?
2. Which population is this test designed for?
3. How much time is required to administer it?
4. Provide a brief description of this assessment.
5. What is the reliability of the SAFE–T assessment?
6. What is the validity of the SAFE–T assessment?
7. What functional inference can be deduced from Emmanuel's score of moderate?
8. What additional standardized assessment can be used in this case? Why?

INTERPROFESSIONAL RELATIONSHIP AND EFFECTIVE INTRAPROFESSIONAL COLLABORATION

1. Identify the other professions that would make up the care team. Explain the focus of each.
2. Identify the roles of the occupational therapy assistant (OTA) that could be used in the occupational therapy process for this case.
3. Identify interventions that can be assigned to the OTA for this case. Justify your selections.

BILLING AND CODING

1. Identify the *International Classification of Diseases (ICD)* codes for Emmanuel's diagnoses.
2. For this case, identify at least two *Current Procedural Terminology (CPT®)* codes that are most appropriate. Justify your selection.

REIMBURSEMENT SYSTEMS AND DOCUMENTATION

1. Who would be the authorized individuals that you could share the occupational therapy findings with? Explain why.
2. For this case, what forms and frequency of documentation will be required?
3. Which reimbursement system or systems most commonly cover occupational therapy services in this practice setting?

ADVOCACY

1. Which of the following areas of advocacy would be beneficial in this case: patient rights, matters of privacy, confidentiality, informed consent, awareness building, accessing education, or benefits/resources?

2. Create a plan to advocate for this client based on the selected areas of advocacy.

1. How can telehealth be integrated as a component of the occupational therapy process in this case?
2. Before launching telemedicine services, what questions would be essential to ask Emmanuel to determine whether it is appropriate for him to engage in telemedicine services?
3. What are the barriers, obstacles, or challenges you foresee if attempting to integrate telehealth services with this client?

Intervention Plan Formulation and Implementation

INTERVENTION PLAN FORMULATION

Create an intervention plan that includes the following:

1. List this individual's **strengths.**
2. List this individual's **barriers** in occupational performance, performance skills, and performance patterns.
3. Based on the individual's goals, health, performance, and service delivery site, **identify the barriers that will be addressed.**
4. From the barriers identified to be addressed, **formulate goals and objectives.**
5. Identify the focus of each goal and objective as either **create, promote, establish, restore, maintain, modify, or prevent.**
6. Identify the **theoretical basis, model(s) of practice, or frame(s) of reference** that will be used to address each goal and objective.
7. For each proposed goal and objective, describe clearly and precisely the **methods** that will be used. This description should include, but not be limited to, safety considerations, environmental considerations, therapeutic use of self, preparatory activities, activity selection, materials, equipment, and flow.
8. Classify the activities selected in the methods description as either **preparatory, enabling, purposeful, or occupation based.**
9. Explain how each activity can be **graded up or down,** creating the just-right challenge.
10. Provide at least two **primary sources of evidence** to support the intervention plan.

INTERVENTION PLAN IMPLEMENTATION

1. Based on your intervention plan, identify which goals and objectives require **more immediate attention.**
2. Describe your proposed **first treatment session.**
3. As the treatment session is progressing, what is **essential to be observed?**

Transition and Discontinuation

Create a plan for discharge from occupational therapy services in collaboration with Emmanuel and members of the interprofessional team. Review the needs of Emmanuel, caregivers, family members, and significant others. The plan must match needs with available resources and the discharge environment.

REFERENCES

American Medical Association. (2019). *CPT® 2020 professional edition.*

U.S. Department of Health and Human Services, Substance Abuse and Mental Health Services Administration. (2009). *SAFE–T: Suicide Assessment Five-Step Evaluation and Triage.* https://www.samhsa.gov/resource/dbhis/safe-t-pocket-card-suicide-assessment-five-step-evaluation-triage-safe-t-clinicians

World Health Organization. (2019). *International statistical classification of diseases and related health problems* (11th ed.). https://icd.who.int/

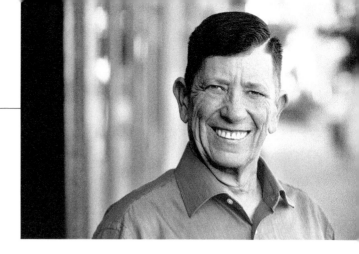

Andres: Alcohol and Substance Use Disorders

DONALD AURIEMMA, MS ED, OTR/L

Andres (he, him, his, himself)

MEDICAL HISTORY

Andres is a 57-year-old Colombian American male who is 5' 10" and weighs 138 pounds. He was electively admitted to the behavioral health unit of his local hospital for treatment of alcohol and substance use disorders. Upon admission, he reported drinking a minimum of a liter of vodka per day and snorting cocaine daily for the past 3 months. His medical history includes relapsing alcohol and substance use disorders for 10 years. Andres reported smoking one pack of cigarettes and drinking up to 10 cups of coffee daily. Surgical history included gender reassignment and multiple facial cosmetic procedures over the past 15 years. Andres has no known allergies.

SOCIAL HISTORY

Andres has worked as an Internal Revenue Service forensic agent for the past 25 years and has been able to maintain employment despite his long history of alcohol and substance use disorders. He lives alone in a one-bedroom rented apartment, which is a 20-minute bus ride from his office; however, he primarily works remotely. Andres had his driver's license revoked 2 years ago as a result of a second driving-while-intoxicated conviction. His current relationship is with Jill, whom he met at an Alcoholics Anonymous meeting. Jill is also currently in a state of relapse. Andres has reported that his alcohol and substance use has strained the relationship with his mother and three siblings and has depleted all his savings and retirement funds. In the past, he spent most of his free time at bars and clubs and in Miami vacationing. Andres identifies as a Pentecostal Christian.

REFERRAL OR PRESCRIPTION

Andres was transferred to an inpatient behavioral health hospital. He has been referred for occupational therapy, physical therapy, social work, psychology, and registered nursing services. The length of stay will be 30 days.

Occupational Therapy Initial Evaluation Findings: Inpatient Behavioral Health Hospital

OCCUPATIONAL PROFILE

Andres's preadmission occupational history and experiences included being independent in all ADLs and all IADLs. Andres holds a bachelor's degree in accounting and a master of business administration degree. As a forensic agent, he reported being extremely skilled at his job and has received several commendations for his outstanding work. His patterns of daily living most commonly included waking up by 10:00 a.m. and working without break until 4:00 p.m., consuming only coffee and cigarettes. Thereafter, he usually showered, went to dinner with friends, and would begin to drink. His drinking would continue when he returned home and only stopped once he fell asleep. Cocaine use was usually added to his drinking each Friday and Saturday evening. Andres reported that if he continues his current lifestyle, he will most likely die young and further hurt his family. Andres's interests include watching detective movies and spending time with his family. He reports his greatest needs are to stop using alcohol and drugs, learn to make better life choices, and try to rebuild his relationship with his mom and three siblings.

ADLs

Regarding self-care, at the time of initial evaluation, Andres presented as well dressed and groomed. He reported being independent in self-dressing, bathing, grooming, feeding, and toileting. Regarding functional mobility, Andres reported performing bed mobility, transfers, and functional ambulation independently.

IADLs

Activities needed that provide day-to-day quality of life and relative independence were explored. Andres reported that he is able to independently manage his home, effectively communicate, shop, and prepare meals. He reported having a negative effect on his mother's emotional health, difficulty managing his finances, and managing and maintaining his health. Regarding rest and sleep, Andres reported being a light sleeper and repeatedly waking throughout the night.

MENTAL FUNCTIONS

Cognitive assessment found Andres to be alert and oriented to person, place, time, and situation, and short- and long-term memory were intact. He was able to follow three-step commands and make his needs known. He reported that his thoughts are filled with relentless cravings for alcohol. He acknowledged the negative effect that alcohol has had on him but reported feeling helpless. He was evaluated using the Revised Clinical Institute Withdrawal Assessment of Alcohol Scale (CIWA–Ar; Sullivan et al., 1989) and received a score of 18. Affect appeared appropriate, and no gross deficits in perception were observed.

SENSORY FUNCTIONS AND PAIN

No gross deficits were observed with visual, hearing, vestibular, taste, smell, proprioceptive, and cutaneous functions. Pain was denied.

CARDIOVASCULAR AND RESPIRATORY SYSTEM FUNCTIONS

No gross deficits were observed.

MOVEMENT FUNCTIONS

Active range of motion in all four extremities, prehension, and in-hand manipulation skills were within functional limits. Mild cerebellar tremors were observed in both hands, the right greater than the left. Andres reported finding it "challenging" at times to manage fine fasteners.

NEUROMUSCULAR FUNCTIONS

Andres was able to maintain static and dynamic sitting and standing balance against maximal external resistance. His sitting and standing tolerance appeared to be sufficient to perform all tasks in his identified roles. His muscle tone was normal.

PLAN FOR DISCHARGE

Andres will be discharged home and referred to a substance abuse counselor, clinical psychologist, and psychiatrist.

Questions and Activities

SAFETY OF CLIENT AND OTHERS: PRECAUTIONS AND CONTRAINDICATIONS

1. Andres is receiving services on a locked behavioral health unit. Compare and contrast this setting with a general medical unit.
2. Create a handout identifying the precautions that must be followed when working with a client who abruptly stops using alcohol and cocaine.
3. Explain the detoxification process that Andres will most likely undergo.
4. To keep Andres and others safe, what other factors should be considered?

OCCUPATIONS: ADLs, IADLs, EDUCATION, WORK, PLAY, SOCIAL PARTICIPATION, AND REST AND SLEEP

1. Given the information provided for this case, identify the areas of occupation that will and will not be addressed. Justify your decisions.
2. In the context of delivering occupational therapy services on a behavioral health unit, will your interaction and intervention with Andres be delivered in a group format, individually, or a combination of both? Explain why.

3. What makes a group led by an occupational therapist distinctly different from one led by a social worker, recreational therapist, or psychologist?
4. What effect does substance or alcohol abuse have on sleep?

PERFORMANCE SKILLS: MOTOR SKILLS, PROCESS SKILLS, AND SOCIAL INTERACTION SKILLS

1. Given the information provided, identify the motor, process, and social interaction skills that affect Andres's occupational performance.
2. Which of these skills would be appropriate to address in this service delivery site? Justify your selection.
3. Which of these skills would be addressed through remediation, compensation, and education?
4. Which of these skills would be addressed through the following intervention approaches: create/promote, establish/restore, maintain, modify, and prevent?

PERFORMANCE PATTERNS: HABITS, ROUTINES, ROLES, AND RITUALS

1. Identify Andres's useful habits, routines, roles, and rituals that support valued occupations. How can you make use of this information?
2. Identify Andres's impoverished habits, routines, roles, and rituals that do not support valued occupations. How can you make use of this information?
3. Identify Andres's dominating habits, routines, roles, and rituals that interfere with valued occupations. How can you make use of this information?

CLIENT FACTORS

Values, beliefs, and spirituality
How can the identified values, beliefs, and spirituality be used in this case?

Body structures
Considering Andres's primary diagnoses, identify the related body structures.

Body functions
1. Identify how the primary diagnoses have affected the function of the identified body structure.
2. Explain the relationships between the structural and functional factors and Andres's current level of occupational performance.

MENTAL FUNCTIONS: AFFECTIVE, COGNITIVE, AND PERCEPTUAL

1. Identify the focus of a psychiatrist, psychologist, social worker, nurse, recreational therapist, and occupational therapist working with a client experiencing alcohol and substance use disorders on a behavioral health unit.
2. Explain the chemical changes that occur in the brain that cause Andres to crave alcohol, cigarettes, and cocaine.
3. Andres and Jill are in a codependent relationship. Explain codependency.
4. Given the information provided, what additional mental function considerations need to be addressed?

NEUROMUSCULOSKELETAL AND MOVEMENT-RELATED FUNCTIONS

1. Given the information provided, identify neuromusculoskeletal and movement-related functions that need to be addressed. Justify your selections.
2. Identify observable signs and reported symptoms that would indicate that Andres is experiencing withdrawal.
3. Identify at least two approaches to address the cerebellar tremors in both of Andres's hands. Evaluate them and select one. Defend your selection.

CARDIOVASCULAR, HEMATOLOGICAL, IMMUNOLOGICAL, AND RESPIRATORY FUNCTIONS

1. Given the information provided, identify cardiovascular, hematological, immunological, and respiratory functions that need to be addressed. Justify your selections.
2. Describe the long-term effects of chronic alcohol, cigarette, and cocaine use on each of the following functions: cardiovascular, hematological, immunological, and respiratory. Identify and justify your sources.

SKIN AND RELATED STRUCTURE FUNCTIONS

What is the long-term effect of nicotine use on the skin?

VOICE AND SPEECH FUNCTIONS

Describe how Andres's diagnoses may affect his voice, speech, and associated occupational performance.

ASSISTIVE TECHNOLOGIES AND DEVICES

1. What assistive technologies or adaptations might be used or made for Andres while he is receiving occupational therapy services on the behavioral health unit? Why?
2. What assistive technologies or adaptations might be recommended for when he returns home? Why?

ETHICAL DECISION MAKING

1. Andres is the first transgender person you have worked with. You have a sincere interest in understanding the process he underwent. Is this a topic that could be broached with Andres? Why or why not? If yes, what would be the guiding principles to do so?
2. You see one of Andres's visitors hand him a cigarette. You are aware that smoking is strictly prohibited in the hospital. How should this situation be addressed?
3. One of your coworkers lets you know that he is one of Andres's drinking buddies. He asked you not to tell anyone. How should this situation be addressed?

PHARMACOLOGY

Andres is currently taking naltrexone.

1. What is the brand name?

2. Does this drug have a high alert status?
3. What is the classification of this drug?
4. What is the indication for this drug?
5. What is the action of this drug?
6. How may this drug affect client participation during a therapy session?

SOCIOCULTURAL, SOCIOECONOMIC, AND DIVERSITY FACTORS AND LIFESTYLE CHOICES

1. Given Andres's profile, how may your own culture and beliefs affect your interaction with him?
2. Based on this self-examination, what area of cultural knowledge do you need to pursue?
3. How can this newly acquired cultural knowledge be integrated for effective outcomes?
4. How can you foster cultural interaction and awareness among your coworkers?
5. Discuss how a lack of understanding in the areas of discrimination and stigma, implicit bias, social identity, or racism may contribute to disparities in the delivery of occupational therapy services in this case.

ASSESSMENT TOOLS AND INTERPRETATION OF RESULTS

1. What is the purpose of the CIWA–Ar?
2. Which population is this test designed for?
3. How much time is required to administer it?
4. Provide a brief description of this assessment.
5. What is the reliability of the CIWA–Ar?
6. What is the validity of the CIWA–Ar?
7. What does a score of 18 indicate?
8. What additional standardized assessment can be used in this case? Why?

INTERPROFESSIONAL RELATIONSHIP AND EFFECTIVE INTRAPROFESSIONAL COLLABORATION

1. Identify the other professions that would make up the care team. Explain the focus of each.
2. Identify the roles of the occupational therapy assistant (OTA) that could be used in the occupational therapy process for this case.
3. Identify interventions that can be assigned to the OTA for this case. Justify your selections.

BILLING AND CODING

1. Identify the *International Classification of Diseases (ICD)* codes for Andres's diagnoses.
2. For this case, identify at least two *Current Procedural Terminology (CPT®)* codes that are most appropriate. Justify your selection.

REIMBURSEMENT SYSTEMS AND DOCUMENTATION

1. Who would be the authorized individuals that you could share the occupational therapy findings with? Explain why.

2. For this case, what forms and frequency of documentation will be required?
3. Which reimbursement system or systems most commonly cover occupational therapy services in this practice setting?

ADVOCACY

1. Which of the following areas of advocacy would be beneficial in this case: patient rights, matters of privacy, confidentiality, informed consent, awareness building, accessing education, or benefits/resources?
2. Create a plan to advocate for this client based on the selected areas of advocacy.

TELEHEALTH

1. How can telehealth be integrated as a component of the occupational therapy process in this case?
2. Before launching telemedicine services, what questions would be essential to ask Andres to determine whether it is appropriate for him to engage in telemedicine services?
3. What are the barriers, obstacles, or challenges you foresee if attempting to integrate telehealth services with this client?

Intervention Plan Formulation and Implementation

INTERVENTION PLAN FORMULATION

Create an intervention plan that includes the following:

1. List this individual's **strengths.**
2. List this individual's **barriers** in occupational performance, performance skills, and performance patterns.
3. Based on the individual's goals, health, performance, and service delivery site, **identify the barriers that will be addressed.**
4. From the barriers identified to be addressed, **formulate goals and objectives.**
5. Identify the focus of each goal and objective as either **create, promote, establish, restore, maintain, modify, or prevent.**
6. Identify the **theoretical basis, model(s) of practice, or frame(s) of reference** that will be used to address each goal and objective.
7. For each proposed goal and objective, describe clearly and precisely the **methods** that will be used. This description should include, but not be limited to, safety considerations, environmental considerations, therapeutic use of self, preparatory activities, activity selection, materials, equipment, and flow.
8. Classify the activities selected in the methods description as either **preparatory, enabling, purposeful, or occupation based.**
9. Explain how each activity can be **graded up or down,** creating the just-right challenge.
10. Provide at least two **primary sources of evidence** to support the intervention plan.

INTERVENTION PLAN IMPLEMENTATION

1. Based on your intervention plan, identify which goals and objectives require **more immediate attention.**
2. Describe your proposed **first treatment session.**
3. As the treatment session is progressing, what is **essential to be observed?**

Transition and Discontinuation

Create a plan for discharge from occupational therapy services in collaboration with Andres and members of the interprofessional team. Review the needs of Andres, caregivers, family members, and significant others. The plan must match needs with available resources and the discharge environment.

REFERENCES

American Medical Association. (2019). *CPT® 2020 professional edition.*

Sullivan, J. T., Sykora, K., Schneiderman, J., Naranjo, C. A., & Sellers, E. M. (1989). Assessment of alcohol withdrawal: The Revised Clinical Institute Withdrawal Assessment for Alcohol Scale (CIWA–Ar). *British Journal of Addiction, 84,* 1353–1357. https://doi.org/10.1111/j.1360-0443.1989.tb00737.x

World Health Organization. (2019). *International statistical classification of diseases and related health problems* (11th ed.). https://icd.who.int/

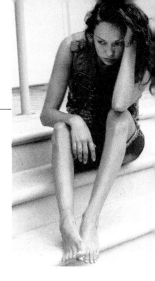

Brianna: Anorexia Nervosa

TIFFANY CORDERO-VELEZ, MS, OTR/L

Brianna (she, her, hers, herself)

MEDICAL HISTORY

Brianna is an 18-year-old Armenian American female who is 5' 10" and weighs 101 pounds. She was taken to the school nurse, who noticed that Brianna appeared "gaunt." She had blotches of dry skin, low blood pressure, and complained of dizziness. The school nurse immediately called Brianna's mom, Kate, and suggested she take Brianna to the pediatrician. While at the pediatrician, Kate was directed to take Brianna to a nearby emergency department (ED) for an evaluation. In the ED, Brianna was evaluated by cardiology and neurology. Findings from both services were unremarkable. At that time, a psychiatric evaluation was ordered and concluded that Brianna was experiencing anorexia nervosa. A recommendation was made for an inpatient stay in the behavioral health unit, which was consented to by Brianna and Kate. Medical history included nondiabetic hypoglycemia, two episodes of fainting, and a history of purging. Since adolescence, Brianna has been below the norm for weight. Brianna reported allergies to eggs, wheat, and nuts.

SOCIAL HISTORY

Brianna is a senior in high school and resides in a small town in South Carolina. She currently lives with her parents and two younger twin sisters. Kate is an accountant, and Brianna's father is a data analyst and is very involved with work, leaving little time to spend with his family. Kate described Brianna as a straight-A student who is internally motivated and highly competitive. She is a cheerleader, president of the student government, and active member of the National Honor Society. However, Brianna's academic performance has recently declined and she has become socially withdrawn. Brianna identifies as a Christian and as bisexual.

REFERRAL OR PRESCRIPTION

Brianna was transferred to an inpatient behavioral health unit. She has been referred for occupational therapy, physical therapy, social work, psychology, and registered nursing services. The length of stay will be 10 days.

Occupational Therapy Initial Evaluation Findings: Inpatient Behavioral Health Unit

OCCUPATIONAL PROFILE

Brianna's preadmission occupational history and experiences included being independent in all ADLs and all IADLs. Brianna works at a local coffee cafe 15 hours per week over 3 days. Her patterns of daily living most commonly included getting up at 6:30 a.m., skipping breakfast, arriving at school by 8:30 a.m., attending classes until 2:30 p.m., and participating in extracurricular activities until 4:30 p.m. Her interests include fashion and going to the gym as often as she can. Brianna used social media platforms as an influencer and uses Instagram™ and TikTok™ to post fitness-related content. She discloses that she is often careful of what she posts because she does not want to show her "bad angles." She values family traditions and prioritizes her appearance. Her current needs are to return to school and the gym as soon as she can.

ADLs

Regarding self-care, findings revealed that Brianna struggled with balancing her ADLs because she spent most of her time in physical activities rather than eating and preparing meals, as a means to avoid eating. She was preoccupied with her weight and body image. She had difficulty choosing what to wear, stating that she feels "fat" and "nothing fits right." Regarding functional mobility, no gross deficits in bed mobility, transfers, and functional ambulation were observed.

IADLs

Activities needed that provide day-to-day quality of life and relative independence were explored. Brianna reported that recently she has been having difficulty concentrating and organizing her assignments and schedule. She sometimes forgot when assignments were due and took exams that she was not prepared for. In food-related activities, Brianna spent most of her time preoccupied with calorie counting. Regarding rest and sleep, the medical chart indicated that Brianna had a history of short sleep duration, low sleep quality, and inadequate time spent in restorative deep sleep and REM sleep stages.

MENTAL FUNCTIONS

Cognitive assessment found Brianna to be alert and oriented to person, place, time, and situation, and short- and long-term memory were intact. Throughout the interview, however, Brianna said she was feeling tired and appeared lethargic. She was able to follow three-step commands and make her needs known. Her affect appeared appropriate, and no gross deficits in perception were observed.

Brianna reported that she is often preoccupied with the thought of food and plans her day in a way to avoid food. She stated that she is careful about how many calories she consumes, trying to limit herself to 500 a day, and that she avoids eating at social events that involve food. She also reported that when she looks in the mirror she thinks she looks "fat" and uses this perception to justify taking diet pills. Brianna has also been spending less time with her friends and engaging in activities that she once enjoyed. Kate reported that Brianna was moody and irritable during family gatherings. In addition, Brianna reported that in school she was having difficulty keeping up with her assignments, making decisions, following directions, and staying awake in class. She was beginning to worry because she knows that she will soon take the SAT for college admissions. Brianna was assessed using the SCOFF (sick, control, one, fat, food) Questionnaire (Morgan et al., 2000) and received a total score of 3.

SENSORY FUNCTIONS AND PAIN

No gross deficits were observed with visual, hearing, vestibular, taste, smell, proprioceptive, and cutaneous functions. Brianna described that her hands often feel cold despite the warm temperatures outside. Kate reports that Brianna would often complain of abdominal pain and constipation when confronted with skipping several meals.

CARDIOVASCULAR AND RESPIRATORY SYSTEM FUNCTIONS

Brianna's resting heart rate was 48 beats per minute, blood pressure was 80/52 mm Hg, and respiration rate was 12 breaths per minute. During the interview, Brianna reported that she had been feeling fatigued and dizzy since her admission to the ED.

MOVEMENT FUNCTIONS

Range of motion and muscle strength in muscle groups in all four extremities were within defined limits (WDL). Fine motor abilities were WDL for grasp formation, pinch formation, and in-hand manipulation.

NEUROMUSCULAR FUNCTIONS

Static and dynamic sitting and standing balance were WDL. Muscle tone was normal, and reflex integration was grossly intact.

PLAN FOR DISCHARGE

Brianna will be discharged home and seen by a community-based psychiatrist and psychologist.

Questions and Activities

SAFETY OF CLIENT AND OTHERS: PRECAUTIONS AND CONTRAINDICATIONS

1. What forms of monitoring are required for Brianna's blood pressure and heart rate levels?
2. Given Brianna's body image, what types of activities should be avoided in therapy?
3. Is Brianna a fall risk? Support your answer.

4. Identify three up-to-date, reliable, and valid sources to obtain precautions for working with clients with anorexia nervosa. Evaluate them, select the strongest source, and justify your selection.
5. Create a handout that identifies the precautions for working with clients with anorexia nervosa.
6. Identify the common emotional reactions associated with challenging a client's strongly held belief that may affect the treatment process.
7. To keep Brianna and others safe, what other factors should be considered?

OCCUPATIONS: ADLs, IADLs, EDUCATION, WORK, PLAY, SOCIAL PARTICIPATION, AND REST AND SLEEP

1. Given the information provided for this case, identify the areas of occupation that will and will not be addressed. Justify your decisions.
2. How will Brianna keep up with her school assignments while in the behavioral health unit?
3. What coping strategies do you anticipate can be used to promote Brianna's performance in her occupations?
4. What are some home and school recommendations that you can give Brianna and her mother to help her complete assignments on time?
5. Brianna avoids eating in the presence of others. How can this behavior be addressed?

PERFORMANCE SKILLS: MOTOR SKILLS, PROCESS SKILLS, AND SOCIAL INTERACTION SKILLS

1. Given the information provided, identify the motor, process, and social interaction skills that affect Brianna's occupational performance.
2. Which of these skills would be appropriate to address in this service delivery site? Justify your selection.
3. Which of these skills would be addressed through remediation, compensation, and education?
4. Which of these skills would be addressed through the following intervention approaches: create/promote, establish/restore, maintain, modify, and prevent?

PERFORMANCE PATTERNS: HABITS, ROUTINES, ROLES, AND RITUALS

1. Identify Brianna's useful habits, routines, roles, and rituals that support valued occupations. How can you make use of this information?
2. Identify Brianna's impoverished habits, routines, roles, and rituals that do not support valued occupations. How can you make use of this information?
3. Identify Brianna's dominating habits, routines, roles, and rituals that interfere with valued occupations. How can you make use of this information?

CLIENT FACTORS

Values, beliefs, and spirituality
How can the identified values, beliefs, and spirituality be used in this case?

Body structures
Considering Brianna's primary and secondary diagnoses, identify the related body structures.

Body functions

1. Identify how the primary and secondary diagnoses have affected the function of the identified body structures.
2. Explain the relationships between the structural and functional factors and Brianna's current level of occupational performance.

MENTAL FUNCTIONS: AFFECTIVE, COGNITIVE, AND PERCEPTUAL

1. Identify the signs and symptoms of anorexia nervosa.
2. Create a plan to develop a therapeutic rapport with Brianna.
3. Brianna has a distorted body image. How may her perception affect her occupational performance?
4. Brianna has reported difficulty with time management. Identify three assistive technologies that may allow her to manage her time more effectively.
5. Given the information provided, what additional mental function considerations need to be addressed?

NEUROMUSCULOSKELETAL AND MOVEMENT-RELATED FUNCTIONS

1. Given the information provided, identify neuromusculoskeletal and movement-related functions that need to be addressed. Justify your selections.
2. How can Brianna's current endurance level affect her occupational performance?
3. Create an exercise program for Brianna based on occupational performance.

CARDIOVASCULAR, HEMATOLOGICAL, IMMUNOLOGICAL, AND RESPIRATORY FUNCTIONS

1. Given the information provided, identify cardiovascular, hematological, immunological, and respiratory functions that need to be addressed. Justify your selections.
2. Explain how low caloric intake can affect vital signs and cognitive function.

SKIN AND RELATED STRUCTURE FUNCTION

What is the physiological explanation of Brianna's dry blotchy skin as it relates to anorexia nervosa?

VOICE AND SPEECH FUNCTIONS

Describe how Brianna's diagnoses may affect her voice, speech, and associated occupational performance.

ASSISTIVE TECHNOLOGIES AND DEVICES

1. What assistive technologies or adaptations might be used or made for Brianna while she is receiving occupational therapy services on the inpatient unit floor? Why?
2. What assistive technologies or adaptations might be recommended for when she returns home? Why?

ETHICAL DECISION MAKING

1. Brianna will miss school during her stay in the behavioral health unit. The psychiatrist calls the school and speaks with the principal to negotiate a plan for an extension on assignments. The principal requests a letter and wants to know what the reason for admission was. What act or law does providing this information violate?
2. As you are walking to Brianna's room to pick her up for group therapy, you hear her purging her breakfast in the bathroom. What is the next step that you should take and who should be notified?
3. After a group therapy session, Brianna tells you that she began to have thoughts of harming herself. She requested that you not disclose this information to anyone as she reiterated that it was "nothing serious." What next steps should you take?

PHARMACOLOGY

Brianna is currently taking Prevacid.

1. What is the generic name?
2. Does this drug have a high alert status?
3. What is the classification of this drug?
4. What is the indication for this drug?
5. What is the action of this drug?
6. How may this drug affect client participation during a therapy session?
7. What foods should Brianna avoid while taking this drug, if any?

SOCIOCULTURAL, SOCIOECONOMIC, AND DIVERSITY FACTORS AND LIFESTYLE CHOICES

1. Given Brianna's profile, how may your own culture and beliefs affect your interaction with her?
2. Based on this self-examination, what area of cultural knowledge do you need to pursue?
3. How can this newly acquired cultural knowledge be integrated for effective outcomes?
4. How can you foster cultural interaction and awareness among your coworkers?
5. What difficulties may Brianna face when she goes home to her family's Armenian traditions around meals?
6. Why is it important to understand Brianna's family cultural traditions around food?
7. Discuss how a lack of understanding in the areas of discrimination and stigma, implicit bias, social identity, or racism may contribute to disparities in the delivery of occupational therapy services in this case.

ASSESSMENT TOOLS AND INTERPRETATION OF RESULTS

1. What is the purpose of the SCOFF Questionnaire?
2. Which population is this test designed for?
3. How much time is required to administer it?
4. Provide a brief description of this assessment.
5. What is the reliability of the SCOFF Questionnaire?
6. What is the validity of the SCOFF Questionnaire?
7. What functional inference can be deduced from Brianna's total score of 3?
8. What additional standardized assessment can be used in this case? Why?

INTERPROFESSIONAL RELATIONSHIP AND EFFECTIVE INTRAPROFESSIONAL COLLABORATION

1. Identify the other professions that would make up the care team. Explain the focus of each.
2. Identify the roles of the occupational therapy assistant (OTA) that could be used in the occupational therapy process for this case.
3. Identify interventions that can be assigned to the OTA for this case. Justify your selections.

BILLING AND CODING

1. Identify the *International Classification of Diseases (ICD)* codes for Brianna's diagnoses.
2. For this case, identify at least two *Current Procedural Terminology (CPT®)* codes that are most appropriate. Justify your selection.

REIMBURSEMENT SYSTEMS AND DOCUMENTATION

1. Who would be the authorized individuals that you could share the occupational therapy findings with? Explain why.
2. For this case, what forms and frequency of documentation will be required?
3. Which reimbursement system or systems most commonly cover occupational therapy services in this practice setting?

ADVOCACY

1. Which of the following areas of advocacy would be beneficial in this case: patient rights, matters of privacy, confidentiality, informed consent, awareness building, accessing education, or benefits/resources?
2. Create a plan to advocate for this client based on the selected areas of advocacy.

TELEHEALTH

1. How can telehealth be integrated as a component of the occupational therapy process in this case?
2. Before launching telemedicine services, what questions would be essential to ask Brianna to determine whether it is appropriate for her to engage in telemedicine services?
3. What are the barriers, obstacles, or challenges you foresee if attempting to integrate telehealth services with this client?

Intervention Plan Formulation and Implementation

INTERVENTION PLAN FORMULATION

Create an intervention plan that includes the following:

1. List this individual's **strengths.**
2. List this individual's **barriers** in occupational performance, performance skills, and performance patterns.

3. Based on the individual's goals, health, performance, and service delivery site, **identify the barriers that will be addressed.**
4. From the barriers identified to be addressed, **formulate goals and objectives.**
5. Identify the focus of each goal and objective as either **create, promote, establish, restore, maintain, modify, or prevent.**
6. Identify the **theoretical basis, model(s) of practice, or frame(s) of reference** that will be used to address each goal and objective.
7. For each proposed goal and objective, describe clearly and precisely the **methods** that will be used. This description should include, but not be limited to, safety considerations, environmental considerations, therapeutic use of self, preparatory activities, activity selection, materials, equipment, and flow.
8. Classify the activities selected in the methods description as either **preparatory, enabling, purposeful, or occupation based.**
9. Explain how each activity can be **graded up or down,** creating the just-right challenge.
10. Provide at least two **primary sources of evidence** to support the intervention plan.

INTERVENTION PLAN IMPLEMENTATION

1. Based on your intervention plan, identify which goals and objectives require **more immediate attention.**
2. Describe your proposed **first treatment session.**
3. As the treatment session is progressing, what is **essential to be observed?**

Transition and Discontinuation

Create a plan for discharge from occupational therapy services in collaboration with Brianna and members of the interprofessional team. Review the needs of Brianna, caregivers, family members, and significant others. The plan must match needs with available resources and the discharge environment.

REFERENCES

American Medical Association. (2019). *CPT® 2020 professional edition.*
Morgan, J. F., Reid, F., & Lacey, J. H. (1999). The SCOFF Questionnaire: A new screening tool for eating disorders. *The BMJ, 319,* 1467. https://doi.org/10.1136/bmj.319.7223.1467
World Health Organization. (2019). *International statistical classification of diseases and related health problems* (11th ed.). https://icd.who.int/

Pediatric Services

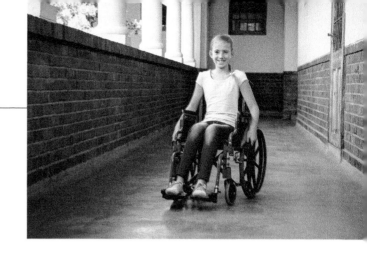

Victoria: Spina Bifida

PAULA STEWART, MS, OTR/L

Victoria (she, her, hers, herself)

MEDICAL HISTORY

Victoria is a 10-year-old Venezuelan American female born full term. She is 4' 4" and weighs 85 pounds. At birth, she was diagnosed with spina bifida (SB) myelomeningocele with comorbidities of hydrocephalus, urinary tract infections, and scoliosis. In early infancy, as a complication of hydrocephalus, Victoria underwent surgery for a shunt placement to drain the fluid. Victoria is transitioning to middle school and will be reevaluated to update her individualized education plan (IEP). She currently receives occupational therapy, physical therapy, and speech therapy services in school and occupational and physical therapy at home. Victoria has no known allergies.

SOCIAL HISTORY

Victoria is a very friendly and cooperative child with a great sense of humor. The majority of family members are bilingual. She is currently in a fifth-grade general education class and gets along well with her classmates. She resides in a two-bedroom basement apartment with her parents and older sister. The apartment is not wheelchair accessible. She recently joined Girl Scouts at her local church. Victoria's family follows the Catholic faith.

INDIVIDUALIZED EDUCATION PLAN

Victoria's IEP has identified the need for occupational and physical therapy services. These services will be provided until she achieves maximal function or ages out.

Occupational Therapy Initial Evaluation Findings: Pediatric Services in the School Setting

OCCUPATIONAL PROFILE

Victoria's preadmission occupational history and experiences included requiring assistance with ADLs and all IADLs. Victoria's parents work at a prominent hotel chain, where her father is a sous chef and her mother is a manager for the housekeeping department. Victoria enjoys playing online video games and watching teen television. Her patterns of daily living most commonly include waking at 7:00 a.m. and being dressed by her parents to save time. She is escorted to the bus by her older sister and arrives at school by 8:30 a.m. Victoria finishes school by 3:00 p.m. and arrives home by 4:00 p.m. A family member is home when she arrives. Her interests, which she shares with her sister, include exploring different types of nail polish and lip gloss. She values spending time with her sister and her family, and she values her friendships from school. Her needs include being able to complete dressing independently in a timely manner and making new friends.

ADLs

Regarding self-care at school, Victoria is able to don and doff her outer garments. Her paraprofessional, however, will place them in and retrieve them from her assigned cubby, which is outside her reach. In the cafeteria, she can make her food selection, which is then brought to the lunch table by her paraprofessional. She is able to independently open containers and feed herself. Victoria requires moderate assistance with toileting. She wears an incontinent garment and can communicate when a change is needed. After toileting, she is able to wash and dry her hands independently. Regarding functional mobility, Victoria uses the wheelchair-accessible stall in the bathroom and transfers with supervision using a sliding method. She uses a lightweight manual wheelchair to move between and in classrooms but requires assistance to open doors. Victoria is able to manipulate items in her book bag and requires minimal assistance to place the bag on the wheelchair.

IADLs

Activities needed that provide day-to-day quality of life and relative independence were explored. Victoria is able to use an accessible computer to perform Internet searches, complete homework and classroom assignments, and send and receive emails. Classroom materials are retrieved by her paraprofessional; however, Victoria tends to keep a messy workspace. Victoria's paraprofessional usually escorts her to the school nurse's office daily, where she receives her medications from the nurse. Victoria is able to use a microwave for small, prepackaged meals at school. Regarding rest and sleep, Victoria's mother reports it takes approximately 1 hour for her daughter to fall asleep, but once asleep, she sleeps well.

MENTAL FUNCTIONS

Victoria is alert and oriented to person, place, time, and situation. She is able to verbally communicate her needs and follow multistep verbal instructions. However, she struggles with spelling, reading, and math at her grade level. Victoria periodically requires reminders to lock her wheelchair brakes.

SENSORY FUNCTIONS AND PAIN

No gross deficits were observed with visual, hearing, vestibular, taste, and smell functions. Victoria has intact cutaneous functions to the upper extremities, but she has diminished cutaneous and proprioceptive sensations to the lumbar spinal nerve (L)2–L4 dermatome distribution. Victoria has no reflexive control over her bowel and bladder. She periodically reports pain in her lower back during prolonged sitting in her wheelchair. Using the Wong-Baker FACES® Pain Rating Scale (Wong-Baker FACES Foundation, 2018), she reports a score of 4. She reports her pain as "feeling like being stabbed with a knife."

CARDIOVASCULAR AND RESPIRATORY SYSTEM FUNCTIONS

No deficits were noted.

MOVEMENT FUNCTIONS

Passive range of motion (PROM), active range of motion, and muscle strength in the upper extremities were in defined limits. Victoria is right-hand dominant. No deficits were found in her fine motor abilities. PROM in both lower extremities were at functional levels. Manual muscle testing (MMT) revealed strength for all muscle groups below the level of the 12th thoracic vertebra was assessed to be 2/5. Victoria has bilateral foot drop and ankle inversion, and she wears bilateral ankle–foot orthotics (AFO) at school. At bedtime, she is placed in a full hip–knee–foot–ankle orthotic.

NEUROMUSCULAR FUNCTIONS

Both lower extremities (BLE) presented with hypotonicity. MMT for static sitting balance was 4–/5, and her dynamic sitting balance was 3+/5. Static standing balance was not assessed. The Bruininks–Oseretsky Test of Motor Proficiency (BOT–2; Bruininks & Bruininks, 2005) was administered, and Victoria's standard score was 31.

PLAN FOR DISCHARGE

Victoria will be periodically reevaluated for the continuation of occupational therapy and other services by the IEP team.

Questions and Activities

SAFETY OF CLIENT AND OTHERS: PRECAUTIONS AND CONTRAINDICATIONS

1. Victoria sits in a wheelchair for the entire school day. What concerns does this situation raise?
2. Identify the risks associated with Victoria's impaired sensory awareness in BLE. How can these risks be mitigated?
3. Create a handout that identities the proper sitting posture in a wheelchair.
4. Victoria is predisposed to osteopenia and muscle atrophy in BLE. Compare and contrast these two conditions.
5. Identify three up-to-date, reliable, and valid sources to obtain precautions for working with clients with spina bifida. Evaluate them, select the strongest source, and justify your selection.
6. Identify the common emotional reactions associated with being wheelchair bound that may affect the treatment process.
7. To keep Victoria and others safe, what other factors should be considered?

PERFORMANCE SKILLS: MOTOR SKILLS, PROCESS SKILLS, AND SOCIAL INTERACTION SKILLS

1. Given the information provided for this case, identify the areas of occupation that will and will not be addressed. Justify your decisions.
2. How can SB affect Victoria's occupations?
3. Which basic ADL deficits should be addressed in the school setting? Explain why.
4. Which areas of functional mobility should be addressed in the school setting? Explain why.
5. Identify the behaviors of the paraprofessional that may hinder the development of Victoria's ADL performance.
6. Which IADL deficits should be addressed in the school setting? Explain why.
7. Identify strategies to facilitate the carryover of skills achieved in school to home.
8. What other areas of occupation would you address? Explain why.

PERFORMANCE PATTERNS: HABITS, ROUTINES, ROLES, AND RITUALS

1. Identify Victoria's useful habits, routines, roles, and rituals that support valued occupations. How can you make use of this information?
2. Identify Victoria's impoverished habits, routines, roles, and rituals that do not support valued occupations. How can you make use of this information?
3. Identify Victoria's dominating habits, routines, roles, and rituals that interfere with valued occupations. How can you make use of this information?

CLIENT FACTORS

Values, beliefs, and spirituality
How can the identified values, beliefs, and spirituality be used in this case?

Body structures
Considering Victoria's primary and secondary diagnoses, identify the related body structures.

Body functions

1. Identify how the primary and secondary diagnoses have affected the function of the identified body structures.
2. Explain the relationships between the structural and functional factors and Victoria's current level of occupational performance.

MENTAL FUNCTIONS: AFFECTIVE, COGNITIVE, AND PERCEPTUAL

1. What are some mental health concerns for a preadolescent with incontinence?
2. How can a transition to a new school affect Victoria's mood and behavior?
3. Victoria requires reminders to lock her wheelchair brakes. Identify three cognitive strategies that can be used to address this oversight. Evaluate them, select one, and defend your choice.
4. Given the information provided, what additional mental function considerations need to be addressed?

NEUROMUSCULOSKELETAL AND MOVEMENT-RELATED FUNCTIONS

1. Given the information provided, identify neuromusculoskeletal and movement-related functions that need to be addressed. Justify your selections.
2. Compare and contrast SB with spinal stenosis.
3. Victoria has significant weakness in BLE. Should this weakness be addressed by an occupational therapist? Support your decision.
4. Given the diagnosis of SB, does Victoria have the potential to attain normal static and dynamic sitting balance? Justify your response.
5. Identify the types of forces that come into play during sliding transfers. How can they be addressed to minimize risk to skin integrity?
6. What biomechanical factors may contribute to Victoria's back pain?
7. Create an exercise program based on occupational performance for Victoria.

CARDIOVASCULAR, HEMATOLOGICAL, IMMUNOLOGICAL, AND RESPIRATORY FUNCTIONS

1. Given the information provided, identify cardiovascular, hematological, immunological, and respiratory functions that need to be addressed. Justify your selections.
2. Identify common cardiac and respiratory comorbidities for people with SB. How may they affect occupational performance?

SKIN AND RELATED STRUCTURE FUNCTIONS

1. What are some skin integrity concerns while wearing an AFO?
2. Identify the factors that can lead to skin breakdown when wheelchair bound.
3. Describe two pressure relief techniques that Victoria can use while seated in her wheelchair at school.

VOICE AND SPEECH FUNCTIONS

Describe how Victoria's diagnoses may affect her voice, speech, and associated occupational performance.

ASSISTIVE TECHNOLOGIES AND DEVICES

1. What assistive technologies or adaptations might be used or made for Victoria while she is receiving occupational therapy services? Why?
2. What assistive technologies or adaptations might be recommended for when she is in class? Why?

ETHICAL DECISION MAKING

1. You believe that Victoria may benefit from a motorized wheelchair. What factors should you consider when recommending this type of technology?
2. Victoria reported a painful blister on her buttocks. How should it best be addressed?
3. Victoria expresses that she is being bullied at school. How should this situation best be addressed?

PHARMACOLOGY

Victoria is currently taking oxybutynin hydrochloride.

1. What is the brand name?
2. Does this drug have a high alert status?
3. What is the classification of this drug?
4. What is the indication for this drug?
5. What is the action of this drug?
6. How may this drug affect client participation during a therapy session?

SOCIOCULTURAL, SOCIOECONOMIC, AND DIVERSITY FACTORS AND LIFESTYLE CHOICES

1. Given Victoria's profile, how may your own culture and beliefs affect your interaction with her?
2. Based on this self-examination, what area of cultural knowledge do you need to pursue?
3. How can this newly acquired cultural knowledge be integrated for effective outcomes?
4. How can you foster cultural interaction and awareness among your coworkers?
5. Discuss how a lack of understanding in the areas of discrimination and stigma, implicit bias, social identity, or racism may contribute to disparities in the delivery of occupational therapy services in this case.

ASSESSMENT TOOLS AND INTERPRETATION OF RESULTS

1. What is the purpose of the BOT–2?
2. Which population is the test designed for?
3. How much time is required to administer it?
4. Provide a brief description of the assessment.
5. What is the reliability of the BOT–2?
6. What is the validity of the BOT–2?
7. What functional inference can be deduced from Victoria's standard score of 31?
8. What additional standardized assessment can be used in this case? Why?

INTERPROFESSIONAL RELATIONSHIP AND EFFECTIVE INTRAPROFESSIONAL COLLABORATION

1. Identify the other professions that would make up the IEP team. Identify the scope of each member.
2. Identify the roles of the occupational therapy assistant (OTA) that could be used in the occupational therapy process for this case.
3. Identify interventions that can be assigned to the OTA for this case. Justify your selections.

BILLING AND CODING

1. Identify the *International Classification of Diseases (ICD)* codes for Victoria's diagnoses.
2. For this case, identify at least two *Current Procedural Terminology (CPT®)* codes that are most appropriate. Justify your selection.

REIMBURSEMENT SYSTEMS AND DOCUMENTATION

1. Who would be the authorized individuals that you could share the occupational therapy findings with? Explain why.
2. For this case, what forms and frequency of documentation will be required?
3. Which reimbursement system or systems most commonly cover occupational therapy services in this practice setting?

ADVOCACY

1. Which of the following areas of advocacy would be beneficial in this case: patient rights, matters of privacy, confidentiality, informed consent, awareness building, accessing education, or benefits/resources?
2. Create a plan to advocate for this client based on the selected areas of advocacy.

TELEHEALTH

1. How can telehealth be integrated as a component of the occupational therapy process into this case?
2. Before launching telemedicine services, what questions would be essential to ask Victoria to determine whether it is appropriate for her to engage in telemedicine services?
3. What are the barriers, obstacles, or challenges you foresee if attempting to integrate telehealth services with this client?

Intervention Plan Formulation and Implementation

INTERVENTION PLAN FORMULATION

Create an intervention plan that includes the following:

1. List this individual's **strengths.**
2. List this individual's **barriers** in occupational performance, performance skills, and performance patterns.

3. Based on the individual's goals, health, performance, and service delivery site, **identify the barriers that will be addressed.**
4. From the barriers identified to be addressed, **formulate goals and objectives.**
5. Identify the focus of each goal and objective as either **create, promote, establish, restore, maintain, modify, or prevent.**
6. Identify the **theoretical basis, model(s) of practice, or frame(s) of reference** that will be used to address each goal and objective.
7. For each proposed goal and objective, describe clearly and precisely the **methods** that will be used. This description should include, but not be limited to, safety considerations, environmental considerations, therapeutic use of self, preparatory activities, activity selection, materials, equipment, and flow.
8. Classify the activities selected in the methods description as either **preparatory, enabling, purposeful, or occupation based.**
9. Explain how each activity can be **graded up or down,** creating the just-right challenge.
10. Provide at least two **primary sources of evidence** to support the intervention plan.

INTERVENTION PLAN IMPLEMENTATION

1. Based on your intervention plan, identify which goals and objectives require **more immediate attention.**
2. Describe your proposed **first treatment session.**
3. As the treatment session is progressing, what is **essential to be observed?**

Transition and Discontinuation

Create a three-paragraph transition summary. In the first paragraph, identify areas of assessment and significant findings. In the second paragraph, identify barriers to be addressed. Justify their selection. In the third paragraph, identify the goals that have been developed.

REFERENCES

American Medical Association. (2019). *CPT® 2020 professional edition.*
Bruininks, R. H., & Bruininks, B. D. (2005). *BOT–2: Bruininks–Oseretsky Test of Motor Proficiency: Manual* (2nd ed.). Pearson Assessments.
Wong-Baker FACES Foundation. (2018). *Wong-Baker FACES® Pain Rating Scale.*
World Health Organization. (2019). *International statistical classification of diseases and related health problems* (11th ed.). https://icd.who.int/

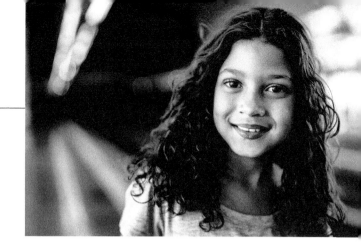

Abigale: Autism Spectrum Disorder

PAULA STEWART, MS, OTR/L

Abigale (she, her, hers, herself)

MEDICAL HISTORY

Abigale is a 9-year-old Peruvian American female who was born weighing 7 pounds, 2 ounces. She was treated as high risk because of advanced maternal age. Abigale was delivered by C-section because of prolonged labor. Her medical history included being placed under bili lights right after birth for 1 day to treat mild jaundice. She was discharged from the hospital at 3 days old as a healthy baby.

By 11 months, her mother expressed concern to the pediatrician about Abigale's development. She reported that Abigale cried inconsolably, was difficult to diaper, did not babble or give eye contact, and was not pulling to stand. Abigale sat and crawled at 8 months, stood at 13 months, and walked at 15 months. At the age of 1, she was diagnosed with autism spectrum disorder (ASD).

Abigale has known allergies. Food allergy testing was conducted at age 7, and after being placed on an elimination diet, allergies to dairy and gluten were identified. School officials were informed and, subsequently, at school she was served only food provided by her family. She is currently taking podophyllum, an herbal supplement.

SOCIAL HISTORY

Abigale is an only child who resides with both of her parents in a private home. Her mother is a stay-at-home mom, and her dad is a restaurant owner. Abigale is in the fourth grade in a self-contained class that includes six children, one teacher, and three paraprofessionals. Abigale's family follows the Roman Catholic tradition.

INDIVIDUALIZED EDUCATION PLAN

Abigale's individualized education plan (IEP) has identified the need for occupational therapy, physical therapy, speech therapy, and special instruction with applied behavioral analysis. Services will be provided until she achieves maximal function or ages out.

Occupational Therapy Initial Evaluation Findings: Pediatric Services in the School Setting

OCCUPATIONAL PROFILE

Abigale's preadmission occupational history and experiences included requiring assistance with ADLs and all IADLs. Her patterns of a daily living most commonly include being awoken by 7:00 a.m., dressed, and transported to school by a school bus staffed with a driver, matron, and paraprofessional. She typically arrives home by 4:30 p.m., has a snack, takes a nap, and then completes homework with the assistance of her mom. On weeknights, Abigale's interests include screen time for an hour. She is usually in bed by 9:00 p.m. On weekends, Abigale is involved with aqua and music therapy. She values cuddle time with her mother. Her mother's current need for Abigale is to dress independently in a timely manner.

ADLs

Regarding self-care, Abigale was independent in toileting skills; however, she required constant supervision to prevent her from turning the faucet on and off, placing items in the toilet, and attempting to run away. Abigale was able to remove food items from the lunch bag and unscrew a top from her water bottle to feed herself; however, she required constant supervision to remain seated and prevent her from grabbing food from other children. Abigale was able to dress but required frequent redirection to stay on task. Regarding functional mobility, no gross deficits in bed mobility, transfers, or functional mobility were observed.

IADLs

Activities needed that provide day-to-day quality of life and relative independence were explored. Abigale required verbal and visual prompts to participate in cleaning up and to manage classroom items, such as placing books on her desk and returning them to her book bag.

MENTAL FUNCTIONS

Abigale was alert and oriented to person, place, and time. She was easily distracted and had moderate difficulty following a one-step verbal command and transitioning from task to task. Abigale requires supervision or redirection of tasks in a timely manner. At times, she has a tantrum if a task is interrupted. She presents with fleeting eye contact as well as limited ability to interact with others and verbally express herself. During the evaluation, she attempted to climb over and crawl under tables as well as run out of the room. Abigale demonstrated a strong preference for routine and had difficulty with novel experiences.

SENSORY FUNCTIONS AND PAIN

No gross deficits were observed with visual, vestibular, taste, smell, and proprioceptive functions. Abigale exhibited several hypersensitive behaviors. She covered her ears in response to loud noises, avoided touching glue, was hesitant walking downstairs, and retreated to a corner when placed in a room with many people. She reported no pain.

CARDIOVASCULAR AND RESPIRATORY SYSTEM FUNCTIONS

No deficits were noted.

MOVEMENT FUNCTIONS

Active range of motion and passive range of motion were within defined limits in all extremities. Abigale presented with bilateral shoulder strength of 3+/5. Assessment of fine motor skills was assessed using a subtest of the Peabody Developmental Motor Scales (2nd ed.; PDMS–2; Folio & Fewell, 2000), which found that Abigale held a pencil and crayon using a very immature supinate-palmar grasp. She was unable to copy basic vertical, horizontal, and circular lines; trace; color a picture; cut using scissors; and manipulate buttons and laces. She demonstrated the ability to hold a small container with one hand and remove the twist-off top with the other hand. Her fine motor skills appeared to be equivalent to those of a child between ages 18 and 26 months.

NEUROMUSCULAR FUNCTIONS

Static and dynamic sitting balance were 4/5, and static and dynamic standing balance were 4/5. Abigale ambulated using a toe-walking gait pattern. Muscle tone in her trunk and all four extremities was low.

PLAN FOR DISCHARGE

Abigale will be periodically reevaluated for the continuation of occupational therapy and other services by the IEP team.

Questions and Activities

SAFETY OF CLIENT AND OTHERS: PRECAUTIONS AND CONTRAINDICATIONS

1. Given Abigale's impulsivity, what safeguards should be put into place?
2. Abigale has difficulty transitioning. How may this challenge affect the safety of her and those in her class?
3. Abigale has been placed on a strict nutritional diet and can eat only the foods that are sent by her parents. What concerns may you have? What are specific precautions to follow?
4. Create a handout that identifies common foods that contain gluten.
5. Compare and contrast sensory-seeking behavior with sensory-avoiding behavior.
6. Abigale is experiencing a tantrum during a therapy session. How should this situation be handled?
7. Identify three up-to-date, reliable, and valid sources to obtain precautions for working with children with nut allergies. Evaluate them, select the strongest source, and justify your selection.

8. Identify the common emotional reactions associated with medical complications during labor and delivery that may affect the treatment process for both the client and their family.
9. To keep Abigale and others safe, what other factors should be considered?

OCCUPATIONS: ADLs, IADL, EDUCATION, WORK, PLAY, SOCIAL PARTICIPATION, AND REST AND SLEEP

1. Given the information provided for this case, identify the areas of occupation that will and will not be addressed. Justify your decisions.
2. As a school-based therapist, what areas of occupation should you focus on to optimize Abigale's ability to participate in school?
3. How would you ensure that the acquired skills during a treatment session are carried over into the classroom?
4. Abigale is also receiving occupational therapy services in the home. How would the focus of these services differ from occupational therapy services in the school?

PERFORMANCE SKILLS: MOTOR SKILLS, PROCESS SKILLS, AND SOCIAL INTERACTION SKILLS

1. Given the information provided, identify the motor, process, and social interaction skills that affect Abigale's occupational performance.
2. Which of these skills would be appropriate to address in this service delivery site? Justify your selection.
3. Which of these skills would be addressed through remediation, compensation, and education?
4. Which of these skills would be addressed through the following intervention approaches: create/promote, establish/restore, maintain, modify, and prevent?

PERFORMANCE PATTERNS: HABITS, ROUTINES, ROLES, AND RITUALS

1. Identify Abigale's useful habits, routines, roles, and rituals that support valued occupations. How can you make use of this information?
2. Identify Abigale's impoverished habits, routines, roles, and rituals that do not support valued occupations. How can you make use of this information?
3. Identify Abigale's dominating habits, routines, roles, and rituals that interfere with valued occupations. How can you make use of this information?

CLIENT FACTORS

Values, beliefs, and spirituality
How can the identified values, beliefs, and spirituality be used in this case?

Body structures
Considering Abigale's primary and secondary diagnoses, identify the related body structures.

Body functions
1. Identify how the primary and secondary diagnoses have affected the function of the identified body structures.
2. Explain the relationships between the structural and functional factors and Abigale's current level of occupational performance.

MENTAL FUNCTIONS: AFFECTIVE, COGNITIVE, AND PERCEPTUAL

1. Compare and contrast autism with intellectual disability.
2. Create a plan to develop rapport with Abigale.
3. Identify three verbal and three nonverbal strategies to optimize communication with Abigale.
4. Identify three models that can be used to guide you in addressing Abigale's negative behaviors. Evaluate them, select one, and defend your selection.
5. Examine the literature and identify two strategies to minimize impulsiveness.
6. Identify Abigale's areas of hypersensitivity. What recommendations would you make to her classroom teacher to create a classroom that provides a tolerable sensory experience?
7. Given the information provided, what additional mental function considerations need to be addressed?

NEUROMUSCULOSKELETAL AND MOVEMENT-RELATED FUNCTIONS

1. Given the information provided, identify neuromusculoskeletal and movement-related functions that need to be addressed. Justify your selections.
2. Muscle strength in Abigale's shoulder groups is 3+/5. Does this level of strength need to be addressed? Support your decision.
3. Create an exercise program based on occupational performance for Abigale.

CARDIOVASCULAR, HEMATOLOGICAL, IMMUNOLOGICAL, AND RESPIRATORY FUNCTIONS

Given the information provided, identify cardiovascular, hematological, immunological, and respiratory functions that need to be addressed. Justify your selections.

SKIN AND RELATED STRUCTURE FUNCTIONS

Upon initiating therapy with Abigale, you noticed a bruise on her knee. What would be your concern, and what possible action or actions would you take?

VOICE AND SPEECH FUNCTIONS

Describe how Abigale's diagnoses may affect her voice, speech, and associated occupational performance.

ASSISTIVE TECHNOLOGIES AND DEVICES

1. What assistive technologies or adaptations might be used or made for Abigale while she is receiving occupational therapy services? Why?
2. What assistive technologies or adaptations might be recommended for when she is in class? Why?

ETHICAL DECISION MAKING

1. You have only treated Abigale one time; however, a progress report is due for her the following week. What should you do?

2. During the occupational therapy session, Abigale falls and hits her arm. Upon clinical observation, she is able to move her arm and does not appear to be in pain, but she has a bruise. What would be your concern, and what possible action or actions should you take?

3. During a push-in treatment session, Abigale is engaged in a feeding activity while sitting with her peers. You notice that she quickly snatches food from the child next to her and puts it in her mouth. What would be your concern, and what immediate action or actions must be taken?

PHARMACOLOGY

Abigale is currently taking podophyllum, a nutritional supplement.

1. Is there a brand name?
2. Does this supplement have an alert status?
3. What is the classification of this supplement?
4. What is the indication for this supplement?
5. What is the action of this supplement?
6. How may this supplement affect client participation during a therapy session?

SOCIOCULTURAL, SOCIOECONOMIC, AND DIVERSITY FACTORS AND LIFESTYLE CHOICES

1. Given Abigale's profile, how may your own culture and beliefs affect your interaction with her?
2. Based on this self-examination, what area of cultural knowledge do you need to pursue?
3. How can this newly acquired cultural knowledge be integrated for effective outcomes?
4. How can you foster cultural interaction and awareness among your coworkers?
5. Discuss how a lack of understanding in the areas of discrimination and stigma, implicit bias, social identity, or racism may contribute to disparities in the delivery of occupational therapy services in this case.

ASSESSMENT TOOLS AND INTERPRETATION OF RESULTS

1. What is the purpose of the PDMS-2?
2. Which population is the test designed for?
3. Was the subtest used in this case an appropriate selection? Explain.
4. How much time is required to administer it?
5. Provide a brief description of the assessment.
6. What is the reliability of the PDMS-2?
7. What is the validity of the PDMS-2?
8. Is the PDMS-2 a norm-referenced or criterion-referenced assessment tool?
9. What functional inference can be deduced from Abigale's developmental age of 18–26 months?
10. What additional standardized assessment was used or can be used in this case? Why?

INTERPROFESSIONAL RELATIONSHIP AND EFFECTIVE INTRAPROFESSIONAL COLLABORATION

1. Identify the other professions that would make up the care team. Explain the focus of each.
2. Identify the roles of the occupational therapy assistant (OTA) that could be used in the occupational therapy process for this case.

3. Identify interventions that can be assigned to the OTA for this case. Justify your selections.

BILLING AND CODING

1. Identify the *International Classification of Diseases (ICD)* codes for Abigale's diagnoses.
2. For this case, identify at least two *Current Procedural Terminology (CPT®)* codes that are most appropriate. Justify your selection.

REIMBURSEMENT SYSTEMS AND DOCUMENTATION

1. Who would be the authorized individuals that you could share the occupational therapy findings with? Explain why.
2. For this case, what forms and frequency of documentation will be required?
3. Which reimbursement system or systems most commonly cover occupational therapy services in this practice setting?

ADVOCACY

1. Which of the following areas of advocacy would be beneficial in this case: patient rights, matters of privacy, confidentiality, informed consent, awareness building, accessing education, or benefits/resources?
2. Create a plan to advocate for this client based on the selected areas of advocacy.

TELEHEALTH

1. How can telehealth be integrated as a component of the occupational therapy process in this case?
2. Before launching telemedicine services, what questions would be essential to ask Abigale to determine whether it is appropriate for her to engage in telemedicine services?
3. What are the barriers, obstacles, or challenges you foresee if attempting to integrate telehealth services with this client?

Intervention Plan Formulation and Implementation

INTERVENTION PLAN FORMULATION

Create an intervention plan that includes the following:

1. List this individual's **strengths.**
2. List this individual's **barriers** in occupational performance, performance skills, and performance patterns.
3. Based on the individual's goals, health, performance, and service delivery site, **identify the barriers that will be addressed.**
4. From the barriers identified to be addressed, **formulate goals and objectives.**
5. Identify the focus of each goal and objective as either **create, promote, establish, restore, maintain, modify, or prevent.**

6. Identify the **theoretical basis, model(s) of practice, or frame(s) of reference** that will be used to address each goal and objective.
7. For each proposed goal and objective, describe clearly and precisely the **methods** that will be used. This description should include, but not be limited to, safety considerations, environmental considerations, therapeutic use of self, preparatory activities, activity selection, materials, equipment, and flow.
8. Classify the activities selected in the methods description as either **preparatory, enabling, purposeful, or occupation based.**
9. Explain how each activity can be **graded up or down,** creating the just-right challenge.
10. Provide at least two **primary sources of evidence** to support the intervention plan.

INTERVENTION PLAN IMPLEMENTATION

1. Based on your intervention plan, identify which goals and objectives require **more immediate attention.**
2. Describe your proposed **first treatment session.**
3. As the treatment session is progressing, what is **essential to be observed?**

Transition and Discontinuation

Create a three-paragraph transition summary. In the first paragraph, identify areas of assessment and significant findings. In the second paragraph, identify barriers to be addressed. Justify their selection. In the third paragraph, identify the goals that have been developed.

REFERENCES

American Medical Association. (2019). *CPT® 2020 professional edition.*
Folio, M. K., & Fewell, R. (2000). *Peabody Developmental Motor Scales: Examiner's manual* (2nd ed.). PRO-ED.
World Health Organization. (2019). *International statistical classification of diseases and related health problems* (11th ed.). https://icd.who.int/

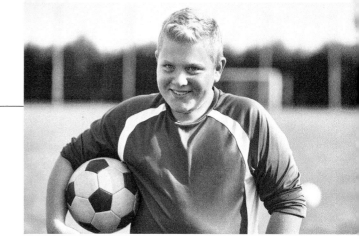

Andrei: Dyslexia

TIFFANY CORDERO-VELEZ, MS, OTR/L; SUSAN QUINTIN, MS, OTR/L;
AND TIFFANY ALMONTE, MS, OTR/L

Andrei (he, him, his, himself)

MEDICAL HISTORY

Andrei is a 13-year-old Belarusian American male who is 5' 5" and weighs 138 pounds. He was diagnosed with a learning disability, dyslexia. He was born full term, weighing 8 pounds, 5 ounces, by normal spontaneous vaginal delivery. Andrei has a medical history of a generalized anxiety disorder. He takes no prescribed medications other than multivitamins, Vitamin D3, and flaxseed oil. Andrei received a comprehensive eye exam, and the results were unremarkable. All milestones were achieved at age level except for expressive language. Andrei has no known allergies.

SOCIAL HISTORY

Andrei and his brother were adopted by his aunt and uncle after the death of his parents 5 years ago. They reside in a six-bedroom home along with three older cousins. The primary language in school is English and at home it is Belarusian. Andrei's uncle is the owner of multiple car dealerships, and his aunt is a manufacturer of women's wigs. He is currently placed in an integrated coteaching seventh-grade class in a private school and is transported by a chauffeur. Andrei reports that he loves music, computers, and electronics. He is good at art, and his interests include karate, dancing, and superheroes. In school, Andrei prefers to work on group assignments, in which he is able to share ideas but is reluctant to contribute any written components. His classmates consider him to be a class clown. Andrei is disruptive at times, lacks motivation, and is easily discouraged and frustrated. Outside of school, Andrei is dedicated to his karate and reports feeling accomplished when he earns new belts. Andrei's family follows the Orthodox Catholic faith.

INDIVIDUALIZED EDUCATION PLAN

Andrei's individualized education plan (IEP) has identified the need for occupational therapy and speech therapy services. These services will be provided until he achieves maximal function or ages out.

Occupational Therapy Initial Evaluation Findings: Pediatric Services in the School Setting

OCCUPATIONAL PROFILE

Andrei's preadmission occupational history and experiences included being independent with all ADLs and requiring assistance with IADLs. His patterns of daily living most commonly include waking at 7:00 a.m., dressing, being driven to school, and having breakfast with his friends at school. His afterschool activities include fencing and karate. Andrei arrives home by 6:30 p.m. Monday through Thursday and before sunset on Fridays. Upon arriving home, he is served dinner and then is assisted by a tutor, whom he is dependent on for helping him complete his homework. In the evenings, his interests include competitive online gaming and social networking through popular social media sites. He values his image and his growing designer watch collection. His current needs are to feel comfortable reading and writing and to no longer be mocked in school.

ADLs

Regarding self-care, Andrei is independent in all self-care activities. Regarding functional mobility, no gross deficits were observed in bed mobility, transfers, or functional mobility.

IADLs

Activities needed that provide day-to-day quality of life and relative independence were explored. According to Andrei's aunt, he is able to independently prepare a snack and walk the dog. Andrei finds texting on his smartphone to be challenging because it takes him a long time to figure out which words are abbreviated and instead prefers to use animated forms of language such as emojis. Regarding rest and sleep, Andrei reported that if he does not get a good night's sleep, he has greater difficulty attending to tasks in school.

MENTAL FUNCTIONS

Andrei was alert and oriented to person, place, time, and situation. He was pleasant and neatly dressed and demonstrated insight into his diagnosis. Andrei has higher-level oral-language skills but difficulty with written language; specifically, reading and spelling in class. Doing these types of tasks commonly results in Andrei having episodes of stomach pain and headaches. Letter reversal has been observed in his handwritten and typed assignments. During a writing task, he was observed putting his head on the desk and fidgeting with his pencil. Andrei reports that he is often frustrated during writing assignments, lacks self-confidence, and projects his frustration onto his peers. As a result, he struggles to maintain positive relationships with peers. For scheduled oral presentations and examinations, Andrei will often feign illness to avoid attending school. Andrei scored 72 on the Oral and Written Language Scales (2nd ed.; OWLS–II; Carrow-Woolfolk, 2011).

SENSORY FUNCTIONS AND PAIN

No gross deficits were observed with visual, vestibular, taste, smell, cutaneous, or proprioceptive functions. Andrei presented with appropriate sensory processing skills. He reported no pain.

CARDIOVASCULAR AND RESPIRATORY SYSTEM FUNCTIONS

No deficits were noted.

MOVEMENT FUNCTIONS

Andrei's range of motion, muscle strength, and endurance were within defined limits. His fine motor skills were age appropriate, and he was able to manipulate classroom tools and instruments.

NEUROMUSCULAR FUNCTIONS

Andrei presented with normal muscle tone, posture, and balance.

PLAN FOR DISCHARGE

Andrei will be periodically reevaluated for the continuation of occupational therapy and other services by the IEP team.

Questions and Activities

SAFETY OF CLIENT AND OTHERS: PRECAUTIONS AND CONTRAINDICATIONS

1. Given that Andrei has dyslexia, what are the most common psychological concerns?
2. What are the most common social concerns for children with dyslexia?
3. How could dyslexia affect self-confidence and academic performance?
4. What are the possible short- and long-term effects of insisting that Andrei read out loud in class?
5. Identify three up-to-date, reliable, and valid sources to obtain precautions for working with clients with dyslexia. Evaluate them, select the strongest source, and justify your selection.
6. Create a handout that identifies precautions for working with clients with dyslexia.
7. Identify the common emotional reactions associated with dyslexia that may affect the treatment process.
8. To keep Andrei and others safe, what other factors should be considered?

OCCUPATIONS: ADLs, IADL, EDUCATION, WORK, PLAY, SOCIAL PARTICIPATION, AND REST AND SLEEP

1. Given the information provided for this case, identify the areas of occupation that will and will not be addressed. Justify your decisions.
2. Identify areas of difficulty that affect Andrei's performance in school.

3. What classroom strategies do you anticipate can be used to increase Andrei's school performance?
4. What home recommendations can be provided for the family and Andrei to decrease his dependence on his tutor for the completion of his homework?
5. When recommending occupational therapy services, what would be the service delivery method (considering frequency, duration, and location) that would promote the least restrictive environment?

PERFORMANCE SKILLS: MOTOR SKILLS, PROCESS SKILLS, AND SOCIAL INTERACTION SKILLS

1. Given the information provided, identify the motor, process, and social interaction skills that affect Andrei's occupational performance.
2. Which of these skills would be appropriate to address in this service delivery site? Justify your selection.
3. Which of these skills would be addressed through remediation, compensation, and education?
4. Which of these skills would be addressed through the following intervention approaches: create/promote, establish/restore, maintain, modify, and prevent?

PERFORMANCE PATTERNS: HABITS, ROUTINES, ROLES, AND RITUALS

1. Identify Andrei's useful habits, routines, roles, and rituals that support valued occupations. How can you make use of this information?
2. Identify Andrei's impoverished habits, routines, roles, and rituals that do not support valued occupations. How can you make use of this information?
3. Identify Andrei's dominating habits, routines, roles, and rituals that interfere with valued occupations. How can you make use of this information?

CLIENT FACTORS

Values, beliefs, and spirituality
How can the identified values, beliefs, and spirituality be used in this case?

Body structures
Considering Andrei's primary and secondary diagnoses, identify the related body structures.

Body functions
1. Identify how the primary and secondary diagnoses have affected the function of the identified body structures.
2. Explain the relationships between the structural and functional factors and Andrei's current level of occupational performance.

MENTAL FUNCTIONS: AFFECTIVE, COGNITIVE, AND PERCEPTUAL

1. Compare and contrast dyslexia with attention deficit hyperactivity disorder.
2. Create a plan to develop rapport and maximize communication with Andrei.
3. Search the literature and identify two strategies to encourage Andrei's active participation during occupational therapy sessions.
4. How could you measure the level of carryover of skills from therapy to Andrei's guardians and teacher?

5. Describe methods or strategies that can be used to increase Andrei's self-efficacy, self-monitoring, and determination.
6. Given the information provided, what additional mental function considerations need to be addressed?

NEUROMUSCULOSKELETAL AND MOVEMENT-RELATED FUNCTIONS

1. Given the information provided, identify neuromusculoskeletal and movement-related functions that need to be addressed. Justify your selections.
2. Is there a correlation between visual impairment and dyslexia? Identify the source used to answer this question.

CARDIOVASCULAR, HEMATOLOGICAL, IMMUNOLOGICAL, AND RESPIRATORY FUNCTIONS

1. Given the information provided, identify cardiovascular, hematological, immunological, and respiratory functions that need to be addressed. Justify your selections.
2. Identify the signs and symptoms that a person may display when experiencing anxiety.

SKIN AND RELATED STRUCTURE FUNCTIONS

During writing tasks, Andrei's skin becomes flushed and sweaty. What could be the cause?

VOICE AND SPEECH FUNCTIONS

Describe how Andrei's diagnoses may affect his voice, speech, and associated occupational performance.

ASSISTIVE TECHNOLOGIES AND DEVICES

1. What school-based assistive technologies or adaptations might be used or made for Andrei while he is receiving occupational therapy services at school? Why?
2. What assistive technologies or adaptations might be recommended for the home? Why?
3. Categorize the recommendations mentioned above as either low or high forms of assistive technology.
4. What websites or online tools can be recommended for Andrei to support his classroom and homework performance?

ETHICAL DECISION MAKING

1. During your therapy session with Andrei, he begins to engage in negative self-talk. At one point, he makes comments about wanting to hurt himself. Identify the necessary steps needed to address this concern, and support your decision.
2. Andrei does not like to be "pulled out" of class for occupational therapy because he feels embarrassed and, at times, he refuses to attend his session. How can this situation be addressed?
3. You overheard Andrei's English teacher say the following to Andrei: "You are lazy, and you do not try hard enough to improve your reading and writing." What would be the best way to address this situation?
4. During the holidays, Andrei's family gives you a very expensive timepiece. How should this gift be addressed?

PHARMACOLOGY

Andrei is currently taking flaxseed oil.

1. Does this oil have a high alert status?
2. What is the classification of this oil?
3. What is the indication for this oil?
4. What is the action of this oil?
5. How may this oil affect client participation during a therapy session?

SOCIOCULTURAL, SOCIOECONOMIC, AND DIVERSITY FACTORS AND LIFESTYLE CHOICES

1. Given Andrei's profile, how may your own culture and beliefs affect your interaction with him?
2. Based on this self-examination, what area of cultural knowledge do you need to pursue?
3. How can this newly acquired cultural knowledge be integrated for effective outcomes?
4. How can you foster cultural interaction and awareness among your coworkers?
5. Discuss how a lack of understanding in the areas of discrimination and stigma, implicit bias, social identity, or racism may contribute to disparities in the delivery of occupational therapy services in this case.

ASSESSMENT TOOLS AND INTERPRETATION OF RESULTS

1. What is the purpose of the OWLS–II?
2. Which population is this test designed for?
3. How much time is required to administer it?
4. Provide a brief description of this assessment.
5. What is the reliability of the OWLS–II?
6. What is the validity of the OWLS–II?
7. What functional inference can be deduced from Andrei's OWLS–II score of 72?
8. What additional standardized assessment can be used in this case? Why?

INTERPROFESSIONAL RELATIONSHIP AND EFFECTIVE INTRAPROFESSIONAL COLLABORATION

1. Identify the other professions that would make up the care team. Explain the focus of each.
2. Identify the roles of the occupational therapy assistant (OTA) that could be used in the occupational therapy process for this case.
3. Identify interventions that can be assigned to the OTA for this case. Justify your selections.
4. Who would be involved in the collaborative process? List four ways to promote collaboration in the team to increase Andrei's functional performance and carryover of intervention.

BILLING AND CODING

1. Identify the *International Classification of Diseases (ICD)* codes for Andrei's diagnoses.
2. For this case, identify at least two *Current Procedural Terminology (CPT®)* codes that are most appropriate. Justify your selection.

REIMBURSEMENT SYSTEMS AND DOCUMENTATION

1. Who would be the authorized individuals that you could share the occupational therapy findings with? Explain why.
2. For this case, what forms and frequency of documentation will be required?
3. Which reimbursement system or systems most commonly cover occupational therapy services in this practice setting?

ADVOCACY

1. Which of the following areas of advocacy would be beneficial in this case: patient rights, matters of privacy, confidentiality, informed consent, awareness building, accessing education, or benefits/ resources?
2. Create a plan to advocate for this client based on the selected areas of advocacy.

TELEHEALTH

1. How can telehealth be integrated as a component of the occupational therapy process into this case?
2. Before launching telemedicine services, what questions would be essential to ask Andrei to determine whether it is appropriate for him to engage in telemedicine services?
3. What are the barriers, obstacles, or challenges you foresee if attempting to integrate telehealth services with this client?

Intervention Plan Formulation and Implementation

INTERVENTION PLAN FORMULATION

Create an intervention plan that includes the following:

1. List this individual's **strengths.**
2. List this individual's **barriers** in occupational performance, performance skills, and performance patterns.
3. Based on the individual's goals, health, performance, and service delivery site, **identify the barriers that will be addressed.**
4. From the barriers identified to be addressed, **formulate goals and objectives.**
5. Identify the focus of each goal and objective as either **create, promote, establish, restore, maintain, modify, or prevent.**
6. Identify the **theoretical basis, model(s) of practice, or frame(s) of reference** that will be used to address each goal and objective.
7. For each proposed goal and objective, describe clearly and precisely the **methods** that will be used. This description should include, but not be limited to, safety considerations, environmental considerations, therapeutic use of self, preparatory activities, activity selection, materials, equipment, and flow.
8. Classify the activities selected in the methods description as either **preparatory, enabling, purposeful, or occupation based.**
9. Explain how each activity can be **graded up or down,** creating the just-right challenge.
10. Provide at least two **primary sources of evidence** to support the intervention plan.

INTERVENTION PLAN IMPLEMENTATION

1. Based on your intervention plan, identify which goals and objectives require **more immediate attention.**
2. Describe your proposed **first treatment session.**
3. As the treatment session is progressing, what is **essential to be observed?**

Transition and Discontinuation

Create a three-paragraph transition summary. In the first paragraph, identify areas of assessment and significant findings. In the second paragraph, identify barriers to be addressed. Justify their selection. In the third paragraph, identify the goals that have been developed.

REFERENCES

American Medical Association. (2019). *CPT® 2020 professional edition.*

Carrow-Woolfolk, E. (2011). *Oral and Written Language Scales, second edition (OWLS–II).* Western Psychological Services.

World Health Organization. (2019). *International statistical classification of diseases and related health problems* (11th ed.). https://icd.who.int/

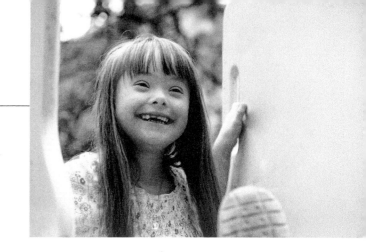

Dara: Down Syndrome

IVY RENTZ, EdD, MSA, OTR/L

Dara (she, her, hers, herself)

MEDICAL HISTORY

Dara is a 5-year-old British American female who is 4' 3" and weighs 77 pounds. She has been diagnosed with Down syndrome (DS). Her medical history includes an atrioventricular septal defect and Hirschsprung disease. She was born full term, weighing 7 pounds, 6 ounces, by normal spontaneous vaginal delivery to a mother of advanced maternal age. Dara's development milestones were significantly delayed. She sat up at 12 months, crawled at 20 months, stood at 3 years, and began walking at 4 years. Dara has no known allergies.

SOCIAL HISTORY

Dara resides with her mother and stepfather, ages 44 and 49, respectively, in a three-bedroom high-rise cooperative apartment building along with her two stepbrothers, ages 16 and 18 years. Dara's mother is a freelance advertising consultant, and her stepfather is a blog editor. Dara's parents share the responsibility of dropping her off at and picking her up from school. Dara attends a school that specializes in students with ongoing medical needs. Dara's parents follow a Pentecostal Christian faith.

INDIVIDUALIZED EDUCATION PLAN

Dara's individualized education plan (IEP) has identified the need for occupational therapy, physical therapy, and speech therapy. Services will be provided until she achieves maximal function or ages out.

Occupational Therapy Initial Evaluation Finding: Pediatric Services in the School Setting

OCCUPATIONAL PROFILE

Dara's preadmission occupational history and experiences included requiring assistance with ADLs and all IADLs. Her patterns of daily living most commonly include being awoken by 7:00 a.m., being dressed and fed by one of her parents, and then being driven to school. Dara is picked up from school at 2:45 p.m. by one of her parents. Once home, she has a snack and takes a nap. After dinner, she completes her homework with her mom and is read a story by her dad. She is in bed by 8:00 p.m. On Saturday mornings, Dara participates in hippotherapy. On Sundays, she attends church with her family. Her parents value providing Dara with the opportunity to live a life as independently as possible. Dara's interests include watching children's programs on the television. Her parents' current need for Dara is to use a spoon and cup independently.

ADLs

Regarding self-care, Dara is able to drink from a sippy cup and feed herself finger food. She requires hand-over-hand (HOH) assistance to drink from a cup and to use a spoon and fork. With minimal assistance, she can doff pullover tops and elastic-waist pants, but maximal assistance is needed to don them. She requires maximal assistance in donning and doffing her backpack. She requires HOH assistance when manipulating large, adapted pencils and crayons. She is unable to manipulate scissors. Dara is not toilet trained and wears elastic-waist diapers. Regarding functional mobility, Dara is able to independently transfer on and off desk chairs, the cafeteria bench, and the school toilet. She can ambulate independently throughout the classroom but requires supervision for safety throughout the school. Her gait is wide based, and she uses a step-to-step pattern when ascending and descending stairs. Activities needed that provide day-to-day quality of life and relative independence were explored. Dara requires maximal assistance to place items in her cubby and to manage books and materials on or in her desk.

MENTAL FUNCTIONS

Dara presents with impaired attention, judgment, sequencing, planning, and problem solving. She is able to follow one-step commands with periodic prompts and demonstrations. She scored a 49 on an Intelligence Quotient examination administered by the school psychologist. Her affect is generally pleasant, and she is commonly observed smiling and giggling. She consistently responds to simple one-step commands. Her expressive language is limited to one- or two-word responses.

SENSORY FUNCTIONS AND PAIN

No gross deficits were observed with visual, taste, smell, and proprioceptive functions. No indications of pain were observed, and none were indicated by the use of the Wong-Baker FACES® Pain

Rating Scale (Wong-Baker FACES Foundation, 2018). Dara presented with vestibular insecurity during engagement in rapid gross body movements such as playing on a swing or slide.

CARDIOVASCULAR AND RESPIRATORY SYSTEM FUNCTIONS

Dara presents with labored breathing during rigorous outdoor play.

MOVEMENT FUNCTIONS

Dara presents with hypermobility in all joints of all extremities. Muscular strength in all extremities is within functional limits. Observed functional movements appear to be slow and lack precision.

NEUROMUSCULAR FUNCTIONS

Dara presents with low tone throughout the trunk, all extremities, and hands. The Beery–Buktenica Developmental Test of Visual–Motor Integration (6th ed.; Beery VMI–6; Beery et al., 2010) was administered. In the area of visual–motor integration, Dara received a raw score of 6, a standard score of 61, and a percentile rank of 0.9%.

PLAN FOR DISCHARGE

Dara will be periodically reevaluated for the continuation of occupational therapy and other services by the IEP team.

Questions and Activities

SAFETY OF CLIENT AND OTHERS: PRECAUTIONS AND CONTRAINDICATIONS

1. Create a handout that identifies precautions for working with a client with DS.
2. Because Dara has a diagnosis of an atrioventricular septal defect, what precautions and contraindications should be followed?
3. Given Dara's cognitive deficits, what safety issues should be considered?
4. Identify three up-to-date, reliable, and valid sources to obtain precautions for working with clients with Hirschsprung disease. Evaluate them, select the strongest source, and justify your selection.
5. Identify the common emotional reactions associated with not being toilet trained that may affect the treatment process?
6. To keep Dara and others safe, what other factors should be considered?

OCCUPATIONS: ADLs, IADL, EDUCATION, WORK, PLAY, SOCIAL PARTICIPATION, AND REST AND SLEEP

1. Given the information provided for this case, identify the areas of occupation that will and will not be addressed. Justify your decisions.

2. What adaptive strategies should be used to facilitate independence in using an open cup, spoon, and fork?
3. What adaptive strategies should be used to facilitate independence in using pencils and crayons?
4. Identify an alternative form of communication that Dara could use to indicate a need for toileting.

PERFORMANCE SKILLS: MOTOR SKILLS, PROCESS SKILLS, AND SOCIAL INTERACTION SKILLS

1. Given the information provided, identify the motor, process, and social interaction skills that affect Dara's occupational performance.
2. Which of these skills would be appropriate to address in this service delivery site? Justify your selection.
3. Which of these skills would be addressed through remediation, compensation, and education?
4. Which of these skills would be addressed through the following intervention approaches: create/promote, establish/restore, maintain, modify, and prevent?

PERFORMANCE PATTERNS: HABITS, ROUTINES, ROLES, AND RITUALS

1. Identify Dara's useful habits, routines, roles, and rituals that support valued occupations. How can you make use of this information?
2. Identify Dara's impoverished habits, routines, roles, and rituals that do not support valued occupations. How can you make use of this information?
3. Identify Dara's dominating habits, routines, roles, and rituals that interfere with valued occupations. How can you make use of this information?

CLIENT FACTORS

Values, beliefs, and spirituality
How can the identified values, beliefs, and spirituality be used in this case?

Body structures
Considering Dara's primary and secondary diagnoses, identify the related body structures.

Body functions
1. Identify how the primary and secondary diagnoses have affected the function of the identified body structures.
2. Explain the relationships between the structural and functional factors and Dara's current level of occupational performance.

MENTAL FUNCTIONS: AFFECTIVE, COGNITIVE, AND PERCEPTUAL

1. Compare and contrast Down syndrome with Fragile X syndrome.
2. What strategies would you use to improve Dara's ability to understand directions?
3. People with an IQ score of 49 present with difficulties in expressive language. Identify compensatory strategies to maximize communication.
4. Identify and explain two strategies that can be used to improve Dara's ability to attend. Cite your source or sources.
5. Given the information provided, what additional mental function considerations need to be addressed?

NEUROMUSCULOSKELETAL AND MOVEMENT-RELATED FUNCTIONS

1. Given the information provided, identify neuromusculoskeletal and movement-related functions that need to be addressed. Justify your selections.
2. Dara cries and avoids play-based activities that involve rapid gross body movements. How may this behavior be addressed?
3. Identify grasp patterns that are expected for a 5-year-old. Identify your source.

CARDIOVASCULAR, HEMATOLOGICAL, IMMUNOLOGICAL, AND RESPIRATORY FUNCTIONS

1. Given the information provided, identify cardiovascular, hematological, immunological, and respiratory functions that need to be addressed. Justify your selections.
2. Compare and contrast cardiac distress with respiratory distress.
3. Identify the school-based activities that may place the greatest cardiac demand on Dara's cardiovascular system.
4. Based on your findings, identify which school-based activities need to be closely monitored or avoided.

SKIN AND RELATED STRUCTURE FUNCTIONS

During treatment sessions, you notice that Dara has bruises, scratches, and minor abrasions to her arms and legs. What would be the concern and what possible actions would you take?

VOICE AND SPEECH FUNCTIONS

Describe how Dara's diagnoses may affect her voice, speech, and associated occupational performance.

ASSISTIVE TECHNOLOGIES AND DEVICES

1. What assistive technologies or adaptations might be used or made for Dara while she is receiving occupational therapy services at school? Why?
2. What assistive technologies or adaptations might be recommended for when she is at home? Why?

ETHICAL DECISION MAKING

1. Dara requires adult supervision outside of the classroom. You observe her frequently going to the water fountain alone in the hallway. How should this situation be addressed?
2. During lunchtime, you notice that most of Dara's food remains uneaten. Who should this situation be reported to? Why?
3. Dara has a peanut allergy and is often unaware of what items contain peanuts or similar ingredients. After accidental ingestion, what steps should be taken to prevent future accidents?

PHARMACOLOGY

Dara is currently taking acebutolol.

1. What is the brand name?
2. Does this drug have a high alert status?

3. What is the classification of this drug?
4. What is the indication for this drug?
5. What is the action of this drug?
6. How may this drug affect client participation during a therapy session?

SOCIOCULTURAL, SOCIOECONOMIC, AND DIVERSITY FACTORS AND LIFESTYLE CHOICES

1. Given Dara's profile, how may your own culture and beliefs affect your interaction with her?
2. Based on this self-examination, what area of cultural knowledge do you need to pursue?
3. How can this newly acquired cultural knowledge be integrated for effective outcomes?
4. How can you foster cultural interaction and awareness among Dara's teachers, parents, and other members of the IEP team?
5. Discuss how a lack of understanding in the areas of discrimination and stigma, implicit bias, social identity, or racism may contribute to disparities in the delivery of occupational therapy services in this case.

ASSESSMENT TOOLS AND INTERPRETATION OF RESULTS

1. What is the purpose of the Beery VMI–6?
2. Which population is this test designed for?
3. How much time is required to administer it?
4. Provide a brief description of this assessment.
5. What is the reliability of the Beery VMI–6?
6. What is the validity of the Beery VMI–6?
7. What functional inference can be deduced from Dara's standard score of 61 and percentile rank of 0.9%?
8. What additional standardized assessment can be used in this case? Why?

INTERPROFESSIONAL RELATIONSHIP AND EFFECTIVE INTRAPROFESSIONAL COLLABORATION

1. Identify the other professions that would make up the care team. Explain the focus of each.
2. Identify the roles of the occupational therapy assistant (OTA) that could be used in the occupational therapy process for this case.
3. Identify interventions that can be assigned to the OTA for this case. Justify your selections.

BILLING AND CODING

1. Identify the *International Classification of Diseases (ICD)* codes for Dara's diagnoses.
2. For this case, identify at least two *Current Procedural Terminology (CPT®)* codes that are most appropriate. Justify your selection.

REIMBURSEMENT SYSTEMS AND DOCUMENTATION

1. Who would be the authorized individuals that you could share the occupational therapy findings with? Explain why.

2. For this case, what forms and frequency of documentation will be required?
3. Which reimbursement system or systems most commonly cover occupational therapy services in this practice setting?
4. Dara is expected to transition to a 12:1:2 classroom setting. What does this ratio represent?

ADVOCACY

1. Which of the following areas of advocacy would be beneficial in this case: patient rights, matters of privacy, confidentiality, informed consent, awareness building, accessing education, or benefits/resources?
2. Create a plan to advocate for this client based on the selected area(s) of advocacy.

TELEHEALTH

1. How can telehealth be integrated as a component of the occupational therapy process in this case?
2. Before launching telemedicine services, what questions would be essential to ask Dara and her parents to determine whether it is appropriate for her to engage in telemedicine services?
3. What are the barriers, obstacles, or challenges you foresee if attempting to integrate telehealth services with this client?

Intervention Plan Formulation and Implementation

INTERVENTION PLAN FORMULATION

Create an intervention plan that includes the following:

1. List this individual's **strengths.**
2. List this individual's **barriers** in occupational performance, performance skills, and performance patterns.
3. Based on the individual's goals, health, performance, and service delivery site, **identify the barriers that will be addressed.**
4. From the barriers identified to be addressed, **formulate goals and objectives.**
5. Identify the focus of each goal and objective as either **create, promote, establish, restore, maintain, modify, or prevent.**
6. Identify the **theoretical basis, model(s) of practice, or frame(s) of reference** that will be used to address each goal and objective.
7. For each proposed goal and objective, describe clearly and precisely the **methods** that will be used. This description should include, but not be limited to, safety considerations, environmental considerations, therapeutic use of self, preparatory activities, activity selection, materials, equipment, and flow.
8. Classify the activities selected in the methods description as either **preparatory, enabling, purposeful, or occupation based.**
9. Explain how each activity can be **graded up or down,** creating the just-right challenge.
10. Provide at least two **primary sources of evidence** to support the intervention plan.

INTERVENTION PLAN IMPLEMENTATION

1. Based on your intervention plan, identify which goals and objectives require more immediate attention.
2. Describe your proposed first treatment session.
3. As the treatment session is progressing, what is essential to be observed?

Transition and Discontinuation

Create a three-paragraph transition summary. In the first paragraph, identify areas of assessment and significant findings. In the second paragraph, identify barriers to be addressed. Justify their selection. In the third paragraph, identify the goals that have been developed.

REFERENCES

American Medical Association. (2019). *CPT® 2020 professional edition.*

Beery, K. E., Buktenica, N. A., & Beery, N. A. (2010). *The Beery–Buktenica Developmental Test of Visual–Motor Integration: Administration, scoring, and teaching manual* (6th ed.). Pearson.

Wong-Baker FACES Foundation. (2018). *Wong-Baker FACES® Pain Rating Scale.*

World Health Organization. (2019). *International statistical classification of diseases and related health problems* (11th ed.). https://icd.who.int/

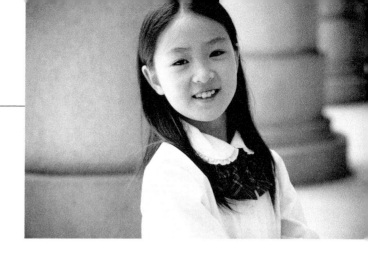

Chi-Ling: Cerebral Palsy

PAULA STEWART, MS, OTR/L

Chi-Ling (she, her, hers, herself)

MEDICAL HISTORY

Chi-Ling is a 10-year-old Taiwanese American female who is 4' 10" and weighs 98 pounds. She was diagnosed at age 4 months with hemiplegic cerebral palsy (CP) affecting her left upper and left lower extremities. She was born full term, weighing 5 pounds, 1 ounce, by a complicated vaginal delivery. Chi-Ling has a medical history of seizure disorder, which is controlled through medications, and a history of constipation, which is treated with Pedia-Lax. No surgical history was reported. Chi-Ling sat at 10 months, crawled at 13 months, and walked at 16 months. She recently started her menstrual cycle. She has no known allergies.

SOCIAL HISTORY

Chi-Ling is a fifth-grader who attends public school and receives occupational therapy, physical therapy, and speech–language pathology services. She is an only child and resides with both her parents in a private home. Their house has 6 steps to enter the first floor and 12 steps to access the second floor. She and her family are practicing Taoists. Her mother works part-time in a department store, and her father is a full-time computer technician. Chi-Ling enjoys helping her father in the kitchen when cooking meals. She enjoys watching television and using social media to connect with her friends and family abroad. She also enjoys taking selfies and often uses her mother's tablet to watch online videos. Chi-Ling avoids outdoor physical activities.

PRESCRIPTION OR REFERRAL

Chi-Ling was referred by her pediatrician for non–school based occupational therapy services, which will be delivered in her home. Services are expected to last until the maximal potential is achieved.

Occupational Therapy Initial Evaluation Findings: Community-Based Pediatric Services

OCCUPATIONAL PROFILE

Chi-Ling's preadmission occupational history and experiences included requiring assistance with ADLs and IADLs. Her patterns of daily living most commonly include being awoken by her mother at 6:30 a.m., dressing with assistance, eating a cold breakfast, and boarding the school bus by 7:30 a.m. She arrives at school by 8:00 a.m. and returns home by 3:30 p.m. Her father meets her at the bus, provides her with an afternoon snack, and assists with homework while her mother starts her shift at work. In the evenings, she values the time cooking with her father and socializing with her friends on social media. Her interests include playing with her mother's makeup and watching music videos. Her current goals are to be able to dress and bathe without the assistance of her parents. Her parents stated that their main concerns were her weakness to the left side of her body, which affects her ability to play with her peers and to independently care for herself.

ADLs

Regarding self-care, Chi-Ling is able to feed herself using a fork or spoon with her right hand but has difficulty with bilateral cutting. She is able to drink from an open cup and sip from a straw. She tolerates eating foods of various textures but often coughs when consuming thin liquids. Chi-Ling brushes her teeth and requires minimal assistance for applying toothpaste. She requires moderate assistance to wash her unaffected side and prefers to take baths over showers. She can don and doff pull-on and pull-over garments but requires moderate assistance for managing fasteners. She prefers to wear slip-on shoes. Her mother reported that Chi-Ling is unable to adequately secure her menstrual pad and is uncomfortable when assistance is offered. Chi-Ling is able to toilet independently but reports feeling uncomfortable when having to use a public restroom. Regarding functional mobility, Chi-Ling is able to independently roll right to left and transition between supine and sit. She is able to transfer independently with the use of a posterior walker on and off from a sofa, chair, and toilet, but she requires contact guard assistance to and from the tub.

IADLs

Activities needed that provide day-to-day quality of life and relative independence were explored. Chi-Ling is able to assist her father with meal preparation but requires moderate assistance to open containers and transport large items from the refrigerator to the stove. She is able to manage a smart device and often uses the voice-to-text feature to search the Internet. Chi-Ling is aware of her medication schedule but is unable to open her medication bottle. Regarding rest and sleep, Chi-Ling has difficulty sleeping through the night and often awakes multiple times. Her parents report her bedtime is typically at 8:00 p.m.; however, they report that "we are concerned that she is addicted to her phone" because they frequently find her using it to access social media for hours at a time. Upon waking, she is irritable and drowsy.

MENTAL FUNCTIONS: AFFECTIVE, COGNITIVE, AND PERCEPTUAL

Chi-Ling was alert and oriented to situation, person, place and time. She was able to follow multiple-step commands. She provided intermittent eye contact and was apprehensive about initiating activities, but she was responsive to verbal prompts. No perceptual deficits were noted.

SENSORY FUNCTIONS AND PAIN

No deficits were noted in vision, auditory, and gustatory functions. During play-based activities that required swift movements, an increase in left-side muscle tone was observed. Noxious smells elicited the same response. Hypertactile sensitivity was noted on her left upper extremity when in contact with objects that were not in her visual field. During static sitting and standing activities, Chi-Ling was observed assuming asymmetrical postures with greater weight bearing toward her unaffected side. No pain was reported.

CARDIOVASCULAR AND RESPIRATORY SYSTEM FUNCTIONS

No deficits were noted.

MOVEMENT FUNCTIONS

Passive and active range of motion were within normal limits in the right upper and lower extremities. In the left upper and lower extremities, there was a mild increase in muscle tone. The Modified Ashworth Scale (Ashworth, 1964) indicated a score of 1. Left-foot clonus was also noted. Chi-Ling tended to use her right side more than her left. When she was presented with activities that required her to use both sides of her body, she would sometimes use her left side as a stabilizer. In the areas of grasping and visual–motor skills, Chi-Ling was able to sort basic shapes on a shaped board, place pegs in peg holes, and hold a pencil with a gross static tripod grasp but had writing challenges in spacing and letter formation. She exhibited difficulty in performing bilateral tasks, such as cutting with scissors. She was assessed with the Beery–Buktenica Developmental Test of Visual–Motor Integration (6th ed.; Beery VMI–6; Beery et al., 2010), and her standard score was 82.

NEUROMUSCULAR FUNCTIONS

Chi-Ling's static sitting was good, and her dynamic sitting was fair (F)+. Her static standing balance was F+, and her dynamic standing was F. Upon exertion, she was noted to exhibit a mild asymmetrical tonic labyrinthine reflex and a tonic labyrinthine reflex, which became more prevalent when she was excited. Movement in the left upper and lower extremities was limited in accuracy, speed, and overall motor coordination.

PLAN FOR DISCHARGE

Chi-Ling will be discharged to the care of her parents and will continue to receive school-based services.

Questions and Activities

SAFETY OF CLIENT AND OTHERS: PRECAUTIONS AND CONTRAINDICATIONS

1. Because Chi-Ling is a minor, can services be rendered without the presence of her parents? Explain your response.
2. What type of consent, and from whom, is required for this case?
3. Because Chi-Ling presents with decreased balance, what are the safety concerns you anticipate?
4. Identify three up-to-date, reliable, and valid sources to obtain precautions for working with children with CP. Evaluate them, select the strongest source, and justify your selection.
5. Create a handout that identifies the precautions to use when working with children who ambulate with a walker.
6. Identify the common emotional reactions associated with movement difficulties that may affect the treatment process.
7. To keep Chi-Ling and others safe, what other factors should be considered?

OCCUPATIONS: ADLs, IADL, EDUCATION, WORK, PLAY, SOCIAL PARTICIPATION, AND REST AND SLEEP

1. Given the information provided for this case, identify the areas of occupation that will and will not be addressed. Justify your decisions.
2. Compare and contrast Chi-Ling's roles and occupations.
3. Would it be appropriate to address sleep with Chi-Ling? Why or why not?
4. How could the presence of primitive reflexes affect ADL performance? How can these effects be best addressed?
5. Identify the type of strategy that Chi-Ling presently uses when dressing with pull-over or pull-up garments.
6. What strategies can be provided to facilitate Chi-Ling's use of both hands when manipulating her most commonly used technologies? Support your strategies.

PERFORMANCE SKILLS: MOTOR SKILLS, PROCESS SKILLS, AND SOCIAL INTERACTION SKILLS

1. Given the information provided, identify the motor, process, and social interaction skills that affect Chi-Ling's occupational performance.
2. Which of these skills would be appropriate to address in this service delivery site? Justify your selection.
3. Which of these skills would be addressed through remediation, compensation, and education?
4. Which of these skills would be addressed through the following intervention approaches: create/promote, establish/restore, maintain, modify, and prevent?

PERFORMANCE PATTERNS: HABITS, ROUTINES, ROLES, AND RITUALS

1. Identify Chi-Ling's useful habits, routines, roles, and rituals that support valued occupations. How can you make use of this information?
2. Identify Chi-Ling's impoverished habits, routines, roles, and rituals that do not support valued occupations. How can you make use of this information?
3. Identify Chi-Ling's dominating habits, routines, roles, and rituals that interfere with valued occupations. How can you make use of this information?

Values, beliefs, and spirituality
How can the identified values, beliefs, and spirituality be used in this case?

Body structures
Considering Chi-Ling's primary and secondary diagnoses, identify the related body structures.

Body functions
1. Identify how the primary and secondary diagnoses have affected the function of the identified body structures.
2. Explain the relationships between the structural and functional factors and her current level of occupational performance.

MENTAL FUNCTIONS: AFFECTIVE, COGNITIVE, AND PERCEPTUAL

1. Create a plan to maximize rapport and socialization with Chi-Ling.
2. Search the literature and identify two strategies to address her phone "addiction." Summarize each strategy.
3. Explain the relationship between sleep hygiene and mental function. Identify your sources.
4. Search the literature, and identify and explain two strategies to maximize the carryover of skills that Chi-Ling learned in therapy to her parents.
5. Given the information provided, what additional mental function considerations need to be addressed?

NEUROMUSCULOSKELETAL AND MOVEMENT-RELATED FUNCTIONS

1. Given the information provided, identify neuromusculoskeletal and movement-related functions that need to be addressed. Justify your selections.
2. Compare and contrast spastic diplegia, spastic paraplegia, and spastic quadriplegia.
3. Identify strategies that can be used to address postural instability.
4. Identify strategies that can be used to address motor control.
5. Identify Chi-Ling's numerical grades assigned to her static and dynamic sitting balance. Explain each grade.
6. Identify Chi-Ling's numerical grades assigned to her static and dynamic standing balance. Explain each grade.

CARDIOVASCULAR, HEMATOLOGICAL, IMMUNOLOGICAL, AND RESPIRATORY FUNCTIONS

1. Given the information provided, identify cardiovascular, hematological, immunological, and respiratory functions that need to be addressed.
2. Identify the typical ranges for heart rate, blood pressure, and respiration rate for children of Chi-Ling's age. Name and justify your source.

SKIN AND RELATED STRUCTURE FUNCTIONS

1. Upon clinical observation, you notice mild muscle tightness of the wrist and digit flexors of Chi-Ling's left hand. What would be the concern and what possible actions would you take?

2. What hygienic considerations should be made to address skin integrity during the menstrual cycle?

VOICE AND SPEECH FUNCTIONS

Describe how Chi-Ling's diagnoses may affect her voice, speech, and associated occupational performance.

ASSISTIVE TECHNOLOGIES AND DEVICES

What assistive technologies or adaptations might be used or made for Chi-Ling while she is receiving occupational therapy services? Why?

ETHICAL DECISION MAKING

1. During a treatment session, Chi-Ling reports that she is being touched in school by her paraprofessional and it makes her feel "weird." How must this situation be addressed?
2. During a treatment session with Chi-Ling, you notice an odor of marijuana in the household. How should this situation be addressed?
3. During a treatment session, Chi-Ling's mother states that she needs to go to the store, which leaves only you and Chi-Ling in the home. How should this situation best be addressed?

PHARMACOLOGY

Chi-Ling is currently taking Pedia-Lax.

1. What is the generic name?
2. Does this drug have a high alert status?
3. What is the classification of this drug?
4. What is the indication for this drug?
5. What is the action of this drug?
6. How may this drug affect client participation during a therapy session?

SOCIOCULTURAL, SOCIOECONOMIC, AND DIVERSITY FACTORS AND LIFESTYLE CHOICES

1. Given Chi-Ling's profile, how may your own culture and beliefs affect your interaction with her?
2. Based on this self-examination, what area of cultural knowledge do you need to pursue?
3. How can this newly acquired cultural knowledge be integrated for effective outcomes?
4. How can you foster cultural interaction and awareness among your coworkers?
5. Discuss how a lack of understanding in the areas of discrimination and stigma, implicit bias, social identity, or racism may contribute to disparities in the delivery of occupational therapy services in this case.

ASSESSMENT TOOLS AND INTERPRETATION OF RESULTS

1. What is the purpose of the Beery VMI–6?
2. Which population is the test designed for?
3. How much time is required to administer it?

4. Provide a brief description of the assessment.
5. What is the reliability of the Beery VMI–6?
6. What is the validity of the Beery VMI–6?
7. Is the Berry VMI–6 a norm-referenced or criterion-referenced assessment tool?
8. What functional inference can be deduced from the Beery VMI–6 standard score of 82?
9. What additional standardized assessment was used or can be used in this case? Why?

INTERPROFESSIONAL RELATIONSHIPS AND EFFECTIVE INTRAPROFESSIONAL COLLABORATION

1. Identify the other professions that would make up the care team. Explain the focus of each.
2. Identify the roles of the occupational therapy assistant (OTA) that could be used in the occupational therapy process for this case.
3. Identify interventions that can be assigned to the OTA for this case. Justify your selections.

BILLING AND CODING

1. Identify the *International Classification of Diseases (ICD)* codes for this client's diagnoses.
2. For this case, identify at least two *Current Procedural Terminology (CPT®)* codes that are most appropriate. Justify your selection.

REIMBURSEMENT SYSTEMS AND DOCUMENTATION

1. Who would be the authorized individuals that you could share the occupational therapy findings with? Explain why.
2. Who would be the unauthorized individuals that you could not share the occupational therapy findings with without written permission? Explain why.
3. For this case, what forms of documentation will be required?

ADVOCACY

1. Which of the following areas of advocacy would be beneficial in this case: patient rights, matters of privacy, confidentiality, informed consent, awareness building, accessing education, or benefits/resources?
2. Create a plan to advocate for this client based on the selected areas of advocacy.

TELEHEALTH

1. How can telehealth be integrated as a component of the occupational therapy process in this case?
2. Before launching telemedicine services, what questions would be essential to ask Chi-Ling to determine whether it is appropriate for her to engage in telemedicine services?
3. What are the barriers, obstacles, or challenges you foresee if attempting to integrate telehealth services with this client?

Intervention Plan Formulation and Implementation

INTERVENTION PLAN FORMULATION

Create an intervention plan that includes the following:

1. List this individual's **strengths.**
2. List this individual's **barriers** in occupational performance, performance skills, and performance patterns.
3. Based on the individual's goals, health, performance, and service delivery site, **identify the barriers that will be addressed.**
4. From the barriers identified to be addressed, **formulate goals and objectives.**
5. Identify the focus of each goal and objective as either **create, promote, establish, restore, maintain, modify, or prevent.**
6. Identify the **theoretical basis, model(s) of practice, or frame(s) of reference** that will be used to address each goal and objective.
7. For each proposed goal and objective, describe clearly and precisely the **methods** that will be used. This description should include, but not be limited to, safety considerations, environmental considerations, therapeutic use of self, preparatory activities, activity selection, materials, equipment, and flow.
8. Classify the activities selected in the methods description as either **preparatory, enabling, purposeful, or occupation based.**
9. Explain how each activity can be **graded up or down,** creating the just-right challenge.
10. Provide at least two **primary sources of evidence** to support the intervention plan.

INTERVENTION PLAN IMPLEMENTATION

1. Based on your intervention plan, identify which goals and objectives require **more immediate attention.**
2. Describe your proposed **first treatment session.**
3. As the treatment session is progressing, what is **essential to be observed?**

Transition and Discontinuation

Create a three-paragraph transition summary. In the first paragraph, identify areas of assessment and significant findings. In the second paragraph, identify barriers to be addressed. Justify their selection. In the third paragraph, identify the goals that have been developed.

REFERENCES

American Medical Association. (2019). *CPT® 2020 professional edition.*

Ashworth, B. (1964). Preliminary trial of carisoprodol in multiple sclerosis. *Practitioner, 192,* 540–542.

Beery, K. E., Buktenica, N. A., & Beery, N. A. (2010). *The Beery–Buktenica Developmental Test of Visual–Motor Integration: Administration, scoring, and teaching manual* (6th ed.). Pearson.

World Health Organization. (2019). *International statistical classification of diseases and related health problems* (11th ed.). https://icd.who.int/

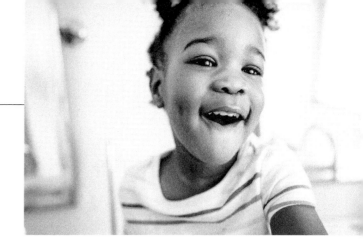

Dion: Fetal Alcohol Syndrome

CAROL BROWN-WASSINGER, MS, OTR/L

Dion (she, her, hers, herself)

MEDICAL HISTORY

Dion is a 2.5-year-old Liberian American female who was diagnosed with fetal alcohol syndrome (FAS) at her 12-month wellness check-up. She is currently 2' 5" and weighs 45 pounds. Her mother has a history of alcohol use disorder but claims she stopped drinking when she found out she was pregnant. There were no complications during pregnancy or delivery. Dion's past medical history includes being born full term by natural delivery, weighing 5.8 pounds. She weighed 19 pounds at the check-up and had a below average occipitofrontal circumference with the presence of facial dysmorphia. Dion's facial features are present with a smooth philtrum, a thin vermillion border, and small palpebral fissures. There is no history of seizures, ear infections, or allergies. Dion is not taking any medications but takes a choline supplement as recommended by her pediatrician. Dion rolled from supine to prone at 4 months, sat up unsupported at 7.5 months, crawled at 6 months, and walked independently at 18 months. She has no known allergies.

SOCIAL HISTORY

Dion lives with her 25-year-old mother, 54-year-old maternal grandmother, and 28-year-old maternal aunt on the fourth floor of an apartment building with an elevator. Dion's grandmother and aunt assist with child care. Dion's mother has been sober since her pregnancy and currently is enrolled in a local technical training program to become a medical biller and coder. She also works part-time as a sales associate. Dion's grandmother is a registered nurse, and her aunt is an emergency medical technician. Dion's father, who is 22, does not live with the family and struggles with alcohol use disorder. He is not an active participant in his daughter's life. Although there is a park at the corner, Dion's family does not take her there because of criminal activity. Once a month, the family takes Dion to an indoor amusement center to play and interact with other children. Dion's family practices the African Methodist Episcopal Zion faith.

REFERRAL OR PRESCRIPTION

Dion was referred for early intervention (EI) services for occupational therapy, which will be delivered in a developmental center. Services will be provided until she achieves maximal function or ages out.

Occupational Therapy Initial Evaluation Findings: Early Intervention Pediatric Services

OCCUPATIONAL PROFILE

Dion's preadmission occupational history and experiences included requiring assistance with ADLs and all IADLs. Her patterns of daily living most commonly include being awoken by 7:00 a.m. and dressed and fed by her grandmother. Dion is taken to day care so she may socialize with peers and receive developmental services. She arrives at the center by 8:30 a.m. and returns home by 3:30 p.m. Her interests include watching cartoons and playing games on a tablet device. Her mother values being able to provide the developmental services that Dion requires and reported that her current need is for Dion "to be more like children her age."

ADLs

Regarding self-care, Dion can drink from an open cup with frequent spillage but mainly uses a sippy cup. She can feed herself with a spoon but prefers to finger feed. Dion can doff her socks and pull-over shirts and untie her laces but is unable to take off any other items. She is dependent on donning all garments. Dion is not toilet trained and does not indicate when she needs toileting. Regarding functional mobility, she has no gross deficits in bed mobility, transfers, or functional ambulation on level surfaces. She ascended and descended stairs in a nonreciprocal pattern while holding onto a rail.

IADLs

Activities needed that provide day-to-day quality of life and relative independence were explored. Dion often tries to remove her car seat restraint, which overwhelms her caregivers. She is able to swipe and answer her mother's smartphone. Regarding rest and sleep, it has been identified that Dion experiences fragmented sleep with elevated nonrespiratory arousal indices.

MENTAL FUNCTIONS: AFFECTIVE, COGNITIVE, AND PERCEPTUAL

Dion presented with fleeting eye contact. She inconsistently followed one- or two-step commands and was easily distracted by visual and auditory stimuli. She frequently required redirection to stay on task. Dion exhibited separation anxiety when her mother was not in arm's reach and had difficulty being seated and would frequently stand.

SENSORY FUNCTIONS AND PAIN

Deficits were noted in vestibular, tactile, auditory, and olfactory functions. Dion demonstrated quick and abrupt movements that resulted in bumping into objects, tripping, and occasionally falling. She demonstrated avoidance in touching rice, Play-Doh, shaving cream, and lotion as well as when presented with strong odors. Dion eats a limited menu of items from home such as cereal, muffins, chicken nuggets, fries, and yogurt. She was distracted by auditory stimuli during the evaluation, often stopping to see where sounds were coming from or asking, "What was that?" According to her mother, Dion becomes upset around loud noises such as fire trucks and will cover her ears. No pain was reported.

CARDIOVASCULAR AND RESPIRATORY SYSTEM FUNCTIONS

No deficits were noted.

MOVEMENT FUNCTIONS

Passive and active range of motion for all extremities was within functional limits. The Peabody Developmental Motor Scales (2nd ed.; PDMS–2; Folio & Fewell, 2000) was administered. For the test's Grasping subtest, her results were raw score of 37, standard score of 4, and description of poor. For the test's Visual–Motor Integration Skills subtest, her results were raw score of 90, standard score of 7, and description of below average. Dion scored a 73 on the test's composite Fine Motor Quotient. Regarding grasp, Dion demonstrated a right-hand preference but throughout the evaluation demonstrated a variety of immature grasp patterns. She also demonstrated difficulty with stabilizing objects with her nonpreferred hand. Dion used a three-jaw chuck grasp pattern to pick up 1-inch blocks and attempted unsuccessfully to use the same pattern to pick up small pellets. She was able to string four large beads but required stabilization of her trunk, forearms, and wrists on the table for support. During the graphomotor portion of the evaluation, Dion alternated between a fisted grasp and brush grasp pattern when holding a marker. She was able to imitate horizontal and vertical strokes, but the lines were angled. Dion was unable to independently hold scissors with a thumb-up grasp or to snip paper. She was able to complete a five-piece insert puzzle and imitate a tower of 10 blocks.

NEUROMUSCULAR FUNCTIONS

Dion presented with low muscle tone in her trunk and extremities. When seated at the table, she presented with a rounded back and a posterior pelvic tilt with a wide base of support. Protective reactions are intact but delayed in all directions when seated upright on a vestibular board.

PLAN FOR DISCHARGE

Dion will continue to receive EI services until she maximizes function or reaches age 3 years.

Questions and Activities

SAFETY OF CLIENT AND OTHERS: PRECAUTIONS AND CONTRAINDICATIONS

1. Identify the common comorbidities associated with FAS.
2. When traveling in a car, in which location and position should Dion's car seat be set?

3. In your state, when would it be appropriate to discontinue the current use of a car seat with Dion? Cite your source.
4. Given Dion's hypersensitivity to smell and touch, what considerations should be made during the occupational therapy process?
5. Identify three up-to-date, reliable, and valid sources to obtain precautions for working with children with FAS. Evaluate them, select the strongest source, and justify your selection.
6. Identify the common emotional reactions associated with FAS that may affect the treatment process.
7. To keep Dion and others safe, what other safety factors should be considered?

PERFORMANCE SKILLS: MOTOR SKILLS, PROCESS SKILLS, AND SOCIAL INTERACTION SKILLS

1. Given the information provided, identify the motor, process, and social interaction skills that affect Dion's occupational performance.
2. Which of these skills would be appropriate to address in this service delivery site? Justify your selection.
3. Which of these skills would be addressed through remediation, compensation, and education?
4. Which of these skills would be addressed through the following intervention approaches: create/promote, establish/restore, maintain, modify, and prevent?

PERFORMANCE PATTERNS: HABITS, ROUTINES, ROLES, AND RITUALS

1. Identify Dion's useful habits, routines, roles, and rituals that support valued occupations. How can you make use of this information?
2. Identify Dion's impoverished habits, routines, roles, and rituals that do not support valued occupations. How can you make use of this information?
3. Identify Dion's dominating habits, routines, roles, and rituals that interfere with valued occupations. How can you make use of this information?

CLIENT FACTORS

Values, beliefs, and spirituality
How can identified values, beliefs, and spirituality be used in this case?

Body structures
Considering Dion's primary and secondary diagnoses, identify the related body structures.

Body functions
1. Identify how the primary and secondary diagnoses have affected the function of the identified body structures.
2. Explain the relationships between the structural and functional factors and her current level of occupational performance.

MENTAL FUNCTIONS: AFFECTIVE, COGNITIVE, AND PERCEPTUAL

1. Compare and contrast FAS with child developmental delay.
2. Describe the correlation between intelligence quotient and FAS.

3. How can Dion's separation anxiety impede her daily activities?
4. Explain the effect of Dion's sleep hygiene on her mental functions.
5. Identify strategies that can be used to maximize Dion's attention.
6. Given the information provided, what additional mental function considerations need to be addressed?

NEUROMUSCULOSKELETAL AND MOVEMENT-RELATED FUNCTIONS

1. Given the information provided, identify neuromusculoskeletal and movement-related functions that need to be addressed. Justify your selections.
2. Provide a probable explanation of why Dion leaned on the table during the performance of fine motor activities.
3. Dion exhibits a rounded back posture. How could it affect her socialization?
4. Explain in biomechanical terms how Dion's sitting posture may affect her handwriting.
5. Create an exercise program based on occupational performance for Dion.

CARDIOVASCULAR, HEMATOLOGICAL, IMMUNOLOGICAL, AND RESPIRATORY FUNCTIONS

1. Given the information provided, identify cardiovascular, hematological, immunological, and respiratory functions that need to be addressed.
2. Identify the typical ranges for heart rate, blood pressure, and respiration rate for children of Dion's age.

SKIN AND RELATED STRUCTURE FUNCTIONS

1. What are the common skin concerns with children who are not toilet trained?
2. Given Dion's sitting posture, which structure may be at greater risk for skin breakdown?

VOICE AND SPEECH FUNCTIONS

Describe how Dion's diagnoses may affect her voice, speech, and associated occupational performance.

ASSISTIVE TECHNOLOGIES AND DEVICES

What assistive technologies or adaptations might be used or made for Dion while she is receiving occupational therapy services? Why?

ETHICAL DECISION MAKING

1. Does toilet training fall within the scope of practice in occupational therapy?
2. Dion's mother reports that Dion's father would like to observe a therapy session. What steps must be taken given this request?
3. Toward the end of the school day, you informed the teacher's aide that Dion is soiled and needs to be changed. The aide states, "Just leave her; she will be going home soon." How should this situation best be addressed?

PHARMACOLOGY

Dion is currently taking a choline supplement.

1. What is the brand name?
2. Does this nutrient have a high alert status?
3. What is the classification of this nutrient?
4. What is the indication for this nutrient?
5. What is the action of this nutrient?
6. How may this nutrient affect client participation during a therapy session?

SOCIOCULTURAL, SOCIOECONOMIC, AND DIVERSITY FACTORS AND LIFESTYLE CHOICES

1. Given Dion's profile, how may your own culture and beliefs affect your interaction with her?
2. Based on this self-examination, what area of cultural knowledge do you need to pursue?
3. How can this newly acquired cultural knowledge be integrated for effective outcomes?
4. How can you foster cultural interaction and awareness among your coworkers?
5. Discuss how a lack of understanding in the areas of discrimination and stigma, implicit bias, social identity, or racism may contribute to disparities in the delivery of occupational therapy services in this case.

ASSESSMENT TOOLS AND INTERPRETATION OF RESULTS

1. What is the purpose of the PDMS–2?
2. Which population is this test designed for?
3. How much time is required to administer it?
4. Provide a brief description of this assessment.
5. What is the reliability of the PDMS–2?
6. What is the validity of the PDMS–2?
7. Is the PDMS–2 a norm-referenced or criterion-reference assessment tool?
8. What functional inference can be deduced from Dion's fine motor quotient score of 73?
9. What additional standardized assessment can be used in this case? Why?

INTERPROFESSIONAL RELATIONSHIP AND EFFECTIVE INTRAPROFESSIONAL COLLABORATION

1. Identify the other professions that would make up the care team. Explain the focus of each.
2. Given your state's policies and procedures on EI services, can OTAs play a role in the delivery of EI occupational therapy services?
3. Identify the roles of the occupational therapy assistant (OTA) that could be used in the occupational therapy process for this case.
4. Identify interventions that can be assigned to the OTA for this case. Justify your selections.

BILLING AND CODING

1. Identify the *International Classification of Diseases (ICD)* codes for Dion's diagnoses.
2. For this case, identify at least two *Current Procedural Terminology (CPT®)* codes that are most appropriate. Justify your selection.

REIMBURSEMENT SYSTEMS AND DOCUMENTATION

1. Who would be the authorized persons you could share the occupational therapy findings with? Explain why.
2. Who would be the unauthorized persons you could not share the occupational therapy findings with without written permission? Explain why.
3. For this case, what forms of documentation will be required?

ADVOCACY

1. Which of the following areas of advocacy would be beneficial in this case: patient rights, matters of privacy, confidentiality, informed consent, awareness building, accessing education, or benefits/ resources?
2. Create a plan to advocate for this client based on the selected areas of advocacy.

TELEHEALTH

1. How can telehealth be integrated as a component of the occupational therapy process in this case?
2. Before launching telemedicine services, what questions would be essential to ask Dion's mother to determine whether it is appropriate for Dion to engage in telemedicine services?
3. What are the barriers, obstacles, or challenges you foresee if attempting to integrate telehealth services with this client?

Intervention Plan Formulation and Implementation

INTERVENTION PLAN FORMULATION

Create an intervention plan that includes the following:

1. List this individual's **strengths.**
2. List this individual's **barriers** in occupational performance, performance skills, and performance patterns.
3. Based on the individual's goals, health, performance, and service delivery site, **identify the barriers that will be addressed.**
4. From the barriers identified to be addressed, **formulate goals and objectives.**
5. Identify the focus of each goal and objective as either **create, promote, establish, restore, maintain, modify, or prevent.**
6. Identify the **theoretical basis, model(s) of practice, or frame(s) of reference** that will be used to address each goal and objective.
7. For each proposed goal and objective, describe clearly and precisely the **methods** that will be used. This description should include, but not be limited to, safety considerations, environmental considerations, therapeutic use of self, preparatory activities, activity selection, materials, equipment, and flow.
8. Classify the activities selected in the methods description as either **preparatory, enabling, purposeful, or occupation based.**
9. Explain how each activity can be **graded up or down,** creating the just-right challenge.
10. Provide at least two **primary sources of evidence** to support the intervention plan.

INTERVENTION PLAN IMPLEMENTATION

1. Based on your intervention plan, identify which goals and objectives require **more immediate attention.**
2. Describe your proposed **first treatment session.**
3. As the treatment session is progressing, what is **essential to be observed?**

Transition and Discontinuation

Create a three-paragraph transition summary. In the first paragraph, identify areas of assessment and significant findings. In the second paragraph, identify barriers to be addressed. Justify their selection. In the third paragraph, identify the goals that have been developed.

REFERENCES

American Medical Association. (2019). *CPT® 2020 professional edition.*
Folio, M. K., & Fewell, R. (2000). *Peabody Developmental Motor Scales: Examiner's manual* (2nd ed.). PRO-ED.
World Health Organization. (2019). *International statistical classification of diseases and related health problems* (11th ed.). https://icd.who.int/

Appendix A. Educator's Guide

This educator's guide is a practical reference resource for academic and clinical educators using this text as a dynamic instructional tool in developing occupational therapy students' interpersonal, professional, clinical, and critical reasoning skills as they prepare for entry-level practice.

Universal Themes Presented Throughout the Text

This text includes the following themes:

- The interrelationship of the uniqueness of the individual, practice setting, length of stay, diagnosis, available resources, and discharge plan must remain in focus.
- Varied views help identify what works best in treating diverse individuals, contributing to effective development of critical thinking.
- Personal reflection contributes to the development of occupational therapy practitioners for contemporary practice.

Tenets

TENET: DIVERSITY, EQUITY, AND INCLUSION

A tenet of this text is the intentional integration of diversity, equity, and inclusion (DEI) principles as a guiding framework for developing critical thinking skills related to the occupational therapy process through a variety of practice areas and client populations. Academic and clinical educators can incorporate this text as an instructional strategy to promote students' cultural humility, foster awareness, and build competency. Each case gives students the opportunity to critically acknowledge their own implicit and explicit biases and discuss grounded strategies with their instructors, supervisors, and peers through a collaborative process.

TENET: INTERDISCIPLINARY AND INTRADISCIPLINARY PRACTICE

A tenet of this text involves occupational therapy students learning principles of intradisciplinary and interdisciplinary practice through a variety of practice areas and client populations. Through facilitation and modeling, students explore the integration of teamwork through a multi-contextual model, expand interpersonal and soft skills, learn the intricacies of conflict resolution, and appreciate of the versatility of leadership skills.

TENET: FROM CLASSROOM TO PRACTICE

A tenet of this text is balancing occupational therapy theory and practice. This balance is an important aspect of the developing student and entry-level practitioner and is outlined through the intentional inclusion of the *Occupational Therapy Practice Framework: Domain and Process* (4th ed.; *OTPF–4;* American Occupational Therapy Association, 2020) and a variety of practice areas and client populations. Academic and clinical instructors can integrate guiding questions from case studies through the lens of the *OTPF–4* domain and process to allow students to bridge their own understanding and interpretation of theory and practice.

Section I. Acute Care

Dominant themes in Section I, "Acute Care," include

- use of the medical model,
- acknowledgement of a fast-paced environment,
- short length of stays,
- prioritizing which problems or barriers to address, and
- transition planning.

Cases have been designed to present the medical history, social history, referral or prescription, and initial evaluation findings of diverse individual. Questions and activities then guide critical thinking. Case content can be matched to Accreditation Council of Occupational Therapy Education (ACOTE®; 2018) standards, course outcomes, or learning objectives (see Table A.1). Portions of a case, or a case in totality, can be assigned, depending on course need. In addition, text content can be used to unify courses being offered during a semester, or interconnect past, present and future courses. Case questions and activities have been constructed to parallel Bloom's Taxonomy of Learning (Bloom et al., 1956). This section focuses on principles of safety, promotes interdisciplinary practice, emphasizes addressing outcomes related to functional and discharge readiness, and highlights the value of therapeutic education.

Section II. Outpatient Rehabilitation

Dominant themes in Section II, "Outpatient Rehabilitation," include

- acknowledging that the individuals receiving services live in community,
- use of biomechanical and medical models,
- use of bottom-up approaches, and
- interspersed treatment sessions.

Cases have been designed to present the medical history, social history, referral or prescription, and initial evaluation findings of diverse individual. Questions and activities then guide critical thinking. Case content can be matched to ACOTE (2018) standards, course outcomes, or learning objectives. Portions of a case, or a case in totality, can be assigned, depending on course need. In addition, text content can be used to unify courses being offered during a semester, or interconnect past, present, and future courses.

The section highlights lengths of stay, frequency and duration of services, clinical emphasis of community reintegration, and outcomes focused on enhancing functional engagement in community-oriented IADLs.

Section III. Rehabilitation Unit or Rehabilitation Hospital

Dominant themes introduced in Section III, "Rehabilitation Unit or Rehabilitation Hospital," include

- transfers from another unit or facility;
- hospital-based facilities;
- individuals demonstrating potential for functional improvement;
- individuals who are medically stable;
- short-term, intense therapy; and
- a focus on skills needed to return home.

Cases have been designed to present the medical history, social history, referral or prescription, and initial evaluation findings of diverse individual. Questions and activities then guide critical thinking. Case content can be matched to ACOTE (2018) standards, course outcomes, or learning objectives. Portions of a case, or a case in totality, can be assigned, depending on course need. In addition, text content can be used to unify courses being offered during a semester, or interconnect past, present, and future courses. This section emphasizes principles of length of stay, reimbursement-specific documentation, biomechanical and rehabilitative frames of references, interdisciplinary and intradisciplinary approaches to care, and occupational-centered outcomes.

Section IV. Subacute Rehabilitation

Dominant themes introduced in Section VI, "Subacute Rehabilitation," include

- transfers from another unit or facility,
- typically non hospital–based facilities,
- individuals demonstrating potential for functional improvement,
- individuals who are medically stable,
- extended periods of less intense therapy, and
- a focus on skills needed to return home.

Cases have been designed to present the medical history, social history, referral or prescription, and initial evaluation findings of diverse individual. Questions and activities then guide critical thinking. Case content can be matched to ACOTE (2018) standards, course outcomes, or learning objectives. Portions of a case, or a case in totality, can be assigned, depending on course need. In addition, text content can be used to unify courses being offered during a semester, or interconnect past, present, and future courses. This section emphasizes principles of discharge planning, client- and occupation-centered goal development, occupational adaptation and therapeutic educational approaches to care, and strategies on measuring functional outcomes.

Section V. Skilled Nursing Facility or Long-Term Care

Dominant themes introduced in Section V, "Skilled Nursing Facility or Long-term Care," include

- transfers from another unit, facility, or community;
- individuals who are unable to live in the community independently;
- facilities serving as residences;
- individuals who demonstrate potential for limited functional improvement;
- individuals who are medically stable; and
- a focus on comfort and maintenance.

Cases have been designed to present the medical history, social history, referral or prescription, and initial evaluation findings of diverse individual. Questions and activities then guide critical thinking. Case content can be matched to ACOTE (2018) standards, course outcomes and or learning objectives. Portions of a case, or a case in totality, can be assigned, depending on course need. In addition, text content can be used to unify courses being offered during a semester, or interconnect past, present, and future courses. This section emphasizes principles of maintenance and restorative care, holistic consideration of mental health needs through a traditional rehabilitative lens, principles of geriatric care and occupational adaptation, interdisciplinary and intradisciplinary care, consideration of hospice and palliative care.

Section VI. Home and Community Health

Dominant themes introduced in Section VI, "Home and Community Health," include

- interfacility transfers;
- individuals who are residing in the community;
- understanding the homebound status and its impact on occupations;
- multiple services and managing expectations;
- individuals who demonstrate potential for functional improvement;
- medical stability and perceived health and wellness outlooks;
- short-term, intermittent therapy delivered in the home;
- a focus on skills needed for independent living; and
- accessing community resources.

Cases have been designed to present the medical history, social history, referral or prescription, and initial evaluation findings of diverse individual. Questions and activities then guide critical thinking. Case content can be matched to ACOTE (2018) standards, course outcomes, or learning objectives. Portions of a case, or a case in totality, can be assigned, depending on course need. In addition, text content can be used to unify courses being offered during a semester, or interconnect past, present and future courses. This section emphasizes principles of community-centered interventions, community reintegration, socioeconomic factors related to disparities and resources, case management, familial and nontraditional support systems, and exploration of contemporary community-centered and culturally sensitive resources.

Section VII. Behavioral Health

Dominant themes introduced in Section VII, "Behavioral Health," include

- individuals who may be considered a danger to self or others,
- individuals who may be hospitalized with or without their consent,
- skills development,
- establishing positive health habits and promoting wellness,
- developing positive routines from a DEI approach to practice, and
- exploring benefits of using community resources that are important to the client.

Cases have been designed to present the medical history, social history, referral or prescription, and initial evaluation findings of diverse individual. Questions and activities then guide critical thinking. Case content can be matched to ACOTE (2018) standards, course outcomes, or learning objectives. Portions of a case, or a case in totality, can be assigned, depending on course need. In addition, text content can be used to unify courses being offered during a semester, or interconnect past, present and future courses. This section emphasizes principles of safety and quality of life, positive behavioral supports, varying forms of hospitalization and the impact towards recovery, and the micro and macro impacts of mental illness.

Section VIII. Pediatric Services

Dominant themes introduced in Section VIII, "Pediatric Services," include

- migrating through the variety of service delivery sites,
- use of the development model,
- the impact of age on available resources,
- balancing best practices and institutional influences,
- play as an occupation,
- skill acquisitional approaches and DEI principles of practice, and
- acknowledgment of the role of a guardian and or nontraditional care provider.

Cases have been designed to present the medical history, social history, referral or prescription, and initial evaluation findings of diverse individual. Questions and activities then guide critical thinking. Case content offers can be matched to ACOTE (2018) standards, course outcomes, or learning objectives. Portions of a case, or a case in totality, can be assigned, depending on course need. In addition, text content can be used to unify courses being offered during a semester, or interconnect past, present, and future courses. This section emphasizes development and contextual influence, academic and occupational-centered practice, expansion of the student's occupational profile through a DEI lens, and the integration of pediatric practice from a sociocultural and institutionally inclusive approach.

Bloom's Taxonomy

ACADEMIC EDUCATORS

The "Questions and Activities Guiding Critical Thinking" parts of this text were carefully crafted using Bloom's Taxonomy, a hierarchical classification of different levels of thinking (Bloom et al., 1956; see Table A.1). Course instructors can use this organizational hierarchy to

- systematically require deeper thinking of students,
- support course learning goals and objectives,
- classify learning goals,
- provide structure to the teaching and learning process,
- create lesson plans,
- assess students' comprehension of course materials, and
- foster intellectual growth.

CLINICAL EDUCATORS

The "Questions and Activities Guiding Critical Thinking" parts of this text were carefully crafted using Bloom's Taxonomy (see Table A.1). Clinical educators can use this organizational hierarchy to

- systematically require deeper levels of knowledge, greater skill, and appropriate attitude from students;
- support fieldwork learning goals and objectives;
- classify learning goals that support entry-level practice;
- provide structure to the teaching and learning process;
- create periodic benchmarks or targets;
- assess students, knowledge, skill, and attitude; and
- foster growth toward entry-level practice.

TABLE A.1. "Questions and Activities Guiding Critical Thinking" According to Bloom's Hierarchical Progression of Learning

Hierarchical Progression of Learning	Remembering	Understanding	Applying	Analyzing	Evaluating	Creating
Learning outcome in the cognitive domain	Students recall or remember information.	Students explain ideas or concepts.	Students use information in a new way.	Students distinguish between different parts or components.	Students justify a stand of decision.	Students produce a new product or point of view.
Look for questions that start with or contain any of these keywords.	list, state, reproduce, repeat, memorize, duplicate, define	explain, describe, select, translate, recognize, locate, report, discuss, classify	choose, interpret, demonstrate, employ, operate, schedule, illustrate,	compare, contrast, criticize, differentiate, discriminate, distinguish, examine, question, test	defend, select, argue, judge, support, evaluate, judge,	create, design, construct, develop, formulate, write
Classification Level	1 Lowest	2	3	3	5	6 Highest

Note. The higher the classification level, the high the level of clinical reasoning skill the student has obtained.

REFERENCES

Accreditation Council for Occupational Therapy Education. (2018). 2018 Accreditation Council for Occupational Therapy Education (ACOTE®) standards and interpretive guide (effective July 31, 2020). *American Journal of Occupational Therapy, 72*(Suppl. 2), 7212410005. https://doi.org/10.5014/ajot.2018.72S217

American Occupational Therapy Association. (2020). Occupational therapy practice framework: Domain and process (4th ed.). *American Journal of Occupational Therapy, 74*(2), 7412410010. https://doi.org/10.5014/ajot.2020.74S2001

Bloom, B. S., Engelhart, M. D., Furst, E. J., Hill, W. H., & Krathwohl, D. R. (1956). *Taxonomy of educational objectives: The classification of educational goals. Vol. Handbook I: Cognitive domain.* David McKay Company.

Appendix B. Matching ACOTE® Standards and Learning Outcomes With Text Questions and Activities Tool

Identify Your Course, Lecture, or Assignment That Addresses a Related ACOTE Standard	B Standard Content Requirement	Learning Outcome	Identify the Page(s), Section(s), and Questions or Activity Numbers You Want to Assign to Your Students
	B 1.0. FOUNDATIONAL CONTENT REQUIREMENTS Program content must be based on a broad foundation in the liberal arts and sciences. A strong foundation in the biological, physical, social, and behavioral sciences supports an understanding of occupation across the lifespan. If the content of the Standard is met through prerequisite coursework, the application of foundational content in the sciences must also be evident in professional coursework.	B.1.1. Human Body, Development, and Behavior B.1.2. Sociocultural, Socioeconomic, Diversity Factors, and Lifestyle Choices B.1.3. Social Determinants of Health B.1.4. Quantitative Statistics and Qualitative Analysis	
	B 2.0. OCCUPATIONAL THERAPY THEORETICAL PERSPECTIVES Current and relevant interprofessional perspectives including rehabilitation, disability, and developmental as well as person/population–environment–occupation models, theories and frameworks of practice. The program must facilitate the development of the performance criteria listed.	B.2.1. Scientific Evidence, Theories, Models of Practice, and Frames of Reference B.2.2. Theory Development	

(Continued)

Identify Your Course, Lecture, or Assignment That Addresses a Related ACOTE Standard	B Standard Content Requirement	Learning Outcome	Identify the Page(s), Section(s), and Questions or Activity Numbers You Want to Assign to Your Students
	B.3.0. BASIC TENETS OF OCCUPATIONAL THERAPY Coursework must facilitate development of the performance criteria listed.	B.3.1. OT History, Philosophical Base, Theory, and Sociopolitical Climate	
		B.3.2. Interaction of Occupation and Activity	
		B.3.3. Distinct Nature of Occupation	
		B.3.4. Balancing Areas of Occupation, Role in Promotion of Health, and Prevention	
		B.3.5. Effects of Disease Processes	
		B.3.6. Activity Analysis	
		B.3.7. Safety of Self and Others	
	B.4.0 REFERRAL, SCREENING, EVALUATION, AND INTERVENTION PLAN The process of referral, screening, evaluation, and diagnosis as related to occupational performance and participation must be client centered; culturally relevant; and based on theoretical perspectives, models of practice, frames of reference, and available evidence.	B.4.1. Therapeutic Use of Self	
		B.4.2. Clinical Reasoning	
		B.4.3. Occupation-Based Interventions	
		B.4.4. Standardized and Nonstandardized Screening and Assessment Tools	
		B.4.5. Application of Assessment Tools and Interpretation of Results	
		B.4.6. Reporting Data	
		B.4.7. Interpret Standardized Test Scores	
		B.4.8. Interpret Evaluation Data	
		B.4.9. Remediation and Compensation	
		B.4.10. Provide Interventions and Procedures	
		B.4.11. Assistive Technologies and Devices	

(Continued)

Identify Your Course, Lecture, or Assignment That Addresses a Related ACOTE Standard	B Standard Content Requirement	Learning Outcome	Identify the Page(s), Section(s), and Questions or Activity Numbers You Want to Assign to Your Students
		B.4.12. Orthoses and Prosthetic Devices	
		B.4.13. Functional Mobility	
		B.4.14. Community Mobility	
		B.4.15. Technology in Practice	
		B.4.16. Dysphagia and Feeding Disorders	
		B.4.17. Superficial Thermal, Deep Thermal, and Electrotherapeutic Agents and Mechanical Devices	
		B.4.18. Grade and Adapt Processes or Environments	
		B.4.19. Consultative Process	
		B.4.20. Care Coordination, Case Management, and Transition Services	
		B.4.21. Teaching–Learning Process and Health Literacy	
		B.4.22. Need for Continued or Modified Intervention	
		B.4.23. Effective Communication	
		B.4.24. Effective Intraprofessional Collaboration	
		B.4.25. Principles of Interprofessional Team Dynamics	
		B.4.26. Referral to Specialists	
		B.4.27. Community and Primary Care Programs	
		B.4.28. Plan for Discharge	
		B.4.29. Reimbursement Systems and Documentation	

(Continued)

Identify Your Course, Lecture, or Assignment That Addresses a Related ACOTE Standard	B Standard Content Requirement	Learning Outcome	Identify the Page(s), Section(s), and Questions or Activity Numbers You Want to Assign to Your Students
	B.5.0 CONTEXT OF SERVICE DELIVERY, LEADERSHIP, AND MANAGEMENT OF OCCUPATIONAL THERAPY SERVICES Context of service delivery includes knowledge and understanding of the various contexts, such as professional, social, cultural, political, economic, and ecological, in which occupational therapy services are provided. Management and leadership skills of occupational therapy services include the application of principles of management and systems in the provision of occupational therapy services to persons, groups, populations, and organizations. The program must facilitate development of the performance criteria listed.	B.5.1. Factors, Policy Issues, and Social Systems B.5.2. Advocacy B.5.3. Business Aspects of Practice B.5.4. Systems and Structures That Create Legislation B.5.5. Requirements for Credentialing and Licensure B.5.6. Market the Delivery of Services B.5.7. Quality Management and Improvement B.5.8. Supervision of Personnel	
	B.6.0. SCHOLARSHIP Promotion of science and scholarly endeavors will serve to describe and interpret the scope of the profession, build research capacity, establish new knowledge, and interpret and apply this knowledge to practice. The program must facilitate development of the performance criteria listed.	B.6.1. Scholarly Study B.6.2. Quantitative and Qualitative Methods B.6.3. Scholarly Reports B.6.4. Locating and Securing Grants B.6.5. Ethical Policies and Procedures for Research B.6.6. Preparation for Work in an Academic Setting	

(Continued)

Identify Your Course, Lecture, or Assignment That Addresses a Related ACOTE Standard	B Standard Content Requirement	Learning Outcome	Identify the Page(s), Section(s), and Questions or Activity Numbers You Want to Assign to Your Students
	B.7.0. PROFESSIONAL ETHICS, VALUES, AND RESPONSIBILITIES Professional ethics, values, and responsibilities include an understanding and appreciation of ethics and values of the profession of occupational therapy. Professional behaviors include the ability to advocate for social responsibility and equitable services to support health equity and address social determinants of health; commit to engaging in lifelong learning; and evaluate the outcome of services, which include client engagement, judicious health care utilization, and population health. The program must facilitate development of the performance criteria listed.	B.7.1 Ethical Decision Making B.7.2. Professional Engagement B.7.3. Promote Occupational Therapy B.7.4. Ongoing Professional Development B.7.5. Personal and Professional Responsibilities	

Source. Standards from ACOTE (2018). Copyright © 2018 by the American Occupational Therapy Association. Used with permission.

Note. ACOTE = Accreditation Council for Occupational Therapy Education; OT = occupational therapy.

REFERENCE

Accreditation Council for Occupational Therapy Education. (2018). 2018 Accreditation Council for Occupational Therapy Education (ACOTE®) standards and interpretive guide (effective July 31, 2020). *American Journal of Occupational Therapy, 72*(Suppl. 2), 7212410005. https://doi.org/10.5014/ajot.2018.72S217

Appendix C. Diversity Represented Through Individuals Presented in Cases

Chapter #	Name	Age	Gender	Sexual Orientation	Nationality	Religion	Disability Status	Race and Ethnicity
1	Juan	67	Male	Homosexual	Guatemalan American	Catholic	Physical	Hispanic/ Latino
2	Song	69	Female	Heterosexual	Korean American	Taoism	Physical, cognitive	Asian
3	Ethan	26	Male	Heterosexual	African American	Black Hebrew Israelite	Physical, sensory	Black
4	Hannah	81	Female	Heterosexual	Chippewa	Ojibwa	Physical	Native American
5	Howie	84	Male	Heterosexual	Filipino	Catholic	Physical	Pacific Islander
6	Florence	69	Female	Asexual	Irish American	Anglican	Physical	White
7	Brian	31	Male	Heterosexual	Native Hawaiian	Buddhist	Physical	Native Hawaiian
8	Yvonne	44	Female	Homosexual	African American	African Methodist Episcopal Church	Physical	Black
9	Chin	62	Male	Heterosexual	Chinese American	Confucianist	Physical	Asian
10	Patricia	36	Female	Heterosexual	Danish American	Evangelical Lutheran	Physical	White
11	Fetu	71	Male	Heterosexual	New Zealander	Presbyterian	Physical, cognitive	Pacific Islander
12	Bianca	47	Female	Heterosexual	Dominican American	Church of Scientology	Physical, sensory	Hispanic/ Latina
13	Derrick	19	Male	Pansexual	Polish American	Agnostic	Physical, cognitive	White

(Continued)

Chapter #	Name	Age	Gender	Sexual Orientation	Nationality	Religion	Disability Status	Race and Ethnicity
14	Sharon	59	Female (Transgender)	Heterosexual	Jamaican	United Church of Christ	Physical, emotional	Black
15	Zachary	75	Male	Heterosexual	Australian	Orthodox Christian	Physical	Pacific Islander
16	Isaura	38	Female	Heterosexual	Puerto Rican	Catholic	Physical, emotional	Hispanic/ Latina
17	Pierre-Louis	82	Male	Heterosexual	Haitian American	Haitian Vodou	Physical	Black
18	Rosalind	51	Female	Homosexual	Ukrainian American	Jewish	Physical, cognitive, sensory	White
19	Aki	91	Male	Heterosexual	Japanese American	Shinto	Physical, cognitive	Asian
20	Ting	72	Female	Heterosexual	Malaysian American	Buddhist	Physical, sensory	Asian
21	Jacob	94	Male	Heterosexual	Israeli	Hasidic Judaism	Physical, cognitive	White
22	Aretha	78	Female	Heterosexual	Trinidadian American	Jehovah Witness	Physical	Black
23	Epa	72	Female	Heterosexual	Polynesian American	Animism	Physical, Sensory	Pacific Islander
24	Mohammad	77	Male	Heterosexual	Iranian American	Sunni Muslim	Physical	White
25	Eileen	57	Female	Heterosexual	Irish American	Catholic	Physical	White
26	José	81	Male	Heterosexual	Salvadoran American	Dominican Santeria	Physical, sensory	Hispanic/ Latino
27	Katrina	38	Female	Heterosexual	Georgian American	Russian Orthodox	Physical, cognitive	White
28	Ivy	66	Female	Homosexual	Nigerian American	Baptist	Physical	Black
29	Zoran	63	Female	Heterosexual	German American	Yazidi	Emotional, physical	White
30	Gabriela	22	Female	Heterosexual	Honduran	Catholic	Emotional	Black/ Hispanic

(Continued)

Chapter #	Name	Age	Gender	Sexual Orientation	Nationality	Religion	Disability Status	Race and Ethnicity
31	Samuel	62	Male	Heterosexual	African American	Born Again Christian	Emotional	Black
32	Emmanuel	31	Male	Heterosexual	Moroccan American	Shia Muslim	Behavioral	Black
33	Andres	57	Male	Heterosexual	Columbian American	Pentecostal Christian	Behavioral	Hispanic/Latino
34	Brianna	18	Female	Bisexual	Armenian American	Christian	Behavioral	White
35	Victoria	10	Female	Unassigned	Venezuelan American	Catholic	Physical, sensory	Hispanic/Latina
36	Abigale	10	Female	Unassigned	Peruvian American	Roman Catholic	Cognitive, physical	Hispanic/Latina
37	Andrei	13	Male	Homosexual	Belarusian American	Russian Orthodox Catholic	Cognitive, sensory	White
38	Dara	5	Female	Unassigned	British American	Pentecostal Christian	Intellectual, Physical	White
39	Chi-Ling	10	Female	Unassigned	Taiwanese American	Yinguidoa	Physical, sensory	Asian
40	Dion	2.5	Female	Unassigned	Liberian American	African Methodist Episcopal Zion	Cognitive, sensory, physical	Black